UHB Trust Library

D1351520

38.50
30/10/03
WC 680

TROPICAL INFECTIOUS DISEASES

This book is due for return on or before the last date shown below.

- 8 DEC 2006

UHB TRUST LIBRARY
WITHDRAWN FROM STOCK

This book is dedicated to our children,
Suran, Lakmalie, Joel and Trishe
who have joined us in the medical fraternity.

TROPICAL INFECTIOUS DISEASES

EPIDEMIOLOGY, INVESTIGATION, DIAGNOSIS AND MANAGEMENT

By

RANJAN L. FERNANDO
MBBS, MD, MRCP (London), FRCP (Edin),
FACEM, FRACP
Senior Consultant Physician, Military Hospital, Liverpool, NSW
Former Director of Accident and Emergency Medicine
The Liverpool Hospital and Senior Lecturer, University of NSW, New South
Wales, Australia

SUJATHA S. E. FERNANDO
MBBS, MSc (Lon), FRSTM&H, DCP, FRCPA, MIAC
Senior Consultant Pathologist, Quinn Pathology Services, Kensington, NSW
Former Director of Anatomical Pathology
South Western Area Pathology Service
Liverpool and Senior Lecturer, School of Pathology
University of NSW, New South Wales, Australia

ANTHONY S.-Y. LEONG
MBBS, MD (Adelaide), FRCPA, FRCPath, FCAP,
Honorary FHKCPath, FHKAM (Pathol)
Medical Director, Hunter Area Pathology Services, Newcastle
Professor and Head, Discipline of Anatomical Pathology
University of Newcastle, New South Wales, Australia

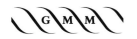

© 2001

Greenwich Medical Media Limited
137 Euston Road
London
NW1 2AA

ISBN **1 900 151 39 1**

First published 2001

Apart from any fair dealing for the purposes of research or
private study, or criticism or review, as permitted under the UK
Copyright Designs and Patents Act 1988, this publication may
not be reproduced, stored, or transmitted, in any form or by any
means, without the prior permission in writing of the publishers,
or in the case of reprographic reproduction only in accordance
with the terms of the licences issued by the appropriate
Reproduction Rights Organisations outside the UK. Enquiries
concerning reproduction outside the terms stated here should be
sent to the publishers at the London address printed above.

The rights of RL Fernando, SSE Fernando and T S-Y Leong to
be identified as authors of this work has been asserted by them
in accordance with the Copyright, Designs and Patents Act 1988.

The publisher makes no representation, express or implied, with
regard to the accuracy of the information contained in this book
and cannot accept any legal responsibility or liability for any
errors or omissions that may be made.

A catalogue record for this book is available from the British
Library.

Visit our website at: www.greenwich-medical.co.uk

Typeset by Saxon Graphics Ltd, Derby

Printed by Alden Press, Ltd

CONTENTS

PREFACE

Young maidens of AD 1600 were well aware of the dangers of infectious diseases. Rosalind had asked:

> 'Alas, what danger will it be to us maids as we are to travel so far?'
> (William Shakespeare, *As You Like It*, Act 7, Scene 3).

The need for preventive measures was reflected by the warning:

> 'The girls of Italy take heed of them'
> (*idem*, *All's Well That Ends Well*, Act 2, Scene 1).

The advent of relatively inexpensive air travel, transcontinental trains and ocean liners has made international travel within the reach of many. Today, two-thirds of travellers visit the tropics and are exposed to diseases not prevalent in their normal habitat. In geographic terms, the 'tropics' is confined to latitudes 23° 27′ N (Tropic of Cancer) and 23° 27′ S (Tropic of Capricorn); however, in relation to infectious diseases, the 'tropics' includes South East Asia, Korea, Japan, Northern Australia, the tropical belts of the Pacific, Central America and the Caribbean. Tropical Africa embraces the entire continent with the exception of South Africa, and the Mediterranean littoral from Spain to Israel is also part of the 'medical tropics'.

Most of the tropical infections are parasitic although there are some bacterial, rickettsial and viral infections that are endemic to the tropics and must also be considered. Zoonotic parasites form a substantial proportion of parasitic diseases in humans and the list of parasite species which infect man in both advanced and less-developed regions of the world are made up of more than 300 species of helminths alone. With the emergence of immunodeficiency conditions including the acquired immunodeficiency syndrome (AIDS), poorly known pathogens previously thought to be of minor importance, such as cryptosporidia and microsporidia, have emerged as important causes of significant human disease. Some parasites may be common but because their adult or larval stages are sequestrated in the tissues of the host and consequently rarely encountered, they are often not readily recognized or identified. The clinical manifestations of these infections may be common and non-specific, or they may rarely be completely exotic and defy recognition.

As the world becomes smaller through the efficiency and speed of modern travel, people may become exposed to and contract a wide variety of infections normally prevalent in far-off places. Such diseases are diagnosed only when the travellers return home. Tropical infections may enter temperate countries through their immigrant hosts and these often only become clinically manifest after the hosts arrival in their newly adopted country. In addition, people who have exotic tropical food preferences may be exposed to infections endemic to the tropics.

This book provides coverage of tropical diseases due to parasites including protozoa, nematodes, trematodes, cestodes, acanthocephala and arthropods. It also includes bacteria, rickettsia and viruses common to the tropics. It discusses the epidemiological and clinical aspects of each tropical infectious disease in detail and illustrates the biology and life cycles of the infectious organisms and the pathology caused. The goal of providing a comprehensive coverage is completed by the inclusion of treatment aspects for each disease, making this book suitable for the general practitioner, specialist clinician, parasitologist, pathologist, technician, researcher and student who needs to identify and treat infectious tropical diseases. Above all, the reader is reminded that the question *'Quo vadis? Unde veni?' (Where have you been. And when?)* must be asked when taking a clinical history.

R. L. F.
S. S. E. F.
A. S.-Y. L.
June, 2000

FOREWORD

I have been a clinical colleague of the Fernandos for over ten years in the South Western Sydney Area Health Service and watched with admiration the production of this very useful publication. Both authors qualified in Sri Lanka with honours, obtaining distinction in parasitology. Ranjan had his post graduate physician's training in Colombo and subsequently in Edinburgh and Leeds. He returned to Sri Lanka and was consultant physician treating many patients with tropical diseases. He emigrated to Australia where he brought his expertise to the Emergency Department, Liverpool Hospital Sydney including teaching and training of staff.

Sujatha completed her Internship at Leeds General Infirmary UK. In Sri Lanka she was in charge of the Medical Entomology/Parasitology Department at the Medical Research Institute in Colombo where she contributed to many research projects. She was awarded a W.H.O. Fellowship to the London School of Tropical Medicine and Hygiene where she obtained her MSc with Distinction. Subsequently she trained as an anatomical pathologist in Sydney. She has conducted many lectures, tutorials and workshops, some jointly with her husband, both nationally and internationally at the invitation of learned colleges and scientific societies. Preparation for these is a major factor in producing this book.

Professor Tony Leong is an author of international standing with numerous publications. He helped to make this focused and readable, with up to date referencing and critical review of each chapter.

I am sure that healthcare personnel including medical microbiologists, infectious diseases physicians, nurses, anatomical pathologists, haematologists, parasitologists and general practitioners involved in the diagnosis and treatment of tropical infectious diseases will find this book very valuable.

Rosemary Munro
MBBS, MRCP, FRCPA, FRCPATH, DipBACT, FASM
Director and Associate Professor
Department of Microbiology and Infectious Diseases,
South Western Area Pathology Services and University of New South Wales.
Australia

ACKNOWLEDGEMENTS

We thank Katherine R Kociuba MBBS, FRACP, FRCPA, Consultant in Infectious Diseases, South Western Sydney Area Health Service and Department of Microbiology and Infectious Diseases, South Western Area Pathology Service, Liverpool Hospital, Liverpool for the chapters on melioidosis and donovanosis.

We also acknowledge the contribution made by Suran Fernando, BSc (Med), MBBS (Hon), Medical Registrar in Immunology, St Vincent's Hospital, Sydney to the chapter on tuberculosis.

GENERAL INTRODUCTION

Parasitic and tropical diseases continue to be a significant cause of morbidity and mortality in many countries. In the past they were considered to be only the problems of developing tropical countries, but this is no longer true. With the ready accessibility of rapid travel and the continuous movement of migrants and refugees, often across continents, tropical infectious diseases are a global problem and can pose diagnostic difficulties in countries remote from the site of the endemic disease. Besides international travel and the influx of migrants and refugees into the more affluent countries of the West, the extensive use of immunosuppressive therapy and the advent of the acquired immunodeficiency syndrome (AIDS) have contributed to the prevalence and increasing incidence of tropical infectious diseases in temperate countries. Unfortunately, this area of clinical medicine is relatively neglected in medical curriculum and health professionals in many developed countries receive limited instruction in parasitic and infectious tropical disease. This deficiency is reflected in the failure to include appropriate tropical infectious diseases when considering the differential diagnoses of various clinical presentations. Often, it is the surgical or autopsy pathologist who ultimately renders the unsuspected diagnosis. For example, a diagnosis of amoebic abscess or hydatid cyst in the case of the clinically suspected carcinoma of the liver, toxoplasmic lymphadenitis for the suspected malignant lymphoma, giardiasis for coeliac disease and toxocariasis for retinoblastoma. In addition, opportunistic infections such as pneumocystosis, toxoplasmosis and strongyloidiasis are frequently encountered in the setting of the immunosuppressed patient. Parasitic diseases such as malaria remain one of the major fatal diseases in the world. In Australia, a developed country, malaria is an imported disease and yet more than 1000 cases are diagnosed a year and hydatid disease remains common.

There have been many new developments both in the diagnostic aspects and treatment of parasitic and tropical diseases. While a parasitologist may be very familiar with the life cycle and structure of the parasite, s/he may not be fully cognisant of the variations in clinical presentation and management. It is the aim of this book to provide a comprehensive coverage of all aspects of tropical infectious diseases to help the broad spectrum of health professionals in the diagnosis and treatment of these diseases.

Detailed discussion of the epidemiology, clinical features, diagnosis, parasitology, microbiology, pathology, treatment and prevention of each tropical infectious disease will be supplemented by illustrations to provide easy reading and reference. Because of the limitation of space, coverage cannot be exhaustive, but some diseases such as malaria, tuberculosis and hydatid disease will be described in greater detail because of their relative importance. Illustrative cases are included at the ends of the relevant chapters.

I

Protozoa

1

Introduction

Protozoa are unicellular organisms in which the single cell is highly specialized to perform the functions of respiration, digestion, excretion and reproduction.

Their basic structure comprises a nucleus and cytoplasm. The nucleus is composed of a chromatinic rim or nuclear membrane enclosing a fine network of reticulum with a karyosome (inaccurately called the nucleolus), which is a condensed aggregate of chromatin. The location of the karyosome and the chromatin pattern is helpful in identifying different species of protozoa, e.g. the ciliated protozoan *Balantidium coli* has a micronucleus and macronucleus, whereas haemoflagellates have a kinetoplast or accessory nucleus.

The cytoplasm consists of an ectoplasm and endoplasm. The ectoplasm is the outer transparent layer that performs a protective as well as locomotory and sensory function. The endoplasm is the internal granular part of the cell and performs the nutritive, reproductive and excretory functions. A limiting membrane or plasma membrane binds the entire cell.

Protozoans exist in two main forms: the trophozoite, which is the active, invasive stage; and the cyst, which is the resistant stage that can survive unfavourable conditions.

Reproduction of protozoa may be asexual through binary or multiple fission, sexual through conjugation and syngamy or gametogony.

To survive, protozoa must be transmitted from one host to another. This is achieved by either transforming into the cyst stage or by changing their method of reproduction from asexual to sexual, e.g. in malaria, the sexual cycle or gametogony takes place in the mosquito and the asexual cycle or schizogony takes place in man. This process is known as alternation of generation. In leishmania and trypanosomes the haemoflagellate protozoa metamorphose into the amastigote (or leptomonad) forms and flagellate forms in both the insect and human host by means of asexual reproduction.

A classification of pathogenic protozoa is provided in Table 1 on p4.

Table 1 – Classification of pathogenic protozoa based on locomotive function

Class	Locomotion organ	Principal human pathogens
Mastigophora	flagella	*Leishmania*
		Trypanosoma
		Giardia★
		Trichomonas★
Rhizopoda	pseudopodia	*Entamoeba*
		Naegleria★ and *Acanthamoeba*
Ciliophora	cilia	*Balantidium*
Sporozoa	none	*Plasmodium*★
		Toxoplasma★
		Cryptosporidium★
		Isospora★
		Pneumocystis★

★Infections commonly encountered in Australia.

2

Amoebiasis

PARASITOLOGY

Amoebiasis refers to infection by *Entamoeba histolytica* and is found most frequently in tropical and subtropical regions where the socio-economic status and sanitation are poor. Amoebiasis is indigenous to some developed countries like Australia. In New York, most reported cases of amoebiasis occur among the homosexual population, described with other intestinal parasitic and sexually transmitted diseases as the 'gay bowel syndrome' (Williams *et al.* 1971).

E. histolytica occurs as both trophozoite and cyst stages. The trophozoite is the invasive form; the cyst stage the infective form.

Man acquires infection by ingesting amoebic cyst-contaminated food or water (most outbreaks are water borne) (Fig. 2.1). Rarely, trophozoites can directly invade abraded genital organs ('gay bowel' transmission as in homosexuals). Four metacystic trophozoites are released into the small intestine from each cyst and migrate to the colon where they mature. These trophozoites invade the submucosa probably by releasing digestive enzymes such as protease, hyaluronidase and mucopolysaccharidase. The incubation period varies from 1 to 3 weeks.

Trophozoites measure 12–60 μm and have transparent ectoplasm with pseudopodia. The endoplasm is granular and may contain engulfed cells, particularly red blood cells, which indicate invasive activity (Fig. 2.2). The nucleus has a centrally located karyosome with fine peripheral chromatin (Fig. 2.3). Multiplication is by binary fission. Amoebic cysts measure 10–20 μm and contain two to four nuclei with the identical nuclear structure as trophozoites. In addition, chromatoidal bodies (cigar-shaped, darkly stained or refractile) are present.

Other types of non-pathogenic Entamoebae may be encountered in stools and need to be distinguished from *E. histolytica*. *E. hartmanni* is a smaller species measuring < 12 μm; *E. coli* is larger measuring 10–35 μm, containing two to eight large nuclei with splinter-shaped chromatoidal bodies and eccentrically located karyosomes. *Iodamoeba butschlii* has one nucleus with a large central karyosome and a prominent glycogen vacuole that stains brown with iodine. *Endolimax nana* is small (5–10 μm) with a prominent central karyosome, no peripheral chromatin and clear cytoplasm (Table 2.1).

Infection with *E. histolytica* can be intestinal or extraintestinal.

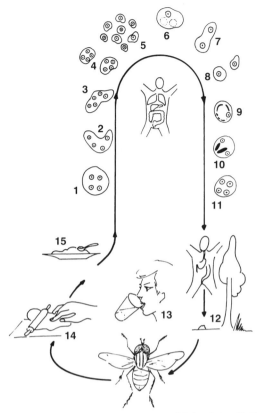

Figure 2.1 – Life cycle and transmission of *E. histolytica*. (1) The mature 4-nucleate cyst enters the alimentary canal; (1–5) the 4-nucleate amoeba that leaves the cyst and divides to form eight individual amoebae; (6–10) multiplication in the intestinal lumen; (9–11) cyst formation; (9) typical uninucleate stage with peripheral chromidial bodies; (10) binucleate cyst with chromidial bodies; (11) mature 4-nucleate cyst; (12–15) possible modes of infection: (13) drinking water contaminated with faeces; (14) by contaminated communal dishes; (15) flies transport cysts from faeces to food.

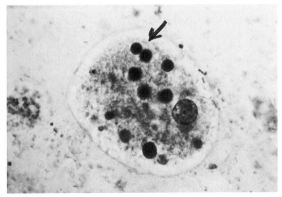

Figure 2.2 – Trophozoite containing a compact, centrally located karyosome. The presence of ingested red blood cells (arrow) is diagnostic of *E. histolytica* (trichrome × 1000).

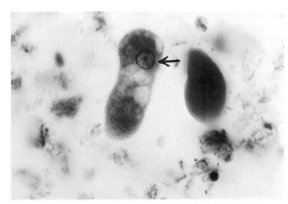

Figure 2.3 – Trophozoite showing the typical nuclear structure of *E. histolytica* with a centrally located, small, compact karyosome and finely granular chromatin distributed evenly over the inner surface of the nuclear membrane (arrow) (trichrome × 1000).

INTESTINAL AMOEBIASIS

Presentation

Intestinal infection with *E. histolytica* results in different clinical patterns, varying from no symptoms to recurrent episodes, fulminant disease or milder forms. Fulminating intestinal amoebiasis usually affects elderly, debilitated patients and the immunosuppressed. Diarrhoea may be mild or severe, with or without blood or mucus. In severe cases with bloody diarrhoea, there may be associated systemic disturbances such as cramping, abdominal pain, fever, anorexia, tenesmus and flatulence. The faecal volume is smaller than in bacillary dysentery. Infrequently, the appendix may be involved, simulating acute appendicitis. Other differential diagnoses include ulcerative colitis, bacillary dysentery and Crohn's disease.

Complications

- Severe dehydration, hypovolaemia and electrolyte imbalance
- Acute haemorrhage and anaemia
- Toxic dilatation of the colon (toxic megacolon)
- Perforation with peritonitis
- Amoeboma (see below)

Amoeboma

There may be no preceding history of amoebiasis. The presentation is that of chronic diarrhoea, anorexia, anaemia, abdominal pain and loss of weight. Up to 5% of patients with intestinal amoebiasis may present with

Table 2.1 – Comparison of cysts/trophozoites of amoebae in stools

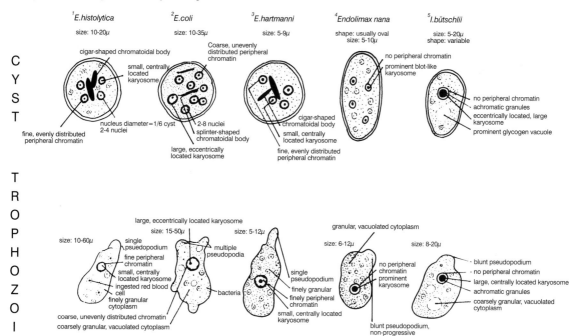

a localized granulomatous reaction in the bowels, which is usually solitary but may be multiple. The tumour-like masses occur in the caecum and rectum and have been mistaken for carcinoma and abdominoperineal resections have been performed. Biopsy and histological examination is necessary for proper distinction.

Pathology

Intestinal amoebiasis produces mucosal ulcerations which are most frequently seen in the caecum, although the ascending colon, sigmoid colon, appendix and, less frequently, the ileum can be involved. Early lesions consist of minute erosions with congestion and oedema of the surrounding mucosa. When fully developed, 'flask-shaped' ulcers with overhanging edges are present (Fig. 2.4) and the intervening mucosa, apart from congestion and oedema, is normal. Sometimes, mucosal inflammation can be generalized and mimics bacillary dysentery. When multiple ulcers are present, the appearance can resemble pseudomembranous colitis.

Microscopically, superficial erosions of the mucosa are filled with inflamed granulation tissue. Trophozoites

are rarely seen in these lesions and serological tests are needed to confirm the diagnosis. Fully developed ulcerated lesions show necrosis with absent or scanty inflammatory reaction with occasional eosinophils. The trophozoites, present at the junction of the necrotic debris and viable tissue, are characteristically surrounded by a clear halo with a tiny central karyosome, delicate nuclear membrane and a 'bubbly' or vacuolated cytoplasm, which sometimes contains ingested red cells (Fig. 2.5). Inflammatory reaction, when present in the adjacent mucosa, consists of plasma cells, lymphocytes, eosinophils and only a few neutrophils. The organisms require distinction from macrophages. The periodic acid-Schiff (PAS) stain is useful to highlight amoebae but macrophages will also be stained so that nuclear details must be studied for correct identification.

Investigations

1. *Stool examination* – diagnosis is based on the finding of motile trophozoites in freshly examined stool or mucosal ulcer smears. Three separate stool samples should be examined. The stools contain pus

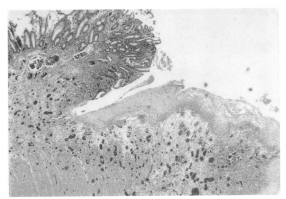

Figure 2.4 – Flask-shaped ulcer caused by *E. histolytica* (H&E × 100).

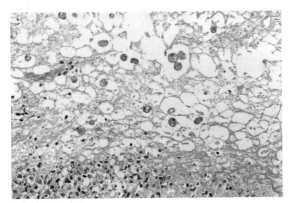

Figure 2.5 – High-power of the 'clear halo' in the trophozoite (H&E × 200).

cells, but in much smaller quantities than in bacillary dysentery. The demonstration of amoebic cysts does not necessarily signify acute infection. The ocular micrometer, a glass disc with linear scale etched on it, is recommended by the WHO for the examination and identification of parasites (González-Ruiz and Bendall 1995). It is useful for the differentiation of the cysts of *E. histolytica* from *E. hartmanni*. Size is the most obvious difference. *E. hartmanni* cysts are 4–8 μm diameter and those of *E. histolytica* are 7.5–15 μm and accurate measurement allows proper distinction.

2. *Serology* – antibodies to *E. histolytica* may be detected in the serum by a variety of immunological methods, e.g. isoenzyme electrophoresis of *E. histolytica* can distinguish the zymodeme pattern of pathogenic or invasive amoebae from non-pathogenic, non-invasive amoebae (Garcia and Bruckner 1993).

3. *Histologic examination* – sigmoidoscopy and biopsy for histologic examination provides definitive diagnosis.

Treatment

Patients with intestinal amoebiasis require rehydration, blood transfusion for haemorrhage, and correction of electrolyte imbalance. Surgery is indicated for peritonitis developing from perforation, and proper resuscitation with fluids, nasogastric intubation, and a combination of antibiotics such as metronidazole, gentamicin and ampicillin are required. In uncomplicated cases, the drugs used should control tissue invasion and eliminate amoebae in the intestinal lumen

Tissue amoebicidals

- Metronidazole 500–750 mg/day for 7–10 days for adults. Children > 12 years adult dose, 7–12 years one-half adult dose, 3–7 years one-third adult dose and infants one-quarter adult dose
- Tinidazole in a single dose 50 mg/kg, which gives almost a 100% cure rate, while others have reported lower cure rates. Adult dose is 2 g
- Paromomycin 30 mg/kg/day for 5 days (Sullam *et al.* 1986)

Tinidazole and metronidazole are best avoided in the first trimester of pregnancy. Tissue amoebicides should be used together with lumen amoebicides for complete eradication.

Lumeinal amoebicidals

- Diloxanide furoate – dose 20 mg/kg/day in divided doses for 10 days, has a very high cure rate. It is generally not indicated for children < 2 years
- Tetracycline 15 mg/kg/day for 10 days. It is generally not indicated for children < 9 years

Successful treatment of intestinal amoebiasis is achieved when three consecutive stool samples, examined 14 days after completion, are negative for *E. histolytica*.

EXTRA-INTESTINAL AMOEBIASIS

Extra-intestinal amoebiasis may occur as amoebic hepatitis, abscesses in the liver, brain or pericardium, cutaneous amoebiasis or pulmonary amoebiasis.

Amoebic hepatitis

Amoebic hepatitis is generally preceded by intestinal disease although there may be no definite preceding history. Unlike a definite abscess, there is no localized lesion. The liver enlargement may be accompanied by fever. Serological tests are usually positive while liver function tests are normal. Amoebic hepatitis occurs in endemic areas and should be suspected particularly in patients with a history of amoebic colitis.

Amoebic liver abscess

This is the commonest extra-intestinal lesion. Amoebic liver abscesses have an insidious onset. A history of preceding intestinal amoebiasis is generally obtainable. There is a long latent period between intestinal infection and liver abscess. The commonest site of the abscess is the right lobe. Presenting symptoms are fever, pain in the right hypochondrium, sometimes referred to the right shoulder tip. Pain may be aggravated by side to side movement and may be pleuritic. The liver is enlarged and tender, with intercostal tenderness on the right side. Abscesses on the left side may present as tender epigastric masses. Clinically, it is not possible to distinguish between an amoebic and non-amoebic liver abscess.

Patients with pleuritic chest pain, enlarged liver, fever and abdominal pain, and a space-occupying lesion on CT and ultrasonography have pyogenic liver abscess, malignancy, congenital hepatic cyst and hydatid disease as differential diagnoses. Differentiation from a primary pyogenic abscess may be difficult as it is often difficult to demonstrate amoebae in the pus. Aspiration, which is not usually done for amoebic liver abscesses, reveals sterile pus. Hepatocellular carcinoma is often associated with chronic liver disease or portal hypertension. Serum α-fetoprotein is usually raised in hepatocellular carcinoma. Hydatid disease may present as a solitary liver abscess. The clinical history and serology for hydatid disease and amoebiasis may distinguish the two conditions.

Complications occur as a result of extension of the liver abscess. The abscess may rupture into the pleural or peritoneal or pericardial cavity, colon or portal vein and hepatic vein with resultant thrombosis.

Investigations

1. *Blood film examination* – white cell count is raised with predominance of polymorphonuclear leukocytes

2. *Stool examination* - generally produces negative results
3. *Chest X-ray* – shows elevation of the right hemi-diaphragm (Fig 2.6). CT scan or ultrasound will reveal one or more space-occupying lesions of the abdomen
4. *Serology* – extra-intestinal amoebiasis generally shows a positive serology with antibodies being present in > 90% of patients with invasive amoebiasis. The serological test was traditionally the amoebic indirect haemagglutination test (IHA) which is positive in 82–98% of patients with symptomatic amoebic colitis but ELISA assays are now producing comparable results

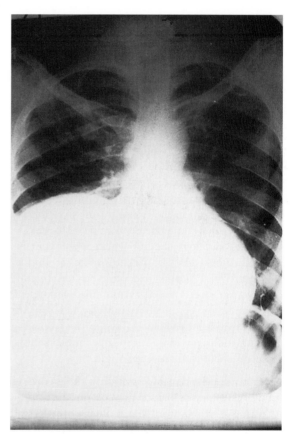

Figure 2.6 – X-ray of an amoebic liver abscess (courtesy Professor C. Kirre, Harare, Zimbabwe).

Pulmonary amoebiasis

Usually secondary to hepatic amoebiasis. It commonly occurs in the right lower lobe of the lung as a result of rupture of a right lobe of the liver abscess. Rupture into the pleural cavity will produce an empyema.

Haematogenous or lymphatic spread can also cause pulmonary amoebiasis.

Cutaneous amoebiasis

Cutaneous amoebiasis is secondary to extension of rectal infection to the perineum or as a result of diagnostic or therapeutic aspiration of liver abscess or empyema, or rupture of an amoebic abscess through the anterior abdominal wall.

Cerebral amoebic abscess

Cerebral amoebic abscesses are very rare and usually solitary. Clinical manifestations are those of a space-occupying lesion or meningitis. Prognosis is poor unless diagnosed and treated early. A CT scan of the brain will demonstrate a space-occupying lesion.

Pathology

Amoebic abscess occurs most frequently in the right lobe of the liver and results from trophozoites from the bowel entering the portal system via the portal veins. In the very early stages, a number of small necrotic foci form in the centres of the liver lobules and these coalesce into one or more big abscesses. As the abscess develops, the liver enlarges and contains grey, ill-defined globular patches up to 25 mm in diameter. These liquefy and coalesce, forming the characteristic ragged abscess cavities filled with viscid, chocolate brown pus (anchovy sauce) which contains necrotic liver tissue and blood. Trophozoites can often be found in this pus as well as in large numbers in the abscess wall but cysts are never found.

Characteristically, the abscess displays three zones: a centre containing yellow or grey opaque material, a mid-zone of stroma and a shaggy outer fibrinous wall invaded by trophozoites. The adjacent liver is oedematous and infiltrated with chronic inflammatory cells. Very rarely, abscesses may calcify and require differentiation from a hydatid cyst.

The pathology of amoebic abscesses in other sites such as lung and brain are similar in appearance. In the brain, the left hemisphere is more frequently involved and abscesses are usually multiple. Gliosis and non-specific inflammation is seen around the abscess. Cutaneous lesions can be ulcerative or condylomatous.

Abscesses in other sites are very similar in appearance. In the brain, the left hemisphere is more frequently involved and abscesses are usually multiple. Gliosis and non-specific inflammation is seen around the area of liquefactive necrosis. In the skin, the lesions can be ulcerative or condylomatous.

Treatment

As a rule, amoebic abscesses in various sites are treated by resection and collections of pus in various spaces such as the pleura are treated by drainage. Specific chemotherapy with amoebicidal drugs should be given in all instances. Pericardial abscesses are associated with very high mortality rate. These are similarly treated with surgical drainage and amoebicidal drugs and the patients should be treated in an intensive care unit.

The drug treatment for extra-intestinal amoebiasis is the same regardless of the site.

- Metronidazole 40 mg/kg/day in three divided doses for 10 days is effective
- Tinidazole 35 mg/kg in divided doses given 12 h apart for 5 days has a high cure rate

In the past, dehydroemetine 1 mg/kg/day maximum 65 mg/day for 10 days was the drug of choice. However, it is more toxic and requires cardiac monitoring.

Tissue amoebicides should be combined with luminal amoebicides for hepatic amoebiasis (see above). Surgical intervention in hepatic amoebiasis is rarely necessary today except for large abscesses and impending rupture. Successful treatment of hepatic amoebiasis is the disappearance of symptoms and signs and reduction in size of the abscess on CT scan within 10 days.

REFERENCES

Garcia LS, Bruckner DA. Intestinal protozoa: amoebae. In Garcia LS, Bruckner DA (eds), *Diagnostic Medical Parasitology*. Washington, DC: American Society for Microbiology, 1993, 6–17

González-Ruiz A, Bendall RP. The use of the ocular micrometer in diagnostic parasitology. *Parasitology Today* 1995; **11**: 83–85

Sullam PM, Slutkin G, Gottlieb AB *et al.* Paromomycin therapy of endemic amoebiasis in homosexual men. *Sexually Transmitted Diseases* 1986; **13**: 151–153

Williams DC, Felman YM, Marr JS *et al.* Sexually transmitted enteric pathogens in male homosexual population. *New York State Journal of Medicine* 1971; **77**: 2050–2052

3

Non-intestinal Amoebiasis

Naegleria Fowleri
  Parasitology
  Presentation
  Pathology
  Investigations
  Treatment
Acanthamoeba
  Parasitology

Granulomatous Amoebic Encephalitis
Acanthamoeba Keratitis
  Presentation
  Pathology
  Investigations
Illustrative Case
References

Non-intestinal amoebiasis is caused by a group of free-living soil amoebae. The two species that cause disease in humans are Acanthamoeba and Naegleria. Acanthamoeba was thought to be the causative agent in the first reported case of primary amoebic meningo-encephalitis in 1965, seen in an Australian patient (Fowler and Carter 1965), but this case was later found to be caused by *Naegleria fowleri* (Bull *et al.* 1968). The distribution of primary amoebic meningo-encephalitis is universal and includes Australia, Belgium, Brazil, Czechoslovakia, the UK, India, New Zealand, Nigeria and the USA (Lowande *et al.* 1980).

NAEGLERIA FOWLERI

Parasitology

Primary amoebic meningo-encephalitis is a very rare infection of the meninges caused by *Naegleria fowleri*. Between 1955 and 1972, 13 probable and confirmed cases of primary amoebic meningo-encephalitis occurred in the Spencer Gulf region of South Australia (Dorsch *et al.* 1983). It was subsequently reported in Queensland, New South Wales, and Western Australia and until 1983, all cases had been fatal (Dorsch *et al.* 1983). Ten pathogenic strains were isolated from the domestic water supply in the northern part of South Australia and *N. fowleri* was isolated from the surface soil in the same area. Its prevalence is universal and up to 1978, > 80 cases had been reported worldwide, of which 38 were from the USA.

Humans acquire the disease by swimming in fresh water lakes and poorly chlorinated outdoor or heated indoor pools, which are contaminated by the parasite. Transmission has been shown to be by water carried through pipelines for several hundred kilometres as some infected patients had never been immersed in water and the only source of infection was pipeline water supply. It was thought chlorine levels had dropped by the time it reached the supply destination allowing growth of the organism. With a chlorine residue of 0.5 mg/litre water the risk of *N. fowleri* infection is negligible. The incidence of the disease is greater during the summer months due to increased water sports and the higher temperatures allow multiplication of the protozoa. The portal of entry is most likely through the nose and the infection has also been reported in people who sniff water before prayers as part of a religious ritual. It has been proven that inhalation of airborne cysts is not a mode of transmission in humans as *N. fowleri* cannot survive desiccation for more than a few minutes (Chang 1978).

The free-living soil amoebae can be found in stagnant fresh water lakes, ponds, hot springs and heated swimming pools. Infection is believed to take place transnasally when diving or engaging in underwater activities. After invading the nasal epithelium, the parasites migrate along the olfactory nerve and pierce the cribriform plate to enter the brain. The infective form of Naegleria is the trophozoite. Naegleria cysts are seldom seen. Since infection is so rapid and fatal, the patient dies before encystment. The cysts will form when there is a depletion of nutrients, changing pH, accumulation of wastes, oxygen deficiency and crowding of cells in culture. When conditions become favourable, excystment occurs and the amoebae digest the mucoid plugs that seal the pores of the cyst wall and squeeze through the pores.

The Naegleria species have a third morphologic form, the flagellate form, the presence of which is the major distinguishing feature from acanthamoeba species. The trophozoites of Naegleria species measure 10–35 μm in greatest dimension with a single blunt pseudopodium. The most characteristic structure is the vesicular nucleus with a large centrally located karyosome. The cytoplasm is coarsely granular with one or more contractile vacuoles, usually located posteriorly. In tissue sections, the amoebae are usually smaller, measuring 8–15 μm with vacuolated cytoplasm. During mitosis, the nucleolus of Naegleria spp. divides into two polar masses and the nuclear envelope persists, whereas the nucleolus and nuclear envelope of acanthamoeba species dissolve completely. The cysts of Naegleria species measure 7–10 μm in diameter with a smooth double cyst wall, whereas that of acanthamoeba species measures 9–27 μm in diameter and show a wrinkled cyst wall. The flagellate form is 10–15 μm in diameter, oval to pear shaped, with a pair of anterior flagella, enabling it to swim very rapidly.

Presentation

The incubation period of *Naegleria fowleri* is 2–15 days. The disease is of acute onset with very rapid progression of signs and symptoms and is associated with a very high mortality rate. It commences with fever associated with severe headache, nausea, vomiting, neck stiffness and fits. There is progressive change in the mental state with confusion, stupor and coma. The clinical picture is identical to pyogenic meningitis. In making the diagnosis, a history of swimming in an indoor or outdoor pool is vital. If more than one person is affected, a common source must be traced.

Pathology

The pathologic changes of primary amoebic meningo-encephalitis are essentially those of a basal meningo-encephalitis with involvement of the cerebrum, cerebellum and spinal cord. There is marked cerebral oedema with uncal herniation. Hyperaemia and patchy cortical haemorrhages associated with necrosis are also seen but a purulent exudate is macroscopically not conspicuous. Necrosis or ulceration is also seen along the route of the passage of the organism that involves the nasal epithelium, olfactory nerve and olfactory bulb.

Microscopically, the changes are similar to bacterial meningo-encephalitis. A fibrinopurulent exudate fills the subarachnoid space and extends into the Virchow-Robin spaces. Trophozoites are found in the purulent exudate. They can be recognized by their round shape, vacuolated cytoplasm, prominent karyosome or nucleolus and the well-delineated nuclear membrane. Quite frequently, the entire nucleus is surrounded by a halo. The parasite should be distinguished from glial cells by their larger size and much smaller nucleus. Special stains such as iron-haematoxylin, Giemsa and trichrome stains help to distinguish the parasite from host cells. *Entamoeba histolytica* is strongly PAS-positive whereas Naegleria spp. are only weakly positive. With progression of the infection, multiple micro-abscesses with vasculitis, thrombosis and focal necrosis occur. In Naegleria infection, organs other than the central nervous system are typically not involved, although positive amoebic cultures have been reported from the lungs, liver and spleen in one patient. It is difficult to distinguish between acanthamoeba and Naegleria in primary amoebic meningo-encephalitis. If cystic forms are also present, it is more indicative of acanthamoeba infection.

Investigations

1. *Lumbar puncture* will demonstrate raised CSF pressure and large numbers of white cells, $> 1700 \times 10^9$/litre, with ~75% neutrophils, the remaining being monocytes and lymphocytes. Stained films will not demonstrate any bacteria, and capsular bacterial antigens are negative. The protein content in the CSF is extraordinarily high, varying from 4 to 6.5 g/litre and the glucose level is low. Hence, a CSF with a very high protein level and negative bacterial antigens in a patient with clinical features of bacterial meningitis should point to an alternative diagnosis and a careful search for motile amoebae in a wet preparation should be performed. This is often negative due to the small numbers of amoebae present. The search for amoebae should include wet microscopy, cytospin preparations with Romanovsky stain and acridine orange. Phase contrast microscopy is preferred. The trichrome stain in alcohol fixed smears will demonstrate the prominent karyosome in red as contrasted with the green cytoplasm of the parasite. Refrigeration of the cerebrospinal fluid (CSF) should be avoided, as should high-speed centrifugation, to avoid damage to the parasite.
2. *Cultures* should proceed simultaneously particularly if amoebae are not identified in the CSF smears. It is important to alert the laboratory of the suspected diagnosis as specialized culture systems are required, e.g. *E. coli* and enterobacter species grow on non-nutrient agar (monoxenic culture) or specialized nutrient broth axenic cultures and need to be performed by a reference or research laboratory. If distinction between Naegleria and acanthamoeba species is necessary, the culture plate can be flooded with distilled water or buffer to induce flagellate transformation, the presence of flagellates indicating the Naegleria species.
3. *Brain biopsy* may reveal amoebic trophozoites. In tissue sections, amoebae are usually found in the deep Virchow-Robin spaces, where inflammation is not as marked as the superficial layer of the brain and the morphology of the parasite is better preserved.
4. *Immunologic tests*, mainly immunofluorescence and immunoperoxidase stains have been used to identify acanthamoeba species.

Treatment

Very little is known of the most effective form of treatment because of the rapidly fatal nature of the disease. A combination of amphotericin B, miconazole and rifampicin has been recommended.

- Amphotericin B (IV and intrathecal) – 1.5 mg/kg/day IV in divided doses for 3 days followed by 1 mg/kg/day for a further 6 days. Intrathecal: 1.5 mg/day for 2 days followed by 1 mg/day every second day for 8 days
- Miconazole (IV and intrathecal) – 350 mg/m² IV three times daily for 9 days. Intrathecal: 10 mg/day for 3 days followed by every second day for 8 days
- Rifampicin (PO) via nasogastric tube, 3 mg/kg three times a day for 9 days

Instructions with regard to IV and intrathecal administration follow strict guidelines given by the drug companies. In addition, co-administration of dexamethasone and phenytoin has been recommended. A more recent successful case was treated as follows (Brown 1994):

- Amphotericin B – 1 mg/kg IVI/day for 9 days
- Rifampicin (through a nasogastric tube) – 10 mg/kg every 12 h
- Amphotericin B – 0.1 mg combined with 0.25 mg dexamethasone in 0.4 ml dextrose and water intrathecal, every second day for a total of 5 days

IV injections of amphotericin produce fever with chills and rigors so that the dose may have to be reduced temporarily. The drug also impairs renal and hepatic function and produces hypocalcaemia and hypotension. In patients with impaired renal function, the dose needs to be reduced. Liposomal amphotericin is less toxic. However, in the management of primary amoebic encephalitis, treatment needs to be aggressive as mortality rate is almost 100%.

All patients should be managed in an intensive care unit where cardiac monitoring, protection of airways, intubation and ventilation can be provided.

ACANTHAMOEBA

Parasitology

Acanthamoeba is a free-living ubiquitous protozoan. Acanthamoeba species has been isolated from fresh water, tap water, swimming pools, air conditioners, sewage and from soft contact lenses. It has also been found in dialysis and dental treatment units, and has been isolated from vegetables, birds, fish and mammals. Only some of these isolated strains are pathogenic. In man acanthamoeba have been found in the throat, nasal cavities, intestines, skin wounds, lungs and cerebral tissue.

The species of acanthamoeba causing granulomatous amoebic encephalitis are *A. castellani*, *A. polyphagia*, *A. culbertsoni*. *A. castellani*, *culbesoni*, *A. hatchetti*, *A. polyphagia* and *A. rhysodes* cause keratitis in contact lens wearers, often attributed to poor contact lens hygiene or the use of contact lens while swimming. Man becomes infected by inhalation of the cysts, or entry of the organism is through open wounds. Acanthamoeba encephalitis has also been seen in patients with AIDS so that this infection should be borne in mind when considering the differential diagnosis of the cerebral complications of AIDS.

There are some differences in the life cycle of acanthamoeba compared with Naegleria. Acanthamoeba has only two stages: trophozoite and cyst. The trophozoite is larger than Naegleria spp. and motility is sluggish. Instead of the broad lobopodia in Naegleria, acanthamoeba forms spiny pseudopods called acanthapodia. It has no flagellate stage. The infective forms are the trophozoites. Cysts of acanthamoeba have also been demonstrated in human tissue. Cysts form under unfavourable conditions and the organism excysts when the environment is favourable. The cysts are distinct from those of Naegleria as instead of a smooth wall, the Acanthomoeba ectocyst is wrinkled. The characteristics of ecto- and endocysts are used to identify the different species of acanthamoeba. The amoebae feed on bacteria such as *E. coli* and other Gram-negative bacilli. Some species engulf *L. pneumophila* and may be a source of *Legionella* infection (Rowbotham 1980). Acanthomoeba cysts are resistant to disinfection and desiccation.

Acanthamoeba can cause a chronic infection in the central nervous system called granulomatous amoebic encephalitis or a serious infection affecting the eyes called Acanthamoeba keratitis. Less common sites of infection include the skin and bone.

Granulomatous amoebic encephalitis

The route of entry of acanthamoeba to the central nervous system is haematogenous, most likely from a focus in the respiratory tract or skin. Oedema, recent haemorrhage and abscesses characterize the brain changes. The areas most affected are the posterior fossa structures, brain stem, thalamus and di-encephalon. The olfactory bulbs and spinal cord are usually spared (Ma *et al.* 1990). Microscopically, a chronic granulomatous reaction with multinucleated giant cells is seen involving blood vessels with prominent necrotizing arteritis and fibrinoid necrosis, and haemorrhage. The trophozoites and cysts are found in the perivascular spaces and in walls of blood vessels. The meningoencephalitis is less purulent in comparison with that due to *N. fowleri*. The panangiitis is due to invasion of vessel walls by amoebae and cysts. Bilateral uncal notching and cerebellar tonsillar herniations from brain swelling may be seen. Other associated pathologic lesions are keratitis, panniculitis and dermatitis.

Presentation

The earliest symptoms are headaches, sporadic fever, nausea, vomiting and lethargy. These are followed by symptoms of meningeal irritation and altered mental status such as confusion, somnolence and irritability. Some patients develop seizures.

Clinical examination will reveal neck stiffness and localizing cerebral signs such as aphasia, hemiplegia and cranial nerve palsy mainly affecting the third and sixth nerves. Papilloedema is often seen. The disease process eventually ends in coma and death. It is a slow process in comparison with primary amoebic encephalitis.

The clinical picture may resemble bacterial meningitis such as that due to tuberculosis, viral encephalitis and space-occupying lesions such as abscess or tumour making correct clinical diagnosis extremely difficult. Predisposing factors such as a chronic illness, alcoholism, malignant disease, diabetes mellitus, liver disease and AIDS are helpful hints and some patients may be immunosuppressed or have had organ transplants.

Investigations

1. *Cerebral CT scan* may show multiple areas of decreased density in the cerebral cortex and white matter similar to infarcts.
2. *Brain biopsy* is useful for the identification of treatable conditions like herpes simplex encephalitis.

3. *Lumbar puncture* reveals CSF with pleocytosis with a predominance of lymphocytes and raised pressure. The protein content is moderately high and glucose concentration is low. Polymorphonuclear leukocyte count may be raised but not as high as in primary amoebic meningo-encephalitis. The CSF is not frankly purulent. Amoebic trophozoites may be present. Light microscopic examination of centrifuged unstained CSF may reveal refractile amoeba especially when they are motile. Acanthamoeba species are sluggish compared with Naegleria. Giemsa or Wright stains can demonstrate the morphology of the amoebae.

4. *Cultures* can be performed from CSF or from brain biopsy tissue but only a few cases have been diagnosed by this method.

5. *Immunofluorescent and immunoperoxidase staining* of brain tissue allows more specific identification of trophozoites and cysts than is possible by light microscopy.

6. *Isoenzyme analysis* is another method to identify pathogenic and non-pathogenic Naegleria and Acanthamoeba.

Treatment

Results of treatment of Acanthamoeba by chemotherapy are most disappointing as with *N. fowleri*. See the section on *N. fowleri*.

ACANTHAMOEBA KERATITIS

Presentation

In the early stage of the disease, the symptoms are non-specific, with recurrent redness and irritation of the eyes. Severe ocular pain, blepharospasm or photophobia, and watery discharge follow this and the visual acuity may be markedly diminished.

On examination, there is multiple, patchy and granular infiltrates of the cornea, and some are ring-shaped. Ulceration and erosion occurs and there may be ciliary injection, bilateral lid oedema and cloudiness of the anterior chamber. These features are invariably mistaken for herpes simplex keratitis.

Pathology

There is destruction of the anterior cornea with acute inflammatory cells in the superficial and middle layers of the stroma of the cornea. Amoebae may be seen infiltrating between the lamellae of the cornea. If keratoplasty has been performed there may be ulceration and formation of descemetocele. Cysts with irregular walls may be identified with special stains and intense inflammation is seen around encysted or necrotic organisms.

Investigations

Diagnosis is established in the following ways:

1. *Corneal scraping* should be obtained for microbiological and morphological studies. Elevated corneal epithelial lines are a clinical feature in corneal infection. When examined cytologically or histologically or by cultures, trophozoites and characteristic double-walled cysts may be found.

2. Corneal biopsies may be required if corneal scrapings are negative. Biopsy to a depth of 1.5–2.0 mm is necessary.

3. Examination of the *contact lens* by light microscopy may reveal amoebic cysts adherent to the lens. A lens fragment may be stained with calcoflour and, when exposed to UV light, the wall of the amoebic cyst fluoresces.

4. *Culture* from contact lens cases and other hardware used for care of lenses and from bottles of homemade saline may provide confirmation of amoebic contamination.

Treatment

Acanthamoebae in the encysted stage are very resistant to chemotherapeutic agents. Acanthamoeba shows wide variation of response to antimicrobial drugs. The drugs that have been used are:

- Propamidine isothionate – 0.1% applied every 1 h to the eye
- Polyhexamethylenbiguanide – 0.02% drops every 1 h
- Gentamicin – drops (1.5%) every 1 h with systemic antibiotics Ciprofloxacin and Intraconazole for ~1 month
- Topical neosporin has also been used. Some patients may require corneal graft and in late, resistant cases, even enucleation

Transmission of infection by contact lenses is preventable. Education on contact lens care and hygiene is necessary. At present several questions remain unanswered. The best disinfectant for contact lenses is not known. Disinfectants have varying effectiveness in that those effective in one type of Acanthamoeba may not be effective in another. Furthermore, commercial disinfectants have not been standardized as to their effectiveness. Laboratory studies have indicated that heat will kill both trophozoites and cysts. However, heating systems are not satisfactory for all types of contact lenses. The washing of contact lenses with tap water, or home-made saline, wearing them for long periods without chemical sterilization, and the use of contact lenses when swimming are practices to be avoided.

ILLUSTRATIVE CASE

A 25-year-old man presented to the ophthalmologist with a painful left eye. He was a contact lens wearer. On examination he was found to have an annular infiltrate in the cornea.

A corneal biopsy revealed ulcerated epithelium with a fibrinopurulent exudate, thickened Bowman's membrane and a stromal infiltrate of fragmenting neutrophils with scattered but numerous amoebic cysts (Fig. 3.1). A diagnosis of acanthamoebic keratitis was rendered.

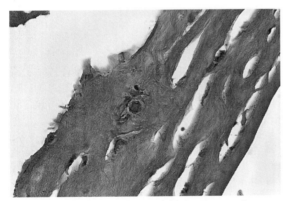

Figure 3.1 – Distorted corneal tissue showing amoebic cysts with the characteristic irregular cyst walls (H&E × 400).

REFERENCES

Brown RL. Successful treatment of primary amoebic meningoencephalitis. *Archives of Internal Medicine* 1991; **151**: 1201–1202

Bull CG, Baro C, Knorr RW. Naegleria identified in amoebic encephalitis. *American Journal of Clinical Pathology* 1968; **50**: 568–574

Chang SL. Resistance of pathogenic Naegleria to some common physical chemical agents. *Applied and Environmental Microbiology* 1978; **35**: 368–375

Dorsch MM, Cameron AS, Robinson BS. The epidemiology and control of primary meningo-encephalitis with particular reference to South Australia. *Transactions of the Royal Society of Tropical Medicine and Hygiene* 1983; **77**: 372–377

Fowler M, Carter RF. Acute pyogenic meningitis probably due to *Acanthamoeba* sp.: a preliminary report. *British Medical Journal* 1965; **2**: 740–742

Lowande RV, MacFarlane JT, Weir WRC *et al.* A case of primary amoebic meningo-encephalitis in a Nigerian farmer. *American Journal of Tropical Medicine and Hygiene* 1980; **29**: 21–25

Ma P, Visvesvara GS, Martinez AJ *et al.* Naegleria and *Acanthamoeba* infections: a review. *Review of Infectious Diseases* 1990; **12**: 490–513

Rowbotham TJ *et al.* Preliminary report on the pathogenicity of *Legionella pneumophila* from fresh water and soil amoebae. *Journal of Clinical Pathology* 1980, **33**: 1179–1183

4

Giardiasis

Parasitology
Presentation
Pathology

Investigations
Treatment
References

PARASITOLOGY

Giardiasis is caused by the flagellated protozoan *Giardia lamblia* (syn. *G. duodenalis* and *G. intestinalis*), the first human intestinal protozoan recognized by Leu von Hauk in 1681. Giardiasis is responsible for most outbreaks of water-borne gastroenteritis and has worldwide distribution, both in tropical and temperate countries. In developing countries it is very common among children < 10 years of age with an estimated prevalence of up to 20%. Its role as a pathogen in tropical areas, where it is highly endemic, is not quite certain. In non-endemic areas it is a cause of illness among travellers from areas of low prevalence.

The cysts of *G. lamblia* are viable for up to 3 months. Infection in man is caused by the ingestion of contaminated water or by the faecal-oral route. Cysts may be present in the stools of asymptomatic people. Patients in highly endemic areas get reinfected within a short period after treatment so that routine treatment is debatable. Some consider it to be a commensal organism. In the USA, 23 outbreaks of waterborne gastro enteritis reported from 1965 to 1977, in several states, were traced to chlorinated unfiltered water reservoirs. Beavers were the main reservoir host. Oral-anal transmission of giardiasis has been reported in male homosexuals as a component of the 'gay bowel syndrome'. Giardiasis is also a sexually transmitted disease causing vaginitis and proctitis. It is common in patients with acquired hypogammaglobulinaemia.

The parasite exists in the cyst and/or trophozoite form in the upper small intestine, particularly the duodenum. The trophozoite is pear shaped with a rounded anterior and pointed posterior end, measuring 12–18 μm in length. The dorsal surface is convex and the ventral surface has a concave sucking disc with a raised ridge at its anterior end, the posterior extremity tapering into a fine tail, terminating in flagella. Altogether there are four pairs of flagella arising from the ventral side of the body. The two oval nuclei are in the anterior end, each consisting of a central karyosome described as 'eyes' which appear unstained in stool preparations (Fig. 4.1). The flagellate swings rapidly, swaying from side to side. The cysts are formed in the lower bowel and may occur in large numbers in the stools. They are oval in shape and measure 10–20 μm in diameter, containing four nuclei, each with a prominent karyosome. In the middle of the cyst, a pair of axostyles is seen with two parabasal bodies across them (Fig. 4.2). The cytoplasm is characteristically retracted from the cyst wall.

Reproduction is by binary fission. The cysts remain viable at 21°C in water for up to 8 days and in stored water at 8°C for up to 5 weeks. They can resist the

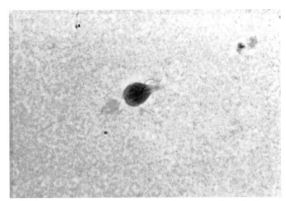

Figure 4.1 – *G. lamblia* trophozoite. The morphological characteristics seen at this magnification are the 'pear shape' and the two unstained nuclei, often described as 'eyes' (iodine stain × 400).

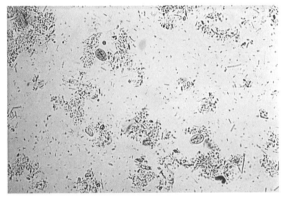

Figure 4.2 – Iodine stain of two *G. lamblia* cysts. While the nuclei are not easily recognized, the dark staining axonemes, running down the middle of the cysts, are recognizable (× 100).

concentration of chlorine normally present in tap water and are killed at 50°C and by 2% iodine solution when allowed to stand for 30 min. The cysts are readily digested by gastric and duodenal juices with resultant excystment of the trophozoite in the duodenum. The trophozoites multiply in the proximal small intestine and encyst again in the distal small intestine and throughout the colon. The cysts are expelled with the stools.

Man is the usual source of infection, although mammals such as dogs, beavers and muskrats can become infected and excrete cysts. Children also excrete large numbers of cysts.

PRESENTATION

Most infections with *G. lamblia* are asymptomatic. The incubation period is 10–14 days. Acute presentations occur with diarrhoea, abdominal pain or discomfort, distension with tenderness, nausea, vomiting and weight loss (Oberhuber and Stolte 1997). The symptoms generally last for a few days but can continue for weeks and months. The stools are foul smelling without blood and pus, and similar to stools in steatorrhoea. In the tropics, acute symptoms are common in malnourished, debilitated children. In the long-standing or chronic cases, malabsorption syndrome develops, similar to coeliac disease. Investigations reveal steatorrhoea, vitamin B_{12} and folate deficiency, xylose malabsorption and lactose intolerance. Even with eradication of the parasite, lactose intolerance persists due to lactase deficiency. An association between giardiasis and allergy has been demonstrated, possibly because infection by this protozoan enhances sensitization towards food antigens due to increased antigen penetration through the damaged bowel mucosa (Di Prisco *et al.* 1998).

PATHOLOGY

There is increased susceptibility to infection in those patients with achlorhydria, blood group A, chronic pancreatitis, protein energy malnutrition or immune deficiency states such as lack of IgA, hypogammaglobulinaemia and AIDS.

Several theories have been postulated to explain the clinical symptoms. Giardia may block the absorptive function of the small intestine, there is competition for nutrients between Giardia and the host or toxic substances may be released. There is some histochemical evidence that microvillous damage is caused by the parasite, leading to deficiencies of disaccharidases. Giardia may enhance sensitization towards food antigens due to increased antigen penetration through the damaged mucosa (Di Prisco *et al.* 1998).

No specific diagnostic features are seen in most small intestinal biopsies. However, enzymatic deficiency can be present in morphologically normal intestinal villi. In severe cases there may be villous atrophy with focal damage of the epithelium, an increased crypt mitotic index, blunting of the villi and acute or chronic inflammation in the intestinal mucosa similar to that seen in coeliac disease. The trophozoites are normally found in the mucus, adherent to the mucus membrane of the duodenum and jejunum, or attached to the mucosal surface. Sometimes superficial invasion of the mucosa is seen. In addition, diffuse nodular hyperplasia of intestinal mucosal lymphoid tissue may be present. Secretory immunoglobulin A deficiency has also been recorded.

The parasite can be seen in haemotoxylin and eosin stained sections of the jejunum (Figures 4.3a and 4.3b). Giemsa or trichrome stains highlight fine structures such as the paired nuclei. The trophozoites also stain with periodic acid Schiff (PAS) stains. Silver stains such as Gomori methenamine silver do not stain *Giardia*.

INVESTIGATIONS

1. Trophozoites can be demonstrated in fluid and biopsy samples obtained from the jejunum and cysts can be found in the stools. Examination of formed stools on 3 separate days is recommended for cysts, whereas trophozoites are found in watery stools. Identification of cysts needs special laboratory competence. Duodenal aspirate and microscopic examination of biopsies for the trophozoite is another routine method of diagnosis.

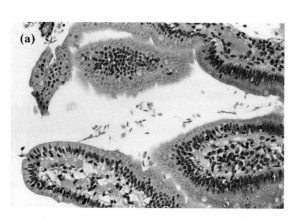

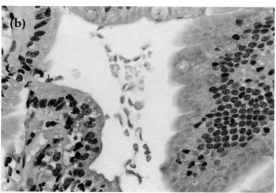

Figure 4.3 – *G. lamblia* trophozoite. (a) H&E × 40; (b) H&E × 100.

2. The Entero test with a nylon yarn partially enclosed in a gelatine capsule, which is retrieved after swallowing, is a very successful way of demonstrating the parasite. Giardia stains purple with Giemsa.

3. The ELISA technique detects specific anti-*Giardia* serum IgM and has a high specificity and sensitivity. Fluorescein-labelled monoclonal antibody tests for identifying *G. lamblia* in stool are more sensitive (Mank *et al.* 1997).

TREATMENT

Resistance to infection by *G. lamblia* may or may not be immunologically mediated. Giardia has the ability to resist expulsion by intestinal peristaltic forces (Owen 1980). The flagella generates a negative pressure in its ventral sucker. Human milk and infant milk formula have been shown to have a lethal effect *in vitro* on *G. intestinalis* and may have a role in producing resistance by targeting the adherence mechanism.

- Metronidazole cures > 90% of symptomatic patients. The dose for adults is 2 g once daily for 3 days or 200 mg thrice daily for 1 week. For children the dose is 20 mg/kg given as a once daily dose for 3 days
- Tinidazole 2 g for an adult is an alternate drug
- Erythromycin has been found useful but other reports have not confirmed this

Patients with pan-hypogammaglobulinaemia require prolonged treatment for 6 weeks.

REFERENCES

Di Prisco MC, Hagel I, Lynch NR *et al.* Association between giardiasis and allergy. *Annals of Allergy Asthma and Immunology* 1998; **81**: 261–265

Mank TG, Zaat JO, Deelder AM *et al.* Sensitivity of microscopy versus enzyme immunoassay in the laboratory diagnosis of giardiasis. *European Journal of Clinical Microbiology and Infectious Diseases* 1997; **16**: 615–619

Oberhuber G, Stolte M. Symptoms in patients with giardiasis undergoing upper gastrointestinal endoscopy. *Endoscopy* 1997; **29**: 716–720

Owen RL. The ultrastructural basis of *Giardia* function. *Transactions of the Royal Society of Tropical Medicine and Hygiene* 1980; **74**: 429–433

Malaria

PARASITOLOGY

Malaria is the infection caused by protozoa of the genus *Plasmodium*. Four species affect humans, namely, *P. vivax*, *P. falciparum*, *P. ovale* and *P. malariae*. A simian parasite, *P. knowlesi*, is also capable of causing human infection.

Malaria is the most widespread parasitic disease in man and is of cosmopolitan distribution. It is still one of the leading fatal diseases in the world. About 300 million people have malaria at any one time and the global death toll is between 1.5 and 2.5 million/year, the mortality rate being highest among children. It is prevalent within the latitudes 60°N and 40°S and seldom occurs

UHB TRUST LIBRARY
QEH

at altitudes > 2000 m. *P. falciparum* is present predominantly in the tropics. *P. vivax* and *P. malariae* are in the temperate zones and *P. ovale*, the rarest, is mainly seen in Africa.

Macassan and other traders introduced malaria to the Northern Territory of Australia and only in 1981 was Australia cleared by the WHO of indigenous malaria. Almost all cases seen in Australia today are imported although the potential for human–mosquito–human transmission from the imported cases and possibility of recurrence of endemic malaria remains as the vector, anopheles species, exists in Australia (Figures 5.1 and 5.2). The vast majority of cases reported in Australia were caused by *P. vivax* but greater numbers of cases are now caused by *P. falciparum*.

The countries where malaria is endemic and most likely to be visited by Australians are shown in Table 5.1.

The life cycle of plasmodium consists of a sexual phase or sporogony in female Anopheline mosquitoes and an asexual phase or schizogony in man (Figure 5.3). The asexual phase occurs in liver cells and erythrocytes.

Sporozoites, which are inoculated by the mosquito into the host, disappear from the circulation within 30 min. Some sporozoites enter hepatocytes, where they undergo development and multiplication, a stage known as pre-erythrocytic schizogony. The tissue schizonts enlarge and the nucleus and cytoplasm divides to form many thousands of merozoites which,

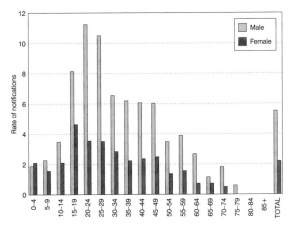

Figure 5.2 – Annual rate of notification of malaria/100 000 population, 1993, by age group and sex in Australia. (Courtesy of Communicable Disease Intelligence Canberra, 18: 22, 31 Oct 1994)

after 6–16 days, rupture the liver cells and invade the circulation where they enter red blood cells.

The incubation periods are: *P. vivax* 6–8 days, *P. malariae* 12–16 days, *P. ovale* 9 days, and *P. falciparum* 5–7 days.

Erythrocytic phase

The merozoites enter red blood cells and develop into ring forms that grow into trophozoites, absorbing haemoglobin and leaving a pigment (haematin or haemozoin – a combination of haemoglobin with protein) known as malaria granules. The trophozoite multiplies by schizogony, dividing into a number of small merozoites, the number varying with the species to form a mature schizont. Merozoites are released by rupture of the red cell membrane allowing further entry into new red cells, particularly young red cells. This erythrocytic phase, called schizogonic periodicity, differs with the species of parasite and is responsible for the febrile paroxysms. In *P. vivax*, *P. ovale* and *P. falciparum* the erythrocytic phase lasts 48 h and in *P. malariae* it is 72 h.

Gametogony

After 1 week, some merozoites give rise to two sexually differentiated forms of gametocytes – male microgamete and female macrogamete – which differ in morphology in the various species of the parasite. These gametocytes are taken up by female anopheline mosquitoes where they undergo the sexual phase.

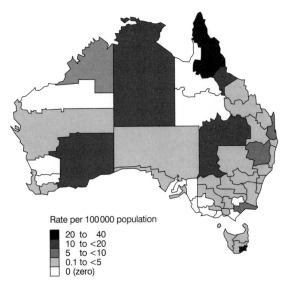

Rate per 100 000 population
- 20 to 40
- 10 to <20
- 5 to <10
- 0.1 to <5
- 0 (zero)

Figure 5.1 – Annual rate of notification of malaria/100 000 population (Courtesy of Communicable Disease Intelligence, 18: 536–537 1994) by statistical division of residence in Australia.

Table 5.1 – Countries where malaria is endemic and most likely to be visited by Australians

Argentina	Haiti	Nigeria	Tanzania
Bahrain	India	Pakistan	Thailand
Bangladesh	Indonesia	Panama	Tunisia
Botswana	Kampuchea	Papua New Guinea	Turkey
Brazil	Kenya	Philippines	Uganda
Celebes	Laos	Rwanda	Vanuatu
Myanmar (Burma)	Malaysia	Saudi Arabia	Vietnam
China Southern	Malawi	Solomon Islands	Zambia
Provinces	Mexico	South Africa	Zimbabwe
Egypt	Nepal	South America	
Ghana	New Hebrides	Sri Lanka	

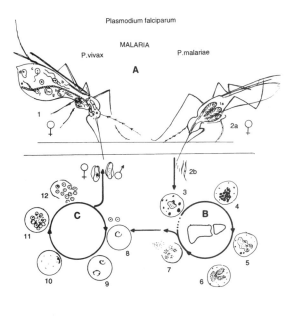

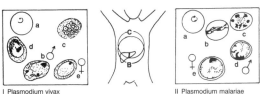

Figure 5.3 – Life cycle of Malaria. A: gametogony in mosquito (1) sporozoites in salivary gland (2a–2b). B: Pre-erythrocytic phase in liver (3–7). C: Erythrocytic phase (8–12).

The male gamete nucleus divides and flagella are formed. They enter the female gamete and fuse to form a zygote that becomes a mobile ookinete. These penetrate between the epithelial cells of the stomach to rest on the outer surface of the stomach wall as an oocyst, of which there may be several hundred in one stomach. In the oocyst, a large number of slender sporozoites form. These burst into the body cavity and enter the salivary glands of the mosquito, ready to be inoculated into a new host at the next blood meal. The duration of the cycle in the mosquito is known as the external incubation period. It varies according to the temperature, being 8–10 days at 28°C and 16 days at 20°C. The cycle cannot be completed at < 15°C.

P. vivax attacks young red blood cells. The ring stage has a vacuole surrounded by a loop of thin cytoplasm and a small round nucleus (Figure 5.4a). The ring enlarges after a few hours, becomes amoeboid and forms a trophozoite (Figure 5.4b). Minute grains of light brown pigment appear in the cytoplasm. The red cell enlarges and becomes pale, containing tiny spots known as Schuffner's dots which stain red with Giemsa or Wright techniques. After 24 h, the nucleus subdivides into daughter nuclei, forming a mature schizont which is the rosette stage with 8–24 merozoites (Figure 5.4c), the total cycle taking 48 h. Gametocytes (Figure 5.4d) appear ~5 days after the schizonts. A full-grown gametocyte occupies the entire red cell, measuring 10–11 μm. The female stains bright blue and the male grey.

P. ovale tends to infect young red blood cells. The morphology resembles *P. vivax* but the rings are smaller. The infected red cell is oval with fimbriated edges and shows dots that stain more deeply, so-called James' dots (Figure 5.5a). The rosette form contains 6–12 merozoites (Figure 5.5b) and the cycle is slightly longer. Gametocytes resemble those of *P. vivax* but are smaller.

P. malariae infects old red cells so that young rings are rare in the peripheral blood (Figure 5.6a). Trophozoites are seen in both mature and young red cells. Amoeboid and band forms are characteristic (Figure 5.6b). The rosette

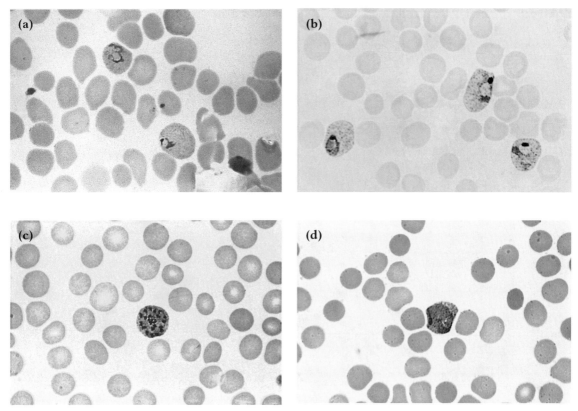

Figure 5.4 – (a) Ring forms of *P. vivax*; (b) early trophozoites of *P. vivax* markedly enlarged red cells containing large amoeboid parasites, pigment and prominent stippling; (c) Schizont of *P. vivax* – this enlarged red cell contains 18 merozoites (usually 12–18 merozoites) and contains a central clump of yellow brown pigmented particles; (d) Gametocyte *P. vivax.*

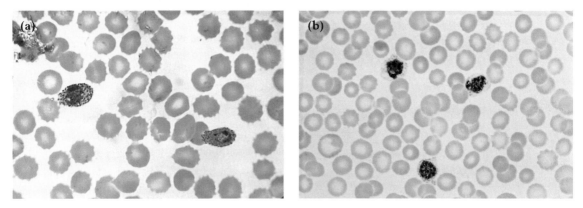

Figure 5.5 – (a) *P. ovale* ring form – compact parasite, brightly staining, contained within a red cell with prominent Schuffner's stippling. The oval shape, present in this case, may not be seen. Also note the presence of a trophozoite; (b) mature schizonts are heavily pigmented and generally produce 6–12 merozoites.

that matures at 72 h, contains 6–12 merozoites. The infected red cell does not enlarge but produces a characteristic stippling (Ziemann's dots). Gametocytes appear after 5–23 days. The male gametocyte has a large nucleus that stains pink and the cytoplasm greenish-grey. The female resembles a large schizont and is spherical, measuring 7 μm, with a deep blue cytoplasm.

P. falciparum attacks both young and mature red cells with preference for the former. The rings are small (1.2 μm) and hair-like with thin cytoplasm and a

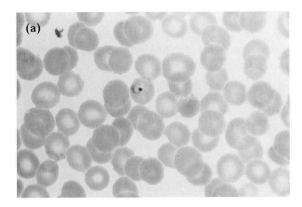

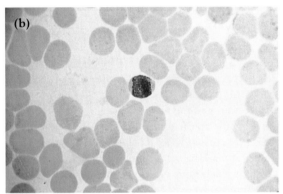

Figure 5.6 – (a) *P. malariae* ring form – a large ring within red cell of normal size and showing no stippling; (b) the band trophozoite most commonly seen in *P. malariae*. Note the bright staining, heavy pigmentation and the absence of enlargement and stippling in the red blood cell.

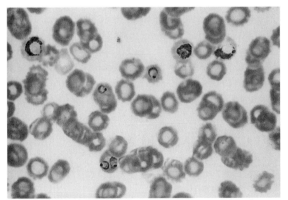

Figure 5.7 - *P. falciparum* – Multiple infection with ring forms.

prominent nucleus, which may be double, and a cytoplasmic vacuole. Multiple infections of red cells are common (Figure 5.7). Only ring forms are found in the blood and the appearance of schizonts is a feature of severe disease and only found in non-immune persons. The red cell is unaltered in size but may show

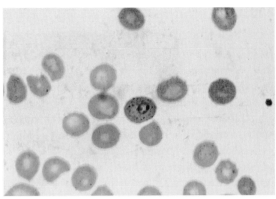

Figure 5.8 – Rings with Maurer's clefts – as *P. falciparum* parasites mature, stippling appears on the red cells in the form of clefts or pits.

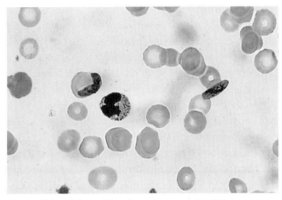

Figure 5.9 – Male and female gametocyte of *P. falciparum*.

spots (Maurer's clefts) (Figure 5.8). The rosette of mature schizont contains 8–32 merozoites. The gametocytes are elongated and crescent shaped (Figure 5.9). They appear after 8–11 days, their numbers occurring in waves, rising and falling for many weeks.

Malaria is transmitted from man to man by female anopheline mosquitoes. Some 60 species are known to be important vectors and are found most frequently in tropical and subtropical regions, the most important being Africa where the major vector is *Anopheles gambiae*. However, malaria can be transmitted in other ways such as transplacentally and by blood transfusion.

PRESENTATION

The clinical features depend on the infecting species. Malaria is mostly uncomplicated as with *P. vivax, ovale* or *malariae*, but it may be complicated as with *P. falciparum*. The progress from uncomplicated to complicated malaria may occur rapidly in *P. falciparum* infection, especially in children.

Malaria is a febrile illness and the fever occurs at the time of rupture of mature schizonts. Classically, a periodicity to the fever is mentioned for different species. However, it may take a few days for this to be established. The periodicity in *P. vivax* and *P. ovale* or benign tertian malaria, classically occurs every 48 h, *P. malariae* or benign quartan malaria, every 72 h and *P. falciparum* or malignant tertian malaria, has a more irregular pattern with intermittent fever or daily paroxysms. The paroxysms often do not fall into a neat pattern due to multiple episodes of infection.

The prodromal symptoms of malaria are not specific. There is a flu-like illness with malaise, muscular discomfort and headache. Next, fever develops with chills and shivering, the temperature rising up to ~40°C. The paroxysms are characterized by a cold phase that lasts up to 1 h resulting in chills and shivering and a cold pale skin. This is followed by a hot phase with flushing of the pale, dry skin. The patient may be incoherent and delirious. This hot phase lasts longer, ~2 h or more and cumulates in drenching sweats, soaking the clothing. The temperature then settles and the patient feels a great relief until the next paroxysm develops. Occasionally there may be abdominal discomfort and diarrhoea. In untreated malaria, the paroxysms of fever may recur over weeks or months before gradually resolving. The spleen may be enlarged.

It is now believed that the incidence of febrile illness rises with parasite densities. It is important to remember that in endemic areas, malaria parasites may be found in the asymptomatic population making it sometimes difficult to interpret its aetiologic role and relevance in a febrile patient. It has been shown that parasitaemia of > 5000/ml was associated with fever, this figure having a sensitivity and specificity of ~90%.

VIVAX MALARIA

The incubation period is ~12–17 days. However, it may be considerably longer in those who have been receiving suppressive chemotherapy during exposure to the infection. The prodromal symptoms, onset and paroxysms are as described above. In the period between the paroxysms, the patient feels well. The spleen is often palpable by the end of the second week of the primary attack. The liver also enlarges and may be palpable during the acute attack. In untreated primary infections, after regular occurrence of paroxysms whose intervals gradually lengthen with diminishing severity, there is spontaneous cure > 2 years. However, after a period of clinical quiescence of several weeks or months, a relapse may occur. The relapse is generally less severe than the initial attack and of shorter duration. It is unusual for relapses to occur after 4–5 years, especially after the patient has left the endemic area. The clinical picture of *P. ovale* is similar to that of *P. vivax*.

There have been a small number of recent reports from India and Sri Lanka of cerebral symptoms associated with *P. vivax* malaria (Mendis and Carter 1995).

PLASMODIUM MALARIA

The incubation period is 20–40 days. Prodromal symptoms are similar to vivax malaria. The onset may be insidious and the primary attack occasionally starts with a quartan periodic fever. The paroxysms are longer that that of vivax. The hot stage may last several hours. After long recurrent infections, especially in children, a nephrotic syndrome may develop. *P. malariae* does not relapse but may be asymptomatic for up to 20 years or more.

FALCIPARUM MALARIA (UNCOMPLICATED)

The incubation period is 8–15 days. Prodromal symptoms can be more severe than vivax infection. The clinical features in the uncomplicated falciparum infection are similar to other forms. However, the clinical features are unpredictable and may end in severe and fatal complications.

FALCIPARUM MALARIA (COMPLICATED)

Cerebral malaria

Cerebral malaria is the most serious complication of falciparum malaria and is associated with a high mortality rate. Patients with falciparum malaria may progress to coma, gradually passing through phases of confusion, delirium, obtundation and finally unarousable coma. Coma may occur suddenly after a convulsion (White and Pukrittayakamee 1993) and is more common in untreated non-immune patients or may be the first indication of an infection. There may be localized neurological signs with unequal pupils, urinary and faecal incontinence. Fundoscopy may reveal cotton wool spots and retinal haemorrhages, although papilloedema is rarely seen. Patients may show abnormal posturing and change in muscle tone. The plantar reflexes may be extensor. Rarely self-limiting cerebellar ataxia has been reported in Sri Lanka.

The coma in falciparum malaria cannot be explained by cerebral oedema alone and there has been controversy as to whether alterations in capillary permeability in the cerebral circulation contributes to the coma and other cerebral complications. Recent studies of capillary permeability in acute falciparum malaria has demonstrated that in severe infections there is a global increase in capillary permeability but only relative to that observed in uncomplicated infections or in the healthy (Roman 1991). In Kenya, children with cerebral malaria who were studied for cerebral haemodynamics revealed no reduction of cerebral blood flow. In some patients there was an increase in velocity of blood flow without the vasospasm that is seen in other encephalopathies. Raised intracranial pressure in children with cerebral malaria had a poor outcome. Possible causes of increased blood flow in cerebral malaria include seizures, anaemia, hyperthermia, tumour necrosis factor induced nitric oxide release, acidosis and hypoxia (Mendis and Carter 1991).

Measurements of regional blood flow, together with autopsy findings showed mechanical obstruction with adherent infected erythrocytes in the microcirculation causing dysfunction of several organs (White 1986). There was also a reduction in the deformability of red cells with intracellular maturation of the parasites. Hence, a multiplicity of factors, together with severe dehydration and probably a very mild degree of fibrin deposition and platelet thromboxane A_2 can lead to loss of tissue viability and hypoxia, accounting for the coma.

Cytokines such as tumour necrosis factor X, interleukin 6 (IL-6), IL-1, are also produced and these enhance adherence of *P. falciparum* infected red cells. Attention has now been focused on the role of nitric oxide in the pathogenesis of cerebral malaria. Nitric oxide has some protective functions such as relaxation of blood vessels, downgrading of cell adhesive molecules and inhibition of endothelial alterations. It has also been demonstrated that nitric oxide blockage in experimental cerebral malaria aggravates the pathology. Nitric oxide can scavenge free radicals. Since cerebral malaria is reversible, it is possible that nitric oxide mediates early changes such as disturbances of neurotransmission and not neurovascular damage. Sequestration of red cells and its role is also not well defined. Monkeys infected with *P. coatneyi* do not develop coma suggesting that sequestration plays an important role (Cerau and de Kossodo 1994). It is postulated that the endothelial cell lesion in cerebral malaria depends on several factors that interact, involving not only the endothelial cell sequestration of parasitized red cells, but also other blood cell types mediated by TNF-X, inducible ICAM-1, ELAM-1 and VCAM-1 that are upgraded in cerebral malaria.

Parasite products are released during paroxysms and are specifically seen in *P. vivax* malaria during the rupture of schizonts. The parasite products induce host cells to produce cytokines. There is evidence to show that a phospholipid glycosyl phosphatidyl inositol is the main TNF-inducing moiety of malarial parasites.

Rosetting is the binding of uninfected erythrocytes to erythrocytes infected with mature parasites. Rosetting is a phenomenon seen specifically in malarial species that sequester such as *P. falciparum*. In Gambia, it has been associated with cerebral malaria, however, it has not been shown in cases in Kenya, Thailand and Papua New Guinea (Al-Yaman 1995).

Acute renal failure

Falciparum malaria may cause acute renal failure from acute tubular necrosis. Hence, regular biochemical investigations and examination of urine for albumin, red cells, casts and the urine output is essential.

Blackwater fever

Acute renal failure can also be precipitated by acute haemolysis with haemoglobinuria and haemoglobinaemia, often described as blackwater fever. Such patients have a history of several bouts of falciparum malaria over a prolonged, irregular period with inadequate treatment with quinine. It occurs generally in endemic areas and in non-immune Caucasians whose erythrocytes are not G6PD deficient. The renal failure is caused by renal ischaemia with tubular necrosis and to some extent, from haemoglobin pigment deposition.

Nephrotic syndrome

Nephrotic syndrome from acute or chronic glomerulo-nephritis may be secondary to immune complex deposits in the glomeruli. *P. falciparum* is generally responsible for the acute form of nephrotic syndrome and *P. malariae* infection for the more chronic form.

Pulmonary oedema

Acute pulmonary oedema results from an increase in pulmonary capillary permeability with normal pulmonary wedge pressure. As in other forms of acute respiratory distress syndrome, it may cause death in adults (White and Pukrittayakamee 1993).

Lactic acidosis and hypoglycaemia

Lactic acidosis due to cellular hypoxia occurs as a direct result of changes in the microcirculation, or due to pulmonary oedema and hypoglycaemia from hyper-insulinaemia in falciparum malaria. Hypoglycaemia is a complication common in children and pregnant women.

Bacterial infections

In African countries, superimposed salmonella infections are common. Patients may develop Gram-negative septicaemia, hence, routine blood cultures are important in patients with cerebral malaria.

Disseminated intravascular coagulation

An association between malaria and low platelet counts is well recognized. However, post-mortem studies do not reveal the presence of platelet microthrombi in patients with cerebral malaria. In vitro platelet activation occurs in patients with severe nonfatal falciparum malaria but is of a low grade and, with treatment, platelet levels return to normal quite soon. Disseminated intravascular coagulation is usually not clinically significant.

Ischaemic skin changes

Peripheral gangrene has been reported as a rare complication in plasmodium infection. This is probably related to tissue sequestration of mature forms of the parasite

with rosette formation causing peripheral microvascular occlusion. Healing is generally complete with recovery from cerebral malaria, especially in children.

Hyperactive malarial splenomegaly

In a very small percentage of patients infected with any species of plasmodium, hyperactive malarial splenomegaly or tropical splenomegaly may develop. The patients usually have had previous bouts of malaria and present with a grossly enlarged spleen. Complications are acute haemolytic anaemia, especially in pregnancy. The cause of the persistent splenomegaly is the aberrant immunological response to the malarial parasite. Action should be taken to completely eradicate the organism, followed by life long chemoprophylaxis. Splenectomy is not indicated as the patients become prone to more frequent bacterial infection and septicaemia. With prolonged chemotherapy the size of the spleen tends to become smaller.

PATHOLOGY

As most fatal cases are caused by falciparum malaria, the pathologic description is essentially derived from this infection. Infection by other plasmodium species causes mild-to-moderate haemolysis, malarial pigment deposition and parasitized red blood cells in internal organs. The severity of falciparum malaria is a function of the large number of merozoites produced during the pre-erythrocytic cycle and the tendency of the parasitized red cells to stick to capillary endothelium. The adherent erythrocytes interfere with the cerebral blood circulation besides causing the retention of red blood cells in the viscera.

Brain

The brain is swollen and heavy with broadening and flattening of the gyri and uncal and tonsillar herniation. There is marked congestion of arachnoid vessels which produces a pink appearance. The selective congestion of the white matter is helpful in distinguishing cerebral malaria from viral encephalitis, which involves mainly the grey matter. Microscopically, the congested vessels contain parasitized erythrocytes that line up along the vascular endothelium – a phenomenon known as margination. The capillaries, which are obstructed by the parasitized erythrocytes, are surrounded by a zone of local softening or necrosis which, in turn, are enclosed by a circle of extravasated red blood cells ('ring haemorrhage'). The so-called Durck's granuloma is a result of a micro-infarct with subsequent local glial proliferation. Demyelination and axonal degeneration are occasionally seen. Ring haemorrhages, Durck's granulomas and demyelination are observed only in lesions > 9 days.

Spleen

The spleen is enlarged to ~500 g in acute malaria but may exceed 1000 g in the chronic stage. The capsule is dark grey-blue and its cut surface is soft and spongy from engorged sinuses filled with parasitized red blood cells and lined by phagocytes containing malarial pigment. Foci of mineralization or Gamna-Gandy bodies can be seen in the fibrotic spleens of chronic cases.

Liver

There is deposition of malarial pigment with a resultant slate grey colour to the enlarged liver. Microscopically, parasitized red blood cells are seen in the sinusoids and malarial pigment in Kupffer cells. In old lesions, malarial pigment gradually shifts into the portal areas. Bile stasis is not a feature, even though the patient might have haemolytic jaundice. Sinusoidal lymphocytosis is present in cases with the tropical splenomegaly syndrome. Tissue macrophages play an important part in the clearance of malaria sporozoites from the circulation. In the spleen, sporozoites are destroyed to a large extent by macrophages. However, sporozoites are able to escape from Kupffer cells and invade the liver parenchyma.

Kidney

The kidneys may be slightly pigmented and mildly enlarged. Malarial pigment is seen in glomeruli and parasites are present in red blood cells in capillaries. There may be a large number of haemoglobin casts in the renal tubules that show tubular necrosis, a characteristic of black water fever. In milder cases, proteinaceous or erythrocyte casts may be seen. In malaria-associated nephrotic syndrome, the glomerulonephritis may be associated with immune complex deposition demonstrable by immunofluorescent staining as well as electron microscopy.

Lungs

The major finding is pulmonary oedema. Uremic changes are evidenced by the presence of hyaline membranes lining the alveolar walls and bronchopneumonia is sometimes seen.

Other organs

Parasitized red blood cells can be seen within vessels throughout the body and a variety of other organs may be grossly affected, especially in falciparum malaria. For example, the bone marrow may be grossly pigmented, placental involvement can be so severe as to cause foetal or maternal death, the heart may be flabby and enlarged with pericardial and endocardial petechiae, and lymph nodes may be hyperplastic and congested with parasitized erythrocytes.

The cause of malarial anaemia, a major cause of mortality in African children, is not clearly defined. It is probably associated with tumour necrosis factor-induced dyserythropoiesis, destruction of red blood cells by free oxygen radicals, splenic hyperactivity and destruction of red cells.

INVESTIGATIONS

1. *Peripheral blood film examination* is the mainstay of diagnosis. Blood should preferably be taken by finger prick. Thick and thin films stained with Giemsa or Wright stains allow identification of the parasites. Thick films are more useful for screening but morphologic details for species identification is better seen in thin films. The possibility of mixed infections must be borne in mind when making the identification.

    The diagnosis of malaria should not be excluded on the basis of a single smear as parasitaemia may be low due to partial suppression by drug treatment. It is extremely important that multiple thick and thin blood films be examined over several days to allow a positive diagnosis. Species identification may be difficult.

2. *Quantitation buffy coat analysis* (QBC, Becton Dickinson, Franklin Lakes, NJ, USA) is performed by filling a microhaematocrit tube coated with Acridine orange centrifuged blood before examination by fluorescence microscopy. Acridine orange induces fluorescence of DNA

present in the sample, including that of malarial parasites. The method does not allow species identification.

3. *An Eliza technique* has been introduced for the identification of *P. falciparum*, but is employed mainly in research. Microtitre wells are precoated with anti-*P. falciparum* monoclonal antibody. If the appropriate antigen is present, it binds to the coated well. Enzyme-labelled antimalaria monoclonal antibody is then added. Colour generated by a chromogen indicates the presence of falciparum malaria antigen.

4. *Serologic tests* are available for epidemiological and research but are not for diagnosis.

PCR and DNA analyses have been devised but are not in clinical use.

Other investigations

These include full haematology screen including coagulation studies, biochemistry profile including liver and renal function tests, arterial blood gases and lactic acid levels, quantitative parasite counts, CT scan on all unconscious patients, followed by CSF examination, routine chest X-ray, ECG and blood culture.

TREATMENT

Uncomplicated malaria

- Treatment with chloroquine is shown in Table 5.2. A consensus recommendation on treatment in Southeast Asia was developed recently (Looareesuwan *et al.* 1998).
- Treatment for chloroquine-resistant malaria is shown in Table 5.3. Quinine infusion should be performed with ECG monitoring and quinine infusion should be stopped if the QT interval is > 25% of base line level. Hypoglycaemia has been reported with IV quinine and regular blood sugar measurements are essential.
- Primaquine is essential to completely eradicate the liver cycle in *P. vivax* and *P. ovale*. G6PD deficient patients may develop haemolysis.
- Mefloquine resistance has been reported in Thailand. Chloroquine resistance to *P. vivax* has been reported in Papua New Guinea and Indonesia.

Treatment of severe falciparum malaria

Severe falciparum malaria is a medical emergency and patients should be treated in an intensive care unit. Airways should be protected. Adequate fluid, resuscitation is essential. Frequent regular check on blood sugar is important. Periodic checks on electrolytes and arterial blood gases will help in the management. Hypotensive patients may require inotropes.

- Specific drug treatment is outlined in Table 5.4.

Adjuvant treatment

Glucose should be administered to prevent hypoglycaemia and prophylactic anticonvulsion drugs should be given. Corticosteroids have not been shown to improve the outcome. There is no definite evidence that exchange transfusion is helpful in seriously ill patients with high levels of parasitaemia. Blood transfusion is indicated if the haemoglobin drops significantly.

Patients with renal failure require haemodialysis and those with non-cardiogenic pulmonary oedema require continuous positive airways pressure.

In blackwater fever, steroids are extremely beneficial to stop the haemolysis. The commencing dose is 60 mg IV hydrocortisone.

Newer drugs for treatment

- Halofantrine has been used in the treatment of chloroquine-resistant malaria at a recommended dose of 8 mg/kg 6-hourly PO, for three doses. It is not recommended for infants and is better absorbed after a fatty meal. Peak plasma level is attained in 6 h with a half-life of 24 h. Asexual ring forms are cleared from blood in 48–72 h. It is recommended that in non-immune patients, the dose be repeated after 2 weeks. Minor side-effects include gastrointestinal symptoms, pruritis, rashes, raised liver enzymes and possible cardiotoxic effects. It should never be used in combination with mefloquine or prescribed for anyone who has been treated with mefloquine. It has no place in prophylaxis because of its variable absorption. It has no action against *P. falciparum* sporozoites or gametocytes.

Table 5.2 – Treatment for *P. vivax, P. ovale, P. malariae* and uncomplicated falciparum infections.

Drug	Adult dose	Childhood dose (do not exceed adult dose)
Chloroquine sensitive:		
Chloroquine (oral)	600 mg base stat dose,	10 mg/kg base stat dose,
	300 mg base 6 h after	5 mg/kg base 6 h after stat dose
	300 mg base days 2 and 3,	5 mg/kg base days 2 and 3,
*Primaquine oral	15 mg daily for 14 days	0.3 mg/kg daily for 14 days

Check for G6PD deficiency used to prevent reinfection in *P. vivax* and *P. ovale*.

Adult dosage 22.5 mg daily for *P. vivax* infection in South East Asia.

Dosage for the Pacific Islands is 30 mg daily for 2 weeks if the patient relapses after primaquine.

Table 5.3 – Treatment for chloroquine-resistant malaria (uncomplicated).

Drug	Adult	Child (do not exceed adult dose)
1. Quinine sulphate oral	600 mg 8-hourly for 7 days	10 mg/kg every 8 h for 7 days
or		
2. Mefloquine oral	750 mg then 500 mg ater 6 h	15 mg/kg in two doses 6 h apart
*1. Tetracycline oral	250 mg 6-hourly for 7 days	NOT for children or pregnant women
or		
*1. Doxycycline oral	100 mg daily for 7 days	NOT for children
or		
*1. Pyrimethamine 25 mg		*6 weeks–1 year, ¼ tablet
Sulphadoxine 500 mg	on day 2	on day 2 one dose
(one tablet) oral	two or three tablets	1–3 years ½ tablet on day 2
	one dose	4–8 years 1 tablet on day 2
		9–14 years 2 tablets on day 2

*Given together with quinine.

Table 5.4 – Specific drug treatment for complicated malaria (*Falciparum malaria*).

Drug	Adult	Child
Quinine (IVI) hydrochloride (cardiac monitoring)	Loading dose 7 mg salt/kg given as a bolus over 30 min by infusion pump dil. in normal saline followed by 10 mg salt/kg over 4 h every 8 h till oral intake	Same regime as adults according to body weight. Do not exceed adult dose
Quinine oral (when oral intake possible)	10 mg salt/kg three times a day for 7 days with	
Tetracycline (for adults only)	4 mg/kg four times a day for 7 days	Not for children or pregnant women
	or	and
Pyrimethamine 25 mg/ sulphadoxine 500 (one tablet)	two or three tablets on day 2	6 weeks–1 year, ¼ tablet 1–3 years ½ tablet 4–8 years 1 tablet 9–14 years 2 tablets

Quinghaosu

This drug had been known for 2000 years in China, and Chinese writings revealed that it was used as an anti-malarial agent. It was rediscovered in 1971 and is an extract of the plant *Artemisia annua* or sweet wormwood used for flavouring vermouth (Lancet 1992). The active chemical is called artemisinin. The derivatives of artemisinin are artemether (an oil-soluble methyl ether) and artesunate (a water-soluble derivative).

These derivatives reduce parasitaemia more rapidly than other antimalarial drugs in studies from China. Clinical trials revealed that fever was shorter and parasite clearance was more rapid than with mefloquine but the recrudescence rate was as high as 10–50% (Looareesuwan *et al.* 1992). This may be explained by rapid drug elimination. Quinghaosu destroys falciparum asexual parasites and acts faster to prevent further development of the early trophozoite. Studies in animals and healthy volunteers indicated that the biologically active metabolite is dihydroartemisinin and both the parent and active metabolite are rapidly eliminated. There has been no local or systemic toxicity in extensive clinical studies. Concerns about toxicity have arisen from animal experiments in which rats and dogs given artemether at several times the human dosage, developed fatal neurotoxicity and with prolongation of QTc interval (Brewer *et al.* 1994). Neuropathological changes occurred in medulla and pons, probably caused by accumulation of a toxic metabolite with multiple doses. However, there was lack of pharmacokinetic details and CNS toxicity may have been due to the disease process. This toxicity has not been recorded in humans. Artemether and oil-soluble methyl ether of artemisinin (quinghaosu) has been shown to be well tolerated and a rapidly effective treatment for severe malaria in children, and is particularly valuable and effective in areas with chloroquine-resistant *P. falciparum* (White *et al.* 1992). In Thailand, oral forms of artesunate at 600 mg for 5 days gave a cure rate of 90%. The cure rate for combined mefloquine and artesunate was 100%.

The preparations available overseas are Artesunate as tablets, capsules and suppositories, aremether as oil based injection for IMI administration, artesunate IV preparation to be dissolved in 5% sodium bicarbonate immediately before injection. The dose regimen is largely empirical as there have been no pharmacokinetic studies.

Adult dosage:

Oral	Artesunate	100 mg stat and 50 mg 12 hourly for 5 days (total 600 mg)
IMI	Artemether	3.2 mg/kg followed by 1.6 mg/kg every 12 h (total 600 mg)
IVI	Artesunate	2 mg/kg IVI bolus followed by 1 mg/kg every 12 h (total 600 mg)

The various preparations of quinghaosu when used alone have a high rate of recrudescence. However, appropriate dose artesunate or artemether used in combination with mefloquine 750 mg 24 h after, followed by a second dose of mefloquine has a very high success rate of recovery from *P. falciparum* and very low rate of recrudescence.

In uncomplicated malaria, the regimen for artesunate or artemether is 300 mg once followed by mefloquine 750 mg 24 h later and 500 mg mefloquine 6 h after the first dose of mefloquine. This combination has a cure rate of 100% (personal communication, Dr T. Harinasula, Faculty of Tropical Medicine, Mahidol University, Bangkok). The same workers also used artemether in severe falciparum malaria at a total dose of 640 mg IM, 160 mg stat and 80 mg/day for 6 days thereafter. A comparative study of artemether IM and quinine IVI found artemether to be superior to quinine.

Artesunate is not a drug for prophylaxis as it has a short half life.

Iron-chelating agents

Malarial parasites require iron for vital cell functions and have a high replication rate but do not have the capacity to mobilize bioavailable iron from the host in spite of the asexual cycle parasites being bathed in blood. Based on this theory, iron chelating agents such as hydroxamate desferioxamine (DFO) have been used successfully on *P. falciparum* both in vitro and in vivo in animals and humans (Gorduek 1993, Mendez 1995).

Exchange transfusion

Although it has been recommended that exchange transfusion be instituted in any non-immune patient with a parasitaemia of > 15%, there is insufficient evidence to allow proper assessment of this form of treatment. Exchange transfusion has its own hazards and will not remove sequestrated red cells, further-more, the removal of parasitized red cells may not be beneficial.

PROPHYLAXIS FOR TRAVELLERS

Malaria is spread through the bite of the female anopheles mosquito that feeds from dusk to dawn. Hence, the first step in prophylaxis is to employ pro-tective measures from the vector such as the wearing of long sleeves and long pants throughout the day especially in rural areas (Schoepke *et al*. 1998). Dark-coloured clothing and perfumes, both of which attract insects, should be avoided. Mosquito coils, which repel mosquitoes, can be used indoors and the applica-tion of repellents containing diethyl-toluamide (DEET) to the clothing and exposed parts of the body is essential. In the absence of air conditioning, the use of mosquito screens and mosquito nets sprayed with permethrin will markedly reduce the risk of mosquito bites, reducing mortality rate in children of 1–4 years by 63% (Wright and Marchand 1995).

Prophylaxic drugs are not 100% effective and are not without side-effects. They should be used with cau-tion and on an individual basis. The choice depends on several factors, namely, the country one is visiting, whether one is residing temporarily in the city, which may be relatively safe, or in the rural area, any history of allergy or other medical conditions, preg-nancy and age.

Chloroquine

In all malarial areas, chloroquine is the drug of choice for prophylaxis. It is safe for use in pregnancy and in children. It can be effectively used even if the person develops infection after leaving the area. It should be stressed that resistance to chloroquine is relative and varies from low to high. There are three recognized levels of resistance to chloroquine. Low level resis-tance is when the parasites disappear from the periph-eral blood following standard chloroquine therapy, but recrudescence occurs within 28 days. Moderate level resistance is when parasitaemia is reduced by > 75% during chloroquine therapy but parasites persist in the peripheral circulation and high level resistance occurs when parasitaemia is reduced by < 75% or is unaffected by standard doses of chloroquine.

Prophylaxis should be commenced 2 weeks before entry to malarious areas (to maintain adequate blood levels) and continued for 4 weeks after departure. This would be effective in eradicating the pre-erythrocytic cycle of vivax and ovale species. Chloroquine acts on the erythrocytic cycle. The recommended weekly adult dose of chloroquine is 300 mg base (500 mg salt). The paediatric dose is 5 mg base/kg body weight, up to a maximum of 300 mg, once a week. It is contraindi-cated in patients with psoriasis, hepatic porphyria and must be used with caution in patients with liver, ocu-lar and renal diseases. Chloroquine-resistant *P. vivax* has been reported in Australia, Papua New Guinea, Indonesia and Thailand (Table 5.5). Where there is a high resistance to chloroquine, an alternative drug has to be considered.

Table 5.5 – Countries known to have chloroquine-resistant malaria

Plasmodium falciparum	
Brazil	Pakistan
China (Hainan Island and Southern Province)	Panama
	Papua New Guinea
	Peru
Colombia	Philippines
India	Rwanda
Indonesia	Solomon Islands
Kampuchea	Thailand
Kenya	Uganda
Laos	Vanuatu
Malawi	Vietnam
Malaysia	Zambia
Myanmar (Burma)	
Plasmodium vivax	
Indonesia	
Papua New Guinea	
Thailand	

Papua New Guinea and Thailand also have species of *P. vivax* known to be resistant to mefloquine.

Doxycycline (DORYX)

This is one of the alternative prophylactic drugs. It is very effective against the pre-erythrocytic stage of *P. falciparum* and against the erythrocytic forms of *P. vivax* and *P. falciparum*. Doxycycline cannot be used in preg-nancy and in children < 8 years as it affects bone and teeth. The dose of doxycycline is 100 mg/day and can be commenced just before visiting an endemic area and should continue for 2 weeks after leaving the area. If a dose is missed, then it should be continued for 4 weeks after returning. The main disadvantage of doxycycline is compliance. The maximum duration for safe use is not known and its minimum effective duration of use in an endemic area is also not known. The main side-effect of doxycycline is photosensitivity and the use of a sunscreen is recommended. Other side-effects include skin reactions, gastrointestinal, hepatic, renal and haematological abnormalities. It is a safe drug and there is no contraindication for its use with suppressive treatment with chloroquine or mefloquine. Doxycycline is the recommended prophylaxis when there is resistance to chloroquine and mefloquine such as encountered in the Thai-Kampuchea and Thai-Myanmar borders.

Mefloquine

Mefloquine has been used for prophylaxis. Although safe and effective for antimalarial prophylaxis in the second half of pregnancy (after 20 weeks), caution must be employed if used in pregnancy. The recommended dose is 250 mg PO once a week, one dose immediately before evening meals 7 days before departure and 28 days after returning. The side-effects of mefloquine are dizziness, anxiety, restlessness or confusion and depression. The drug should not be used when piloting an aircraft or using dangerous machinery and should be stopped if there is depression or confusion. It produces a prolonged QTc interval on ECG and is contraindicated in patients on cardiac drugs and in children < 45 kg weight, although there is no definite reason for the latter. It appears to be safe to use for > 3 months. Mefloquine does not eradicate the liver cycle of *P. vivax* and primaquine has to be used for this purpose. Resistance to mefloquine has been reported in some South East Asian countries. Halofantrine, another drug used in resistant falciparum infection, may interact with prophylactic mefloquine to cause cardiotoxicity.

Other prophylactic drugs

Drugs such as sulphadoxine-pyrimethamine (Fansidar) and Dapsone pyrimethamine (Maloprim) are not recommended because of serious toxic effects. The WHO (1991) advises the use of quinine,

mefloquine halofantrine or, in some parts of the world, sulphadoxine-pyrimethamine or sulphalene-pyrimethamine for self therapy.

MALARIA IN PREGNANCY

It is estimated that 1 billion pregnant women are exposed to malaria. The infection rate appears to be higher in the second trimester and greater in primigravida. The frequency and severity of parasitic diseases generally tend to increase during pregnancy as a result of some degree of immune suppression from increased cortisol levels. There is evidence of both suppression of antibody formation and cell mediated immunity during pregnancy. Anaemia may be a contributing cause. Severe, complicated malaria with cerebral involvement, renal failure and pulmonary oedema occur more commonly in pregnant women.

All species of malaria can infect a pregnant woman; however, *P. falciparum* and *P. vivax* are the most common. Malaria in pregnancy, especially falciparum malaria is also detrimental to the foetus, causing low birth weight in 18.8%, premature labour in 59.6%, abortion in 9.7% and foetal death in 5.7% of the infected. There can be a significant reduction in birth weight of first born child as malaria immunity is lower due to absence of previous infections and the low birth weights may extend to the second and third pregnancies with a high infantile mortality rate.

The morbidity and mortality rate of foetus is the result of ischaemia caused by the large numbers of red cells infected by *P. falciparum*. The parasite crosses the placental barrier and can rarely cause congenital malaria.

Haemolysis is another complication in mother and foetus, resulting in anaemia and hypoxia. In the tropics this is compounded by maternal iron and folic acid deficiency. Haemolysis is partly due to immune destruction of sensitized red cells and depression of erythropoiesis.

Congenital malaria

Congenital malaria is uncommon, however, it may remain undiagnosed for a considerable period. It should be considered in the differential diagnosis of anaemia, jaundice, splenomegaly and fever in an infant whose mother's travel history is unknown. Chloroquine is effective for the infant unless the mother is infected with a chloroquine-resistant strain.

Treatment (Table 5.6)

The essentials of treatment remain the same including those for complications but treatment should be carried out as early as possible to safeguard both foetus and mother. Hospitalization of all pregnant mothers with malaria is essential.

- Chloroquine is the drug of choice in non-resistant falciparum infections and all other types of malaria. If, at any stage, the disease shows no response to chloroquine, quinine should be used either PO in the conscious patient or IV if patient is comatosed, under intensive care monitoring conditions. Intravenous quinine dihydrochloride has been used in pregnant women with severe falciparum malaria with no apparent change in uterine activity despite rising quinine concentrations. Maternal temperature should be reduced to control foetal tachycardia. A close watch on blood sugar is vital as there is increased secretion of insulin in patients with falciparum malaria.

In complicated malaria in pregnancy it is necessary to check the following parameters periodically: full blood count, electrolytes, blood sugar (five base line blood samples at 15-min intervals), lactic acid levels and arterial blood gases.

The treatment for complicated malaria in pregnancy is generally similar to the non-pregnant state with some exceptions. It should be conducted in the setting of an intensive care unit with maternal and foetal monitoring. For peripheral vascular collapse fluid resuscitation and monitoring is performed using a Swan-Ganz catheter. This will allow assessment of the degree of hypovolaemia and non-cardiogenic pulmonary oedema.

In blackwater fever steroid should be promptly employed. This is the only indication for steroid therapy in acute malarial complications. Prednisolone 60 mg/day causes a rapid reduction in the rate of haemolysis. Taper the dose according to response.

Severe anaemia is treated by slow pack cell transfusion.

Chemoprophylaxis

There is no consensus as to the beneficial effect of prophylaxis that is directed at pregnant women who visit or live in endemic areas or women who may become pregnant and are not on oral or any contraceptives while visiting endemic areas. In many regions, routine

Table 5.6 – Treatment regime for malaria in pregnancy.

Type of infection	Drug	Dose
Chloroquine-sensitive falciparum and other type	Chloroquine base 150 mg	600 mg first dose 300 mg 6 h after 300 mg daily for 2 days thereafter
Drug-resistant falciparum	Quinine oral	Quinine 10 mg/kg three times a day for 7–10 days
	plus sulphadoxine 500 mg pyrimethamine 25 mg tablets	Sulphadoxine Pyrimethamine on day 2, two tablets
Severe falciparum infection IVI therapy	Quinine IVI	Loading dose 7 mg/kg over 30 min infusion in normal saline pump then 10 mg/kg in normal saline over 4 h. Eight-hourly. Oral therapy when possible for 7–10 days

Primaquine should not be given in pregnancy for the hepatic cycle of *P. vivax*. It can be given after delivery if the enzyme glucose 6-phosphate dehydrogenase level is adequate to prevent haemolysis.

chemoprophylaxis has been abandoned and is targeted only at special groups such as primigravidae and anaemic women. Chemoprophylaxis (Table 5.7) may reduce transplacental transfer of passive immunity to the foetus but this is controversial. The recommended drugs are:

- Chloroquine is safe for mother and foetus and in the absence of resistance, is the drug of choice. It has been used safely even in high doses for connective tissue disorders such as systemic lupus erythematosus without producing foetal congenital abnormalities. Even with some plasmodial resistance to chloroquine (WHO classification) it is still worth using this drug on a weekly basis.
- Dapsone-pyrimethamine is an alternative drug for chloroquine-resistant falciparum. The major side-effects are blood dyscrasias including agranulocytosis and severe cutaneous reactions. There is very little evidence that dapsone causes congenital malformation.
- There are very few other alternatives for chloroquine-resistant malaria and in each the efficacy and toxicity have to be weighted against the risk of contracting malaria. Pyrimethamine and sulphadoxine have been employed for prophylaxis but toxicity to sulphonamides should be borne in mind and reactions can be very severe such as in the Steven–Johnson's syndrome. Folate replacement is essential with long-term use. In view of possible embryopathic action, the WHO does not recommend its use.
- Mefloquine – there have been initial reservations concerning the use of this drug; however, it has now been cleared of teratogenicity. Prophylactic mefloquine has been used after the 20th week of pregnancy in high endemic areas with 59–94% protection against *P. falciparum* and 100% protection against *P. vivax* with no serious adverse effects on mother or foetus (Nosten *et al.* 1994). Mefloquine has been used in desperate situations such as in refugee camps and when there were no alternative drugs. The side-effects of this drug have been described above. It has been used in combination with quinine for multidrug-resistant *P. falciparum* infection in pregnancy (McGready *et al.* 1998).

VACCINES

There is no effective and safe vaccine for malaria. However, a vaccine for malaria is biologically possible (Abath *et al.* 1998, Holder 1999) and some have been trialled without success. Vaccines are targeted at gametocytes, sporozoites and merozoites. Research on an anti-sporozoite vaccine is in an advanced stage. An effective vaccine should act immediately to kill the sporozoite. Vaccines targeted at gametocytes will only be useful for prevention of malaria. Immune people, when reinfected, have lower levels of parasitaemia due to an antibody response to the erythrocytic stage parasites. Transfer of IgG to human volunteers reduced *P. falciparum* parasitaemia by 99%.

Malarial parasite antigens from life cycle stages have been utilized to develop malaria vaccine components in animals. These include pre-erythrocytic proteins such as C_5 found in large amounts on the surface of sporozoites and SSP_2 in murine malaria, LSA1 in infected hepatocytes; and antigens such as EBA 175 on the surface of merozoites and SERA (Service Repeat Antigen), P_1 or P_{126} in the parasitophorus vacuole. Other avenues of antibody production include those to block the development of the sexual stages of the parasite and to prevent cytoadherence of the parasite (Okenhouse *et al.* 1991, Pye *et al.* 1991).

Multicomponent vaccines have also been investigated. A synthetic polymer SPf66 from *P. falciparum* merozoites and one peptide from the C_5 protein of sporozoites was used to produce a vaccine which delayed or suppressed the onset of parasitaemia in humans challenged with the parasites. SPf66 was found to be safe in a recent trial on 1548 human volunteers, with a protective efficacy of 39% in a study population of all ages (Valero *et al.* 1993) but it is unlikely that SPf66 will be the answer to the global problem of malaria. Malaria vaccines are promising but currently only represent a reality for the future (Tanner *et al.* 1995).

Immunization during pregnancy is controversial. There should be a better understanding of immune mechanisms responsible for the lowered cell-mediated responses observed in pregnancy before prophylactic vaccination is given to pregnant women.

PROGNOSIS

The prognosis of infection with *P. vivax*, *ovale* or *malariae* is excellent with treatment and complications are rare.

Table 5.7 – Prophylaxis in pregnancy.

Type of infection	Drug	Dose
Chloroquine-sensitive plasmodium	Chloroquine 150 mg base	300 mg weekly 2 weeks before and 4 weeks after returning
Drug-resistant falciparum	Mefloquine 250 mg (in special circumstances)	250 mg weekly 1 week before and 4 weeks after returning
	Pyrimethamine 25 mg and sulphadoxine 500 mg	Pyrimethamine 25 mg sulphadoxine 500 mg one tablet weekly

Prognosis in falciparum malaria depends on the clinical presentation and patients presenting in deep coma, multi-organ failure, lactic acidosis, hypoglycaemia, or hyperventilation have a poor prognosis. The presence of more mature parasites in falciparum infection indicates a poor prognosis.

IMMUNITY

Non-immune individuals, such as travellers, suffer most severely from malaria. Severe disease in endemic areas is unusual in the first 6 months of life but thereafter, severe falciparum malaria is common and a major cause of childhood mortality. With repeated infections, immunity develops and malaria is a mild disease by the end of the first decade. During the second decade repeated infections of malaria may even be asymptomatic as a result of immunity. The acquired power of resistance rapidly declines when infection is interrupted for a long period and the patients become susceptible to severe symptoms of the infection. The development of immunity is accompanied by increased circulating gammaglobulin. It is generally believed that maintenance of immunity is largely dependent on the presence of the erythrocyte-phase of the parasite in the blood. Unlike adults, children remain susceptible to infection, perhaps due to immaturity of the immune system.

Virulence in malaria can be secondary to parasite density or to differences in the nature and severity of disease induced by the parasite. It was demonstrated in a model of the cerebral disease in *Babesia canis* in dogs that severity of pathology was dependent on the breed of dog infected. Similarly in humans, genetic differences in the parasite as well as the host may have a role. This is well illustrated by the pattern of mortality in the state of Orissa in India, which has a total population of 4% of the Indian population but a mortality rate of 50% of all malarial deaths in India, suggesting that a very virulent strain of falciparum is responsible.

Some human genetic traits have been described to have immunity to malaria. Those with thalassaemias, sickle-cell disease or who are Duffy-negative homozygous are resistant to *P. vivax* infection. There is a significant association between human MHC Class I allele B53 and protection against both cerebral malaria and anaemia, and there is protection against anaemia in infected persons with MHC Class II allele DR1302.

ILLUSTRATIVE CASE

A 24-year-old female Solomon Islander at 40 weeks gestation ($G_1 P_0$) presented to the Emergency Room in labour and proceeded to normal vaginal delivery of a healthy male (Apgar 9^1, 9^5). The mother had received monthly chloroquine prophylaxis in the Solomon Islands; however, this had ceased on arrival in Australia, 1 month before the birth of the child. She had a normal pregnancy and had no previous treatment for malaria or symptoms of the infection. Investigations of the mother on arrival revealed a normal white cell count 9.0×10^9/litre, haemoglobin of 127 g/litre and mild thrombocytopenia of 141×10^9/litre (normal range 150–400). The blood film was positive for *P. vivax*. Biochemical screen was normal. Hepatitis B surface antigen was positive (HBcAg-negative). G6PD screen was normal. The mother received a course of chloroquine (600 mg PO stat, 300 mg PO at 6 h, then 300 mg PO/day for 2 days), followed by a course of primaquine (15 mg PO/day for 14 days).

37

Mother and baby progressed well and were discharged after 48 h at the request of the mother. The mother and child failed to present for outpatient follow up. Six weeks later the baby was brought to the Emergency Department with a 1-week history of increasing jaundice, dark urine, difficulty feeding and distress. On examination, the baby was afebrile and mildly dehydrated with marked jaundice. Pulse rate was 160 beats/min; respiratory rate was 60/min. A maculopapular rash was noted over the face and torso. Breath sounds were vesicular with scattered crepitations audible. Abdominal examination revealed tender hepatosplenomegaly.

Full blood examination was: white cell count 10.9 × 10⁹/litre (6–18.0); haemoglobin 70 g/litre (95–125); platelet count 81 × 10⁹/litre (150–400). *P. vivax* was seen on thin films. Serum biochemistry was: sodium 138 mmol/litre (137–146); potassium 5.0 mmol/litre (3.5–5.0); chloride 108 mmol/litre (95–105); bicarbonate 17 mmol/litre (24–31); urea 3.2 mmol/litre; creatinine 52 mmol/litre (20–40); aspartate aminotransferase 198 U/litre (20–100); alanine aminotransferase 1440 U/litre (< 54); alkaline phosphatase 374 U/litre (115–460); GGT 70 U/litre (3–30); total bilirubin 429 mmol/litre (0–15); conjugated bilirubin 364 mmol/litre (0–4); protein 55 g/litre (63–80); albumin 33 g/litre (34–45). G6PD screen was normal. VDRL and TPHA non-reactive. HBsAg-negative. Alpha-1-antitrypsin screen normal. Toxoplasma serology-negative. Rubella IgG-positive (maternal), IgM-negative, cytomegalovirus IgG-positive (maternal), IgM-negative.

A diagnosis of neonatal (congenital transmission) vivax malaria complicated by anaemia, thrombocytopenia and hepatitis was made. The baby received chloroquine 40 mg PO/day for 3 days. No other cause for the rash or hepatitis was found. Phenobarbitone 20 mg PO/day for 7 days was given to facilitate recovery from jaundice, and baby was discharged on day 14.

REFERENCES

Abath FG, Montenegro SM, Gomes YM. Vaccines against human parasitic diseases: an overview. *Acta Tropica* 1998; **30**: 237–254

Al-Yaman F *et al*. Human cerebral malaria: lack of significant association between erythrocyte rosetting and disease severity. *Transactions of the Royal Society of Tropical Medicine and Hygiene* 1995; **89**: 55–58

Brewer TG, Peggins JO, Grate SJ, *et al*. Neurotoxicity in animals due to arteether and artemether. *Transactions of the Royal Society of Medicine and Hygiene* 1994; **88 (suppl. 1)**: S33–36

Cerau GE, de Kossodo S. Cerebral malaria, mediators mechanical obstruction or more? *Parasitology Today* 1994; **10**: 408–418

Editorial. *Lancet* 1992; 339

Gorduek VR. Iron chelation as a chemotherapeutic strategy for *Falciparum malaria*. *American Journal of Tropical Medicine and Hygiene* 1993; **48**: 193–197

Holder A. Malaria vaccines. *Proceedings of the National Academy of Sciences, USA* 1999; **96**: 1167–1169

Looareesuwan S, Viravan C, Vanijanonta S *et al*. Randomized trial of artesunate and mefloquine alone and in sequence for acute uncomplicated *Falciparum malaria*. *Lancet* 1992; **339**

Looareesuwan S, Olliaro P, White NJ *et al*. Consensus recommendation on the treatment of malaria in Southeast Asia. *Southeast Asian Journal of Tropical Medicine and Public Health* 1998; **29**: 355–360.

McGready R, Chio T, Hkirijaroen L *et al*. Quinine and mefloquinine in the treatment of multidrug-resistant *Plasmodium falciparum* malaria in pregnancy. *Annals of Tropical Medicine and Parasitology* 1998; **92**: 643–653

Mendis KN, Carter R. Clinical disease and pathogenesis in malaria. *Parasitology Today* 1995; **11**: 2–13

Mendez C. Malaria during pregnancy. A priority area of malaria research and control. *Parasitology Today* 1995; **11**: 178–183

Nosten F, ter Kuile F, Maelankiri L *et al*. Mefloquine prophylaxis prevents malaria during pregnancy. A double blind, placebo-controlled study. *Journal of Infectious Disease* 1994; **169**: 595–603

Okenhouse CF, Klotz FW, Tandon NN, Jamieson GA. Sequestrin a CD36 recognition protein on *Plasmodium falciparum* malaria infected erythrocytes identified by anti-idotype antibodies. *Proceedings of the National Academy of Sciences, USA* 1991; **88**: 3175–3179

Pye D, Edwards SJ, Anders RF *et al*. Failure of recombinant vaccinia virus expressing *Plasmodium falciparum* antigens to protect Saimiri monkey against malaria. *Infection and Immunology* 1991; **59**: 2403–2411

Roman GC. Cerebral malaria. The unsolved riddle. *Journal of Neurological Science* 1991; **101**: 1–6

Schoepke A, Steffen R, Gratz N. Effectiveness of personal protection measures against mosquito bites for malaria prophylaxis in travelers. *Journal of Travel Medicine* 1998; **5**: 188–192.

Tanner M, Teusher T, Alonso PL. SPf66 – the first malarial vaccine. *Parasitology Today* 1995; **11**: 10–13

White NJ. Malaria pathophysiology. *Clinical Tropical Medicine and Communicable Disease* 1986; **1**: 55–90

White NJ, Pukrittayakamee S. Clinical malaria in the tropics. *Medical Journal of Australia* 1993; **159**: 197–202

White NJ, Waller D, Crowley J *et al*. Comparison of artemether and chloroquine for severe malaria in Gambian children. *Lancet* 1992; **339**

World Health Organisation. *International Travel and Health*. Geneva: World Health Organisation, 1991

Wright P, Marchand R. Parasites in Vietnam. *Parasitology Today* 1995; **11**: 68–69

Valero MV, Amador LR, Galindo C *et al*. Vaccination with SPf66, a chemically synthesized vaccine against *Plasmodium falciparum* malaria in Colombia. *Lancet* 1993; **341**: 705–710

Toxoplasmosis

PARASITOLOGY

Toxoplasmosis is caused by *Toxoplasma gondii* that infects almost all mammals and birds. It is probably the most common parasitic infection of felines. Infected adult humans are usually asymptomatic but it is a fatal disease in neonates and immunocompromised patients.

Humans are infected by the ingestion of food (including raw vegetables) or drinking water contaminated by the faeces of cat or other felids, or by consumption of raw or undercooked meat containing oocysts. A second mode of infection is transplacental transmission from mother to foetus. Third, transmission can occur through organ transplants, blood and leukocyte transfusions. The organism can survive for several days in whole concentrated blood kept at 4°C.

Toxoplasma pseudocysts can remain dormant, especially in the brain, for a long time due to immune mechanisms in the host mediated by T-cells. In immunocompromised patients this can break down, resulting in a reactivation of the disease.

The prevalence rate is variable. In certain parts of France the prevalence rate according to serology is > 75% and in the USA it is ~30%. A higher prevalence is associated with AIDS, Hodgkin's disease, leukaemia and immunosuppressed patients. The actual number of clinical cases is few but subclinical infections are common as shown by serological studies in asymptomatic persons. In the USA, the incidence of toxoplasmosis infections during pregnancy is ~0.2–1% (Wong and Remington 1994).

Clinical infection manifests as acquired toxoplasmosis, congenital toxoplasmosis or infection in immunocompromised patients.

During the acute phase of acquired toxoplasmosis there are immunological mechanisms in the host that block the multiplication of the tachyzoites. Host antibodies destroy extracellular tachyzoites whereas cellular immunity plays a part when the parasite is intracellular. However, where immunological defences are poor as in the brain, the parasite can continue to proliferate.

Toxoplasma gondii is a coccidian parasite with a sexual cycle (schizogony and gametogony-isosporin phase) in the intestinal epithelium of its definitive host, the domestic cat. The asexual cycle or toxoplasmic phase occurs in man in which endozoites (tachyzoites) parasitize cells, especially of the reticuloendothelial system, forming pseudocysts in the acute stage and cystozoites or bradyzoites form tissue cysts in the chronic stage. In both stages the trophozoites multiply by endodiogeny or internal budding.

In man, ingested oocysts release sporozoites that enter macrophages in which they form pseudocysts and multiply as endozoites. These cells rupture, releasing the endozoites to infect new macrophages. Endozoites are curved or crescent-shaped organisms, with one rounded end, measuring 4–6 × 2–3 μm. With the Giemsa stain they appear blue with a red or purple nucleus. They are seen enclosed in pseudocysts (which contain up to 100 endozoites) within macrophages. As host immunity develops, the endozoites change their form and become cystozoites, which are elongated sporozoite-like forms, enclosed in a true or tissue cyst whose walls are composed of reactive host tissue. Each tissue cyst can contain thousands of cystozoites.

These cysts can lie dormant for the whole of the host's life and can resist normal refrigeration temperatures and gastric juice. On being ingested by a cat, the cystozoites enter the intestinal epithelial cells where they undergo schizogony and follow the enteric cycle. If the tissue cysts are ingested by another intermediate or prey host they enter macrophages and follow the toxoplasmic cycle as above. Parasites can be transmitted transplacentally in the toxoplasmic phase.

Transmission occurs through ingestion of oocysts from faecal-contaminated soil, ingestion of tissue cysts in the flesh of intermediate host, transplacental blood transfusion, or organ transplantation.

PRESENTATION

Congenital toxoplasmosis

Several factors determine maternal infection and subsequent damage to the foetus. Time of infection during pregnancy is important. It is predicted that foetal infection is 10–15% if the mother is infected in the first trimester, 30% in the second trimester and 60% in the third trimester (Wong and Remington 1994). However, the most severe damage occurs in newborns that acquired the infection in the first trimester and usually results in abortion or stillbirth. Such foetuses have no defensive T-cells to produce IFN-γ that destroys the tachyzoites. Immunological maturity in the latter part of pregnancy results in subclinical, congenital infection so that the infected babies may appear to be normal at birth but will eventually have loss of vision, psychomotor defects or mental retardation. If the mother acquired toxoplasmosis before conception, she can transmit it to the foetus if, at some stage, she becomes immunocompromised. Such cases have been documented in pregnant women with Hodgkin's disease, lymphoma, collagen diseases and those on corticosteroids.

If the neonates survive, they present with cerebral symptoms of convulsions, tremors, paralysis, impaired intellect and behavioural problems. They may be micro- or hydrocephalic. With severe neurological involvement, the neonate usually dies within the first month. Ocular involvement is common. It is bilateral with chorioretinitis and ends in blindness. Strabismus is an early sign of chorioretinitis. Granulomatous inflammation of the choroid occurs secondary to necrotizing retinitis. Chorioretinitis is followed by glaucoma, cataracts and iridocyclitis. Some ocular lesions presenting in the adults may be a reactivation of disease acquired intrauterine. Hepatosplenomegaly with jaundice, thrombocytopenia and purpura may occur. In severe cases there may be pneumonitis, which can be rapidly fatal.

Acquired toxoplasmosis

Acquired toxoplasmosis may be very mild or asymptomatic. Acute infection present as lymphadenopathy with low-grade fever and muscle pain and may be confused with infectious mononucleosis. The enlarged glands are generally painless. Pneumonia with cough and fever may be presenting symptoms. Complications include meningo-encephalitis, hepatitis and myocarditis. Chorioretinitis and uveitis, which tends to be unilateral, can occur in ~1% of patients with acute infection. Chorioretinitis produces pain in the eyes, photophobia and blurred vision. Loss of central vision occurs if the macula is affected. Vision may improve when the inflammation subsides but recurrences are common. The optic fundus shows elevated cotton wool-like patches with indistinct margins. Older lesions have more distinct plaques with black spots of choroidal pigment. The incubation period can be from several days to a month, although symptoms have occurred within 1 week in laboratory-associated infections.

Immunocompromised patients

Patients who have solid organ transplants such as liver, kidney, heart and lung are at risk of reactivation of toxoplasma cysts present in the donor organs (Couvreur 1992, Ambroize-Thomas and Pelloux 1993). In bone marrow transplants there is reactivation of subclinical toxoplasmosis. This is similar to the pathogenesis of toxoplasmosis in patients with AIDS, where recrudescence is invariably the result of a latent infection (Ambroise-Thomas and Pelloux 1993).

Central nervous system involvement is a major complication of toxoplasmosis in this group of patients. The incidence of toxoplasmosis in AIDS patients is between 10 and 15% and is a major cause of encephalopathy among these patients. The symptoms of toxoplasmic encephalitis are fever with chills, headaches, seizures and altered mental states. There is diffuse neurological deficit due to encephalopathy or localizing signs from cerebral mass lesions.

PATHOLOGY

In acute toxoplasmosis the direct action of the endozoites on the cell causes necrosis and parasite antigens cause an antigen antibody reaction with intravascular thrombosis and infarction.

In the chronic stage, tissue cysts rupture to release cystozoites which elicit a host immune reaction with round cell infiltration, granuloma formation and tissue necrosis. Renal involvement has rarely been described with a mesangioproliferative picture.

Lymphadenopathy is seen in acute infections with clusters of epithelioid histiocytes around the follicles and occasionally impinging on enlarged germinal centres (Figure 6.1a and b) Focal distension of the peripheral and medullary sinuses by monocytoid B-cells is also characteristic but parasite pseudocysts are very rarely seen. The reaction is known as the Piringer–Kuchinger reaction.

Toxoplasmic encephalitis may be found in immunosuppressed patients in which there are large areas of cerebral necrosis due to infarction following thrombosis of small vessels. Glial nodules are few or absent but parasites in pseudocysts are more numerous than in the congenital form.

In chronic infections tissue cysts remain dormant until they rupture and the cystozoites are destroyed with the formation of small granulomas. The tissue cysts can be seen virtually in every organ. The central nervous system, the heart and the skeletal muscles are the most common sites in latent infection.

In congenital toxoplasmosis, the infected newborn shows pathologic changes in the heart, liver, lungs and central nervous system. In the heart, parasites enter the muscle cells, forming pseudocysts with no cellular response (Figure 6.2). The lungs show pneumonia with endozoites and mononuclear cells in the bronchioles and congestion. The organisms (bradyzoites) can be demonstrated in smears. The liver demonstrates large areas of necrosis with giant cells. There is hydrocephalus in the brain due to gliosis obstructing CSF flow and encephalitis. Necrosis of brain cells, small scattered infarcts and tissue cysts with tachyzoites are also seen (Figure 6.3a, b and c).

In the acute stage, IgG antibodies measured by the dye complement fixation and specific immunofluorescences, reach their maximum 2 months after infection

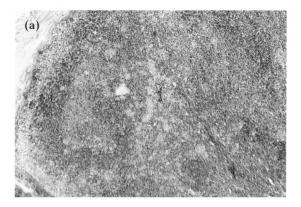

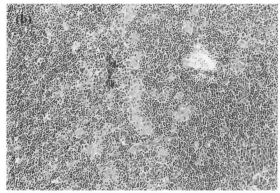

Figure 6.1 – Toxoplasmic lymphadenitis with clusters of histiocytes at the margins of the follicles
a. H&E × 40
b. H&E × 100

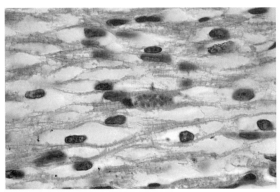

Figure 6.2 – Toxoplasmosis pseudocyst in the cardiac muscle. There is no cellular reaction to the pseudocyst (H&E × 200).

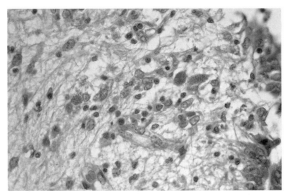

Figure 6.3b – Toxoplasmosis in the brain Tissue cysts with tachyzoites (H&E × 160).

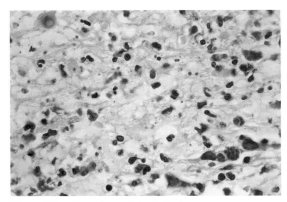

Figure 6.3a – Toxoplasmosis in the brain Necrosis of brain cells and small scattered infarcts (H&E × 250)

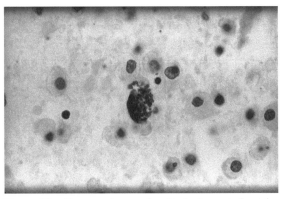

Figure 6.3c – Free toxoplasma tachyzoites broken out of pseudo-cyst in cerebral tissue (H&E × 1000).

and persist probably for life. Cellular immunity occurs in chronic infection and is transferred by lymphocytes. It confers lifelong immunity.

INVESTIGATIONS

1. Isolation of the organism by inoculation of leukocytes, body fluid or tissue specimens into tissue culture. The isolation of *T. gondii* from body fluids implies an acute infection.
2. Demonstration of tachyzoites in tissue sections or smears, or in body fluids such as CSF or amniotic fluid. Demonstration of cysts in the tissues does not differentiate between acute and chronic infection. However, the presence of a large number of cysts in any one organ is highly suggestive of recent infection. Brain biopsy of mass lesions seen on CT scan help in the differential diagnosis of other causes of encephalitis such as cryptococcus, mycobacteria and viral encephalitis. In the

immune-compromised such as the AIDS patient, distinction from malignant lymphoma and other space-occupying lesions is necessary.

Smears of body fluids and touch preparations of tissue are preferably stained by the Giemsa technique that demonstrates the purple red nucleus and blue cytoplasm of the 2–6 μm crescent-shaped trophozoites. However, several morphologically similar protozoa and fungi should be differentiated. The cyst wall stains with Gomori's methanamine silver (GMS) and the amylopectin granules in the cytoplasm of bradyzoites stains with PAS. These reactions readily distinguish toxoplasma from other protozoa which are GMS-negative. Pneumocystis is the only protozoan that shows the same reaction to GMS and PAS but the trophozoites are smaller (1 × 3 μm) and the cyst wall does not stain with haematoxylin and eosin. The size of *Histoplasma capsulata* is similar to toxoplasma trophozoites but it shows a distinct cell border surrounded by a halo.

Its cytoplasm usually contracts to one side, leaving a cup-shaped space and its cell wall is stained by PAS. Leishmania species and *Trypanosoma cruzi* are distinguished from toxoplasma by the presence of a kinetoplast and sarcocystis is characterized by the presence of intracystic septa that can be readily demonstrated by the Wilder stain.

3. There are several serological tests for toxoplasma. They may identify whether the infection is recent or past. However, commercial kits vary in reliability and serological tests should be interpreted with caution. A combination of the various tests listed below will help one obtain a more accurate diagnosis.

   The Gold Standard for the diagnosis of toxoplasmosis is the Sabin–Feldman dye test. It measures IgG antibodies to toxoplasma. It is detectable after 1–2 weeks following infection. The peak of > 1000 IU/ml is at 6–8 weeks. The levels gradually decline. A positive test in a pregnant woman cannot determine whether infection is past or recent, especially if there are no clinical manifestations. A rise in titre is uncommon; hence, other serology tests described below are necessary.

   IgM antibodies detected by ELISA and ISAGA appear in the first 2 weeks of the infection. A negative test rules out a recently acquired infection especially in pregnancy. It should be repeated after 1 week. A positive test, unless there has been a rise in titres of IgG or IgM, is difficult to interpret without further antibody assessment for IgA and IgE antibodies.

   Specific IgA can be detected by ISAGA and ELISA techniques. This test is similar to IgM antibodies after an acute infection. It is more sensitive for the diagnosis of toxoplasmosis in the foetus and newborn.

   IgE antibodies can be detected by ELISA and ISAGA methods. The test becomes positive early in an acute infection. However, it remains positive for a very limited time.

4. Diagnostic nodular, ring or target lesions may be seen in the cortex, white matter or basal ganglia with contrast enhanced CT scans. These lesions may appear after several weeks or CT may be normal in symptomatic patients.

5. The CSF shows pleocytosis and protein content. Tachyzoites may be found in the cytocentrifuged specimen. Cultures should be done for *T. gondii*.

6. In the foetus, amniotic fluid or pre-umbilical foetal blood can be used to detect the parasite or antibodies specific to *T. gondii*. Specific IgM and IgA antibodies are unlikely to appear in the foetus before the 20th week and serological testing should be done after maturation of the immune system. Maternal antibodies should be tested at the same time. β-Human chorionic gonadotrophin estimation should be done on foetal blood to exclude maternal contamination (Wong and Remington 1994).

7. The polymerase chain reaction detects *T. gondii* DNA in body fluids and amniotic fluid. It has an accuracy as high as 100% and is a useful diagnostic tool to determine management of the foetus at an early stage of pregnancy.

8. Foetal abnormalities detected by ultrasonography are ventricular dilatation, hydrocephalus, intracranial calcifications, increase in placental thickness, hepatomegaly and ascites. Hydrocephalus with calcification is highly suggestive of toxoplasmosis but not pathognomonic.

TREATMENT

Adults (non pregnant) and older children who only have lymphadenopathy seldom require specific therapy unless symptoms are severe and persistent. Treatment is indicated if infection is acquired during pregnancy and it is decided for the pregnancy to continue; acquired infection is severe and involves vital organs, the eyes or when it occurs in immunocompetent patients; in immuno-incompetent patients where there is suspicion of toxoplasmosis but imaging or other diagnostic procedures are not conclusive and in laboratory acquired infection because of the high virulence of such cases.

The following chemotherapeutic drugs have been used:

- Pyrimethamine – very effective in combination with sulphadiazine
- Spiramycin – less effective but less toxic. Used in pregnancy but its effectiveness in the foetus is not fully known. It probably diminishes toxoplasmosis transmission through the placenta
- Clindamycin – for choroid and ocular toxoplasmosis
- Cotrimoxazole – for ocular toxoplasmosis

Pyrimethamine/sulphadiazine is more effective than spiramycin in reducing the severity of foetal infection. Pyrimethamine is teratogenic and should not be used in the first trimester. Once commenced on this regimen, treatment must continue up to near term (for details, see Table 6.1). Folic acid 5 mg/day is recommended to prevent bone marrow suppression.

Toxic effect of drugs used in treatment of toxoplasmosis:

- Pyrimethamine – prolonged administration results in inhibition of haematopoiesis with leukopenia and thrombocytopenia. Folinic acid should be given as a supplement. Contraindicated in pregnancy in the first trimester and in patients with megaloblastic anaemia
- Sulphadiazine – hypersensitivity reactions, crystalluria, rashes and Steven–Johnson's syndrome
- Spiramycin – abdominal pains, nausea, vomiting and diarrhoea, skin rashes, vertigo, dizziness and flushing of the face
- Clindamycin – diarrhoea, nausea, skin rashes, neutropenia and jaundice. Severe diarrhoea and enterocolitis (pseudomembranous colitis) may occur due to toxigenic *Clostridium difficile*
- Cotrimoxazole – megaloblastic anaemia, leukopenia and agranulocytosis. Folic acid supplement is recommended. Side-effects of sulpha preparations also apply (see above at sulphadiazine). Not recommended in pregnancy

Therapeutic abortion

Therapeutic abortion should only be considered when foetal infection has been proven. Ultrasonographic demonstration of cerebral abnormalities in the foetus and documentation of early infection during pregnancy (first trimester), help confirm foetal infection (Holdfield *et al.* 1990). Ultrasonography is indicated before consideration of therapeutic abortion and amniocentesis has to be performed at the appropriate time and amniotic fluid examined by PCR.

CONGENITAL TOXOPLASMOSIS AND HIV INFECTION

The congenital transmission rate of *T. gondii* in HIV infected mothers is very much higher compared with normal pregnancies. The chances of reactivation of latent toxoplasmosis and the probability of acquiring the disease for the first time in pregnancy are very high. Infants infected with HIV also invariably have toxoplasma infection. Most infants appear normal at birth, however, their conditions deteriorate rapidly thereafter. Management of the pregnancy is difficult. The options available are termination of pregnancy or prophylaxis in all HIV-positive mothers. Spiramycin is used in the first trimester and pyrimethamine-sulphadiazine or trimethoprim-sulphamethoxazole in the second trimester.

PREVENTION

Infected meat is rendered safe by adequate cooking (70°C). Mutton and pork have a higher incidence of infection than beef. Knives used for cutting meat and vegetables should be washed in hot water. Vegetables, if eaten raw, should be thoroughly washed. Contact with cat faeces should be avoided. Cats should be fed canned or boiled food and not uncooked meats. Pregnant women without toxoplasma antibodies should take extra precautions to avoid contact with cat litter. All organ donors should be screened for toxoplasma antibodies. Blood or leukocyte transfusions from donors who are toxoplasma antibody-positive should not be used. All pregnant mothers should be tested for antibodies at the earliest opportunity or preferably before conception. Education of mothers in antenatal clinics is very important.

There are no vaccines available for humans. Live vaccines to prevent or minimize abortion in sheep have been reported. In the USA where pigs are the main source of infection, a vaccine to prevent cyst formation in pigs is being tried.

Cats may be ideal candidates for vaccination, minimizing transmission to humans and to other animals. Vaccination with T-263 mutant vaccine obtained from brains of infected mice has been tried. The T-263 mutant forms tissue cysts in intermediate hosts, however, there are practical difficulties in obtaining the vaccine (Aranjo 1994)

REFERENCES

Ambroise-Thomas P, Pelloux H. Toxoplasmosis – congenital and in immunocompromised patients. A parallel. *Parasitology Today* 1993; **9**: 61–63

Table 6.1 – Treatment for toxoplasmosis

Drug	Indication	Dosage
Sulphadiazine	Pregnancy if decision to treat (if spiramycin not available)	Loading dose 50–70 mg/kg then 75 mg/kg/day in four divided doses for 14 days. Continue through pregnancy if foetus is infected
Pyrimethamine plus sulphadiazine	In immunocompetent patients with severe infections.★ After first trimester of pregnancy if foetal infection is documented or probability is very high	Pyrimethamine 0.4 mg/kg daily for 21 days, sulphadiazine 10 mg/kg daily for 21 days plus folinic acid. In pregnancy administered till near term
Pyrimethamine plus sulphadiazine	In immunocompromised patients with toxoplasmic encephalitis, 90% recovery	Pyrimethamine loading dose 1.5–2 mg/kg followed by 1–1.5 mg/kg for 21 days or more with sulphadiazine 50 mg/kg in divided doses per day for 21 days or more plus folinic acid
Spiramycin	In pregnancy, may reduce congenital transmission. Probably not effective when foetus is infected.	2–4 g/day. Continue throughout pregnancy
Clindamycin	In ocular toxoplasmosis and immunocompromised patients with pyrimethamine effective toxoplasmic encephalitis	10 mg/kg IV 6 hourly for 6 weeks plus pyrimethamine 0.4 mg/kg daily for 6 weeks
Cotrimoxazole (BACTRIM)	Ocular toxoplasmosis	One tablet trimethoprim 80 mg/sulphamethoxazole 400 mg Adults two tablets twice a day for 21 days. Children: 6–12 years ½ adult dose for 21 days; 2–5 years ⅓ adult dose for 21 days; < 2 years ¼ adult dose for 21 days

★Because of potential toxicity of pyrimethamine to mother and foetus, it should only be used when foetal infection is definitely documented.

Aranjo FG. Immunisation against *Toxoplasma gondii*. *Parasitology Today* 1994; **10**: 358–360

Couvreur J. Toxoplasmosis – congenital and in immunocompromised patients – a parallel. *La Presse Medicale* 1992; **21**: 1569–1574

Holdfield P, Daffos F, Thulliez P *et al*. Foetal toxoplasmosis outcome of pregnancy and infant follow up after *in utero* treatment. *Journal of Paediatrics* 1990; **115**: 765–769

Wong SY, Remington JS. Toxoplasmosis in pregnancy. *Clinical Infectious Diseases* 1994; **18**: 853–862

7

Pneumocystosis

Parasitology
Presentation
Pathology
Investigations

Treatment
Prophylaxis
References

PARASITOLOGY

Pneumocystis carinii pneumonia (PCP) was first described *c.*1910 when an outbreak occurred in malnourished children in Hungary. *P. carinii* is an ubiquitous protozoan pathogen and is found in all age groups of both sexes. Pneumocystosis is one of the leading opportunistic infections, and is prevalent in patients with AIDS, immunocompromised patients, such as renal, liver, heart, lung transplant patients, and those on immunosuppressive therapy. Pneumocystosis is now the leading cause of death in patients in remission from leukaemia and lymphoma. The sporadic form has a global distribution.

The organism is a commensal that has the potential to become an opportunistic pathogen. Human-to-human transmission has been suggested because of outbreaks of pneumocystis pneumonia in hospitals caring for immunocompromised patients. Some workers believe that HIV-positive patients with *P. carinii* pneumonia have introduced the microorganisms into hospitals. It is postulated that ~80% of AIDS patients will develop *P. carinii* infection at some stage of their disease and the infection will be the immediate cause of 25% of all AIDS deaths (Masur *et al.* 1989). From the epidemiology point of view the question arises as to whether prophylactic chemotherapy should be given to those at risk such as solid organ transplant recipients and immunocompromised HIV-positive patients.

The organism exists as trophozoite, cyst and sporozoite forms. The trophozoite varies from 1.5 to 5 μm in greatest dimension with the double membrane measuring 200–300 Å. It possesses a nucleus, mitochondria, rough endoplasmic reticulum, round body and vacuoles. The presence of pseudopodia and filopodia indicates its mobility. In tissue cultures the trophozoite develops through a precyst stage into a thick walled cyst within 4–6 h. The round- or cup-shaped cyst measures 4–6 μm in diameter. The cyst wall is composed of three layers, 0.1–0.3 μm in total thickness. Inside the cyst two nuclear masses develop and multiply into eight sporozoites, often referred to as intracystic bodies (Fig. 7.1). When the cyst matures, the sporozoites exit through one or more sites in the cyst wall. They exit as sporozoites then develop into trophozoites, completing the life cycle.

The mode of transmission is unclear. The general consensus is that it is transmitted from person-to-person through respiratory droplets as the infection can occur in clusters. Another hypothesis is that humans may acquire subclinical infection early in life but pneumonitis develops only when the resistance of the host is lowered.

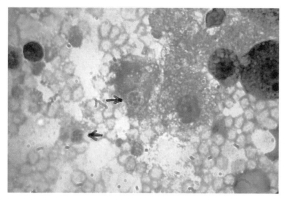

Figure 7.1 – Lung smear with *P. carinii* mature cyst containing eight daughter trophozoites (arrows), often referred to as intracystic bodies (H&E × 1000).

PRESENTATION

The incubation period, based on animal models, is between 4 and 8 weeks. Patients with pneumocystis pneumonia present with fever, shortness of breath and a non-productive cough. In the immunocompromised patient the onset can be abrupt. Physical signs include tachycardia, cyanosis and tachypnoea, but auscultatory signs are few. Since all types of atypical pneumonia such as mycoplasma and Legionella resemble *P. carinii* pneumonia, a definite laboratory diagnosis should be sought.

PATHOLOGY

The pathognomonic feature of pneumocystis pneumonia is the presence of abundant honey-combed foamy material that distends the alveolar spaces. This material stains intensely with eosin and is composed of proteinaceous substance, fibrin complement and immunoglobulins including IgG, IgA and IgM (Fig. 7.2a). Special stains such as GMS and Giemsa will identify the cup-shaped cysts or sporozoites (Fig. 7.2b). By electron microscopy, trophozoites, precyst and empty cysts are also seen in the alveoli. The filling of the alveolar spaces and the heavy interstitial cellular infiltration cause the alveolar-capillary block and severe anoxia in the infected and hyaline membranes that occasionally line the alveolar walls further hamper gas exchange.

In a later stage, the alveolar exudate is organized and forms a spherical mass. Granulomata formed by epithelioid cells and multinucleated giant cells can be seen in some cases and are known as pneumocystosis

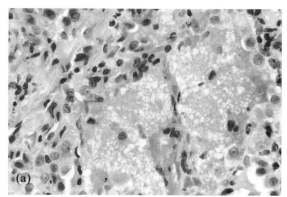

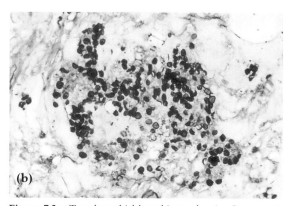

Figure 7.2 – Transbronchial lung biopsy showing *Pneumocystis* cysts, (a) H&E × 40; (b) GMS, × 40.

granulomatosa. The infection may progress to interstitial fibrosis, emphysema, pulmonary calcification and cor pulmonale.

Extrapulmonary pneumocystosis has been reported in ten patients. Hilar lymph nodes were involved and the organisms spread via blood or lymphatics to the liver, spleen, heart, kidney, pancreas, stomach, small intestine, bone marrow, thyroid, adrenal and thymus.

INVESTIGATIONS

1. Chest X-ray reveals diffuse bilateral pulmonary infiltrates. Others that are non-specific include cavitation, cysts, pleural effusion, pneumothorax or an entirely normal X-ray.
2. Specific diagnosis is made by direct and specific identification of the organism. Culture of the organism is not feasible. Sputum examination is seldom helpful. A survey of 249 cases from the US Center for Disease Control, Atlanta, GA, showed the following diagnostic yield: open lung biopsy, 64%; closed lung

biopsy, 51%; lung aspirate, 55%; bronchial biopsy, 62%; bronchial aspirate, 36%. In experienced hands, the positive rate of open lung biopsy can be as high as 97–100%, and for needle biopsy it is 75% (Fig. 7.3a and b). In another study of 171 known or suspected AIDS patients, bronchoscopy with bronchoalveolar lavage and transbronchial biopsy increased the diagnostic sensitivity to 100%.

Open lung biopsy is the method of choice because of its high positive rate and the lower risk of intrapulmonary bleeding. When the tissue is obtained, touch preparations should be made before frozen sections are cut. Touch preparations are air dried before performing a rapid stain such as toluidine blue, Gram-Weigert, Giemsa or cresyl violet. Preparations should be fixed in 95% alcohol if a haematoxylin and eosin stain is used to show the cytologic details of other tissue components.

3. Specific diagnosis is made by indirect immunofluorescence microscopy or enzyme immunohistochemistry using monoclonal antibodies to *P. carinii*. This method is more sensitive than using the methenamine silver staining technique (Kovas *et al.* 1988).

TREATMENT

Patients with *Pneumocystis* pneumonia are often acutely ill and should be treated in an intensive care setting. They are hypoxic and require monitoring, and frequent blood gas analysis. Those who are markedly hypoxic may require assisted ventilation. The two major drugs used in the treatment of *P. carinii* pneumonia are trimethoprim-sulphamethoxazole (co-trimoxazole) and pentamidine isothionate.

- The mode of action of cotrimoxazole on *P. carinii* is not known. However, it is an antifolate compound and can be administered PO or IV. The recommended dose is 20 mg/kg/day trimethoprim and 100 mg/kg/day sulphamethoxazole in four divided doses for 14–21 days. Optimum serum levels of cotrimoxazole should be maintained at 100–150 mmol/ml sulphamethoxazole and 5 mg trimethoprim. It is preferred over pentamidine in non-AIDS patients. IV preparations are available for patients who cannot take PO. Side-effects are leukopenia, fever and rashes, more commonly seen with AIDS patients.
- Pentamidine izothionate acts by several mechanisms that affect cell replication. However, its action on the organism is not well known. It is given by IM or by slow IV injection and is the drug of choice in AIDS patients, given in a dose of 4 mg/kg/day for 14 days. It is administered by nebulizer, 8 mg/kg/day in aerosol particles and has been shown to cure up to 80% of infections with AIDS. Side-effects are painful indurations at injection sites, hypo- or hyperglycaemia, hypocalcaemia, raised liver enzymes, and impaired renal functions.

The response to both these drugs begins around the fourth or fifth dose. Immunosuppressive drugs and corticosteroids need to be tapered to the lowest dose possible.

Mortality of untreated *P. carinii* infection is 100%. The mortality rate in HIV-negative patients on immunosuppressive drugs can be up to 32% despite treatment. More recently, the mortality rate has been reduced to

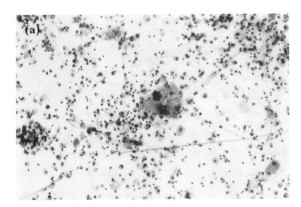

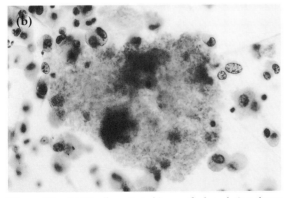

Figure 7.3 – (a) Needle aspirate biopsy of a lung lesion shows the fluffy cotton wool-like and (b) intra-alveolar exudates (Papanicolau stain a. × 100). b. × 400.

32% for HIV patients and 8% for other immunocompromised patients. AIDS patients respond more slowly and may require longer periods of treatment and infection recurs in 25% of cases.

PROPHYLAXIS

In several studies of patients with solid organ transplants, the probability of *P. carinii* infection in various organs was 6% for kidneys, 4.3% for liver and 5% for heart transplants (Kramer *et al.* 1992).

The role for prophylactic cotrimoxazole has been established for several populations at risk of the infection, including HIV and heart–lung transplant patients. However, there are no established clinical trials that show a beneficial role in kidney transplant patients.

Most *P. carinii* infection occurs in the first 6 months after organ transplantation and it is suggested that prophylaxis for 6 months would be beneficial. Nebulized pentamidine may be used as prophylaxis but has been used mainly in extrapulmonary infections.

REFERENCES

Kovas JA, Ng VL, Masur H *et al.* Diagnosis of *P. carinii* pneumonia improved detection in spectrum with use of monoclonal antibodies. *New England Journal of Medicine* 1988; **318**: 589–593

Kramer M, Stoehr C, Leviston N *et al.* Trimethoprim-sulphamethoxazole prophylaxis for *Pneumocystis carinii* infection in heart–lung transplantation. How effective and how long? *Transplantation* 1992; **53**: 586–589

Masur H, Lane C, Joseph A. *Pneumocystis carinii* pneumonia from bench to diagnosis. *Annals of Internal Medicine* 1989; **111**: 813–826

8

Leishmaniasis

Parasitology
Presentation
Pathology
Investigations

Treatment
    Cutaneous leishmaniasis
    Visceral leishmaniasis
Vector and reservoir control
References

PARASITOLOGY

Leishmaniasis is a disease caused by a protozoan haemoflagellate of the genus Leishmania. There are two main types of leishmaniasis, visceral or kala-azar and cutaneous (oriental sore and Espundia). The diseases are endemic in many areas of tropical and subtropical America and are a serious public health problem. It is transmitted by sandflies, Phlebotomus in the Old World and Lutzomyia in the New World. Leishmaniasis has become an important public health problem in Brazil because of increase in the incidence and spread to new areas (Brandon-Filho and Shaw 1994). Leishmaniasis is not endemic in Australia and reported cases have all been imported.

Leishmaniasis can be cutaneous, mucocutaneous or visceral in manifestations and relates to the endemic geographical area and is broadly classified as Old World and New World leishmaniasis

Old World leishmaniasis is found in the dry regions of Afghanistan, India, Asian parts of the former Soviet Union, Middle East, Mediterranean region, East Africa and Namibia. The species responsible are *Leishmania tropica* in India, Afghanistan, Mediterranean Coast and the former Soviet Union; *Leishmania major* (a zoonosis) infects humans sporadically in Middle East, Africa and the former Soviet Union; and *Leishmania aethiopica* (a zoonosis) in Ethiopia, South Yemen, Uganda and Kenya.

New World cutaneous leishmaniasis is caused by several species and subspecies belonging to the subgenera Leishmania and Vianna, and names for the disease varies with geographic locality. Human infections are contracted primarily in zoonotic areas. The subspecies causing New World cutaneous leishmaniasis are *L. mexicana mexicana* (Chiclero ulcer), *L. braziliensis panamanensis* causing various ulcers by metastatic spread, *L. peruviana* (Uta ulcer), *L. braziliensis* (mucocutaneous ulcer), *L. mexicana amazonensis*, *L. garnhami*, *L. venezuelensis*, *L. lainsoni*, *L. colombiensis*, *L. guyanensis*, *L. pifanoi* and *L. infantum*.

Visceral leishmaniasis (kala-azar or dumdum fever) is caused by *L. donovani* complex, *L. donovani*, *L. infantum* and *L. chagasi*. Visceral leishmaniasis is found in the dry regions of the Mediterranean and South America, East Africa, China, India, and the Middle East. Man gets infected through the bite of the female Phlebotomus (Old World) and Lutzomyia (New World) carrying the flagellates. The animal reservoirs in some parts of the world are dogs, rodents and possibly others that can transmit the disease to man via the vector fly. However, it is mostly a man-to-man transmission by the vector. Post-kala-azar dermal leishmaniasis is found mainly in India and Southern Asia, less commonly in Africa, and is secondary to visceral leishmaniasis. About 12 million cases in 80 countries are infected with leishmaniasis. It may be an opportunistic infection in AIDS patients. Patients with HIV are prone to visceral disease and not skin lesions. Leishmania strains behave differently. Some strains are blocked at the skin, producing self-healing lesions of skin. A third strain is supposed to be avirulent in immunocompetent hosts (Gradoni and Gramiccia 1994).

All species of leishmania are morphologically identical and are best classified according to their clinical manifestation, i.e. cutaneous, mucocutaneous and visceral leishmaniasis and epidemiology. *L. donovani*, *L. chagasi* and *L. infantum* cause visceral (syn.: kala-azar, black fever) disease mainly in the Mediterranean basin, Asia, South America and Africa. *L. braziliensis* is the causative organism in mucocutaneous disease (syn: Espundia) seen in Central and South America. *L. tropica* major and *L. tropica* minor cause the oriental or Delhi boil in China, India, Middle East and Africa.

The parasite in human tissue measures 1–3 μm and is the amastigote form, which multiplies in macrophages by binary fission. The infected cells rupture and the parasites are engulfed by other macrophages. When a female phlebotomus bites an infected patient the amastigotes enter the gut of the sandfly and develop into leptomonad or promastigote forms. These multiply by binary fission and migrate from midgut to the pharynx and proboscis of the insect. When the infected sandfly bites a mammalian host or man, the parasite is introduced into the skin, thus completing the life cycle (Fig. 8.1).

PRESENTATION

The incubation period of leishmaniasis varies from 2 to 30 years.

Cutaneous leishmaniasis appears as an erythematous papule, which progresses to a nodule that may ulcerate. The lesions may occur in clusters depending on the number of bites by the sandfly. These lesions are generally painless, even when ulcerated. The border of the ulcer is firm and elevated and regional lymph nodes may be enlarged. They may heal spontaneously with scarring within 12–18 months. The ulcers go by

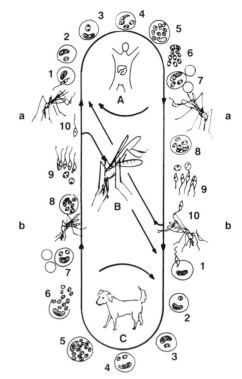

Figure 8.1 – Life cycle of leishmaniasis. (A) Development in man: (1) flagellated leishmania parasite (the so-called leptomonas stage) transmitted by *Phlebotomus* spp. penetrates into an endothelial cell of the host); (2–6) intracellular development in endothelial cells; (7) peripheral blood lymphocyte containing leishmanias. (B) Development in sandflies that are the vectors: (8) leishmania stages in the host cell in the stomach of the sandfly; (9) formation and multiplication of the leptomonas stages; (10) flagellated stage from the proboscis of the sandfly. (C) Development in the reservoir hosts (in dogs, small rodents, etc.) similar to that in man. A transmission by the sandflies can occur in the following manner: (1) from man to man A → B → A; (2) from animal to animal C → B → C; (3) from animal to man C → B → A and vice versa A → B → C

different names in different geographic regions, e.g. *L. mexicana* 'Chiclero ulcer', *L. guyanensis* 'Pian Bois'. Lesions of *L. tropica* major are moist, while those of *L. tropica* minor are dry and crusty. These lesions are called oriental sores. The skin lesions in the New World are called tropical sores. Human cutaneous leishmaniasis caused by *L. donovani* is rare and has been reported in Kenya.

Mucocutaneous leishmaniasis (Espundia) – *L. braziliensis braziliensis* is the cause of mucocutaneous leishmaniasis found mainly in Brazil. The lesion begins as a tropical sore, which is followed by lesions in the mucocutaneous regions such as the nose, lips, mouth, soft palate and larynx. The lesions can erode through the cartilage of the nose and palate. Unlike cutaneous lesions, these do not heal spontaneously.

Visceral leishmaniasis or kala-azar may have an acute onset with fever, gastroenteritis, chronic fatigue, malaise, abdominal pain or infectious mononucleosis-like illness. Patients become cachectic as the disease progresses. There may be lymphadenopathy, hepatosplenomegaly and hyperpigmentation of the skin. The enlarged spleen can occupy the major part of the abdomen. Hepatic involvement causes jaundice. The disease is fatal if untreated, although progression is generally very slow. Recently, a milder form of visceral leishmaniasis has been described in soldiers returning from the 'Desert Storm' in Saudi Arabia with non-specific aches and pains, chronic fatigue, cough and diarrhoea. It is said to be caused by *L. tropica*, which normally causes cutaneous lesions. *L. donovani* has been found in the digestive tracts of 50% of patients with visceral leishmaniasis who are HIV-negative. It has also been reported in HIV patients presenting with diarrhoea, dyspepsia, dysphagia, abdominal pain, epigastric pain, gastrointestinal haemorrhage and rectal discomfort. Longstanding cases of leishmaniasis may rarely cause renal failure due to diffuse tubulopathy, secondary to polyclonal light chains kappa and lambda deposition.

Post-kala-azar dermal leishmaniasis is a disseminated, cutaneous lesion that may appear months or years following treatment, often inadequate, for visceral leishmaniasis. The generalized rash is probably secondary to reinvasion of the skin by *L. donovani*. The dermal lesions vary in their appearance and can be erythematous, hypopigmented macules or nodules which rarely ulcerate. The diagnosis is made by recovering the amastigotes of *L. donovani* from the lesions.

PATHOLOGY

In visceral leishmaniasis the macrophages of the lymphocyte macrophage system of liver, spleen, bone marrow, lymph nodes and connective tissue contain the amastigotes of *L. donovani* called Leishman-Donovan (LD) bodies. The enlarged spleen is firm, often weighing > 1 kg and shows hyperplasia of the red pulp, engorgement by histiocytes and blurring of the white pulp. The liver is also enlarged with the Kupffer cells filled with LD bodies (Fig. 8.2). There is a mononuclear cell infiltrate containing the parasites in the portal tracts

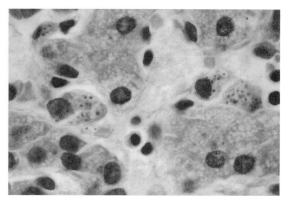

Figure 8.2 – Liver, with the Kupffer cells filled with LD bodies (H&E × 400).

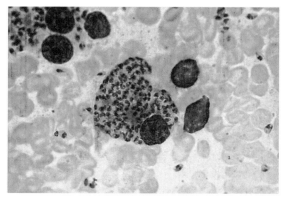

Figure 8.3 – LD bodies within macrophages of bone marrow MGG × 1000.

and in the sinusoids. The bone marrow is hyperplastic and contains LD bodies within macrophages (Fig. 8.3).

Generalized lymphadenopathy is present, especially prominent in the mesenteric lymph nodes. The histology can mimic both toxoplasmosis and malignant histiocytosis. The presence of LD bodies establishes the diagnosis. The interstitial histiocytes of the kidneys, heart and lung can also contain the organisms. However, the parenchymal cells of these organs are spared, a helpful feature to distinguish from Chagas' disease and toxoplasmosis. Although the LD bodies are seen in H&E stained sections, Giemsa stains are more helpful and outline the internal structure of the parasite. Fungal stains such as PAS, Gomori methenamine-silver and Gridley stains will not stain the parasite.

Cutaneous leishmaniasis occurs at the site of the sandfly bite and is characterized by a histiocytic skin reaction which, even in the early stages, contains LD bodies (Fig. 8.4). Later, lymphocytes and plasma cells can also be

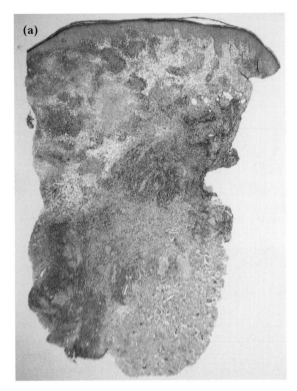

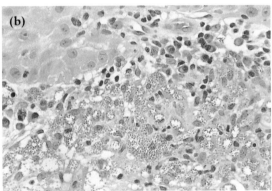

Figure 8.4 – Skin showing histiocytes containing LD bodies (a = H&E × 20) (b = H&E × 400).

seen. As the skin becomes ulcerated and necrotic, a granulomatous response is seen and the LD bodies gradually disappear. When the lesion heals, granulation is replaced by scar tissue. Linear, subcutaneous nodules appear along the lymphatics, which are invaded by the parasite, a feature mimicking sporotrichosis. Disseminated anergic leishmaniasis can resemble lepromatous leprosy, as no necrosis or granuloma formation is seen.

Granulomas and necrosis without healing characterize the mucocutaneous (Espundia) form. This form needs to be distinguished from tuberculosis, sarcoidosis, fungal infections, syphilis and lymphogranuloma venereum. Hence, special stains including acid-fast, fungal, Warthin-Starry and Giemsa stains should be carried out to exclude acid-fast bacilli, fungal and spirochaete infections and donovanosis respectively. Immune complex-mediated glomerular lesions may cause mesangioproliferative glomerulonephritis. Rarely, secondary amyloidosis may be found in the kidney.

INVESTIGATIONS

Morphologic detection of the parasite, culture, identification of the species by enzyme electrophoresis and detection of antibodies by several distinct methods are available. Culture and serological methods are not always available, except in well-established laboratories or reference centres. Identification of the parasite in tissue requires expertise. No single laboratory test is 100% dependable and there can be false-negative results. Combined diagnostic tests produce better diagnostic yield, in comparison with a single test.

1. Fine needle aspirates allow the preparation of smears. These are air-dried and stained with Giemsa, indirect immunofluorescent-monoclonal antibody assays and used for cultures. Cytospin preparations of cellular materials may give better yield than direct smears. This method is extremely useful for leishmania lymphadenitis. The presence of the kinetoplast helps to distinguish leishmania from toxoplasma and histoplasma. The presence of LD bodies exclusively in macrophages helps to distinguish from *Trypanosoma cruzi* which are found in tissue parenchymal cells.

2. Dermal scraping and smears are obtained by making a 3-mm slit in the skin lesion using the back of a scalpel blade to scrape the incision. This smear is used for special stains and for cultures, taking care to avoid contamination. The cut surface of dermal lesions can also be firmly pressed on to glass slides. This specimen is used for staining but is not suitable for cultures.

3. A punch biopsy of 4 mm or a wedge biopsy through the intact skin at the active border produces a specimen for culture of leishmania and other pathogenic organisms. An impression smear can also be made.

4. The smears can be stained with fluorescinated monoclonal antibodies to the amastigotes. There

are several monoclonal antibodies available for the different species of leishmania.

Of all diagnostic methods available, histopathologic examination is the least sensitive with a diagnostic sensitivity of 18% compared with smears from aspirated material which was 57% in one series (Navim *et al.* 1990). Demonstration of intracellular and extracellular amastigotes also depends on the age and type of the cutaneous lesion. Organisms can be demonstrated in early active lesions of ~2–4 months age but may be difficult to demonstrate if lesions are > 1 year. There are relatively few organisms in the mucocutaneous lesions.

Culture is the best method to isolate parasites from aspirates, smears or biopsies; however, it can be done only in specialized centres and takes time.

5. Serological diagnosis takes several forms. Enzyme-linked immunosorbent assay (ELISA) compares favourably with direct morphologic identification. However, the species cannot be identified. The direct agglutination test is of similar sensitivity as ELISA assays. Immunoblot assay using colloid gold conjugated to Protein A and a specific antibody is a rapid method of diagnosis for active visceral disease. Monoclonal and polyclonal antibodies can be used to detect amastigotes, allowing species characterization and dot blots of fluid aspirates or touch blots of infected tissue on nitrocellulose paper and labelled with monoclonal antibodies offers another method of rapid diagnosis.

6. The leishmanin skin test (Montenegro) is not a very useful test. A positive skin test may be interpreted as current or past infection with Leishmania species. The test cross-reacts with trypanosomes and is negative in active disease of a short duration so that a negative result does not exclude the diagnosis of leishmaniasis.

7. The polymerase chain reaction (PCR) and *in-situ* hybridization have been used to amplify DNA sequences of leishmania parasites in biopsy material. It is a rapid and highly sensitive method for diagnosis of visceral leishmaniasis and can be used to monitor therapeutic response (Rossell *et al.* 1992). Recombinant probes, which are specific for individual species, have now been described.

8. Visceral leishmaniasis is diagnosed by direct invasive methods such as splenic aspiration, bone marrow aspirate, liver biopsy, lymph node aspiration or biopsy and by serological tests described above. Splenic aspiration in patients with splenomegaly is the most sensitive method but complications such as bleeding needs to be considered and it is not recommended for the inexperienced operator. Lymph node aspiration or biopsy is a safe procedure with a diagnostic sensitivity of 58–79%. Bone marrow aspiration has a diagnostic sensitivity of 70% and liver biopsy has a diagnostic sensitivity of 77%.

Parasites disappear from spleen and bone marrow during treatment. Regression of splenomegaly is a predictor of cure. Absence of the parasite in bone marrow aspirates and splenic aspirates for those who had positive smears would indicate the success of the treatment.

TREATMENT

Studies in endemic parts of the world reveal a great variability in response to drugs. This behaviour is comparable with the sensitivity of microbial organisms to antibodies in different hospitals and communities. The response to chemotherapy in leishmaniasis varies with different strains of the parasite (El-On *et al.* 1993). Leishmania is an intracellular parasite, which can persist in the presence of a normal host immune response and once the parasite is in the skin or reticuloendothelial system complete eradication is difficult (Saravia *et al.* 1990). Leishmaniasis is also an opportunistic infection in AIDS patients and its presence appears to reduce the efficacy of chemotherapy in AIDS patients. The correct treatment of an imported case of cutaneous or visceral leishmaniasis requires knowledge of the prevalent species of leishmania in the geographical area and its drug sensitivity.

A wide variety of drugs is available including immunotherapy. These are IV or IM, given alone or in combination, and topical applications. In cutaneous leishmaniasis, physical methods such as localized heat and cryotherapy are employed and immunotherapy with or without chemotherapy may be given for both cutaneous and visceral leishmaniasis.

Most of the parenteral drugs are toxic. Some cases of cutaneous leishmaniasis may heal spontaneously with time, and it may be difficult to interpret the efficacy of the drug. However, there is definite benefit from chemotherapy especially in expanding lesions which otherwise cause disfiguration.

Cutaneous leishmaniasis

Topical treatment

- Paromomycin ointment, 15% strength, a non-toxic aminoglycoside, twice daily for 10 days
- Intralesional pentavalent antimonials at 8-day intervals has been effective
- Methylbenzethonium chloride 12% in soft paraffin. Duration of application depends on the strain of parasite
- Heat and cryotherapy are other forms of local therapy used with varying success

The cutaneous lesions should be kept clean with local antiseptics.

Parenteral treatment

- Pentavalent antimonial compounds – the mechanism of action of this group of compounds is very complex and probably through the inhibition of phosphofructokinase. The US Center for Disease Control and Prevention, Atlanta, GA, recommends the use of one of either stibogluconate or meglumine antimonate. Dosage of pentavalent antimony/kg body weight given IVI daily for 20 days. Treatment is commenced at 5 mg on first day and increased to maximum total dose of 850 mg/day if tolerated (WHO 1984). Patients should be monitored during therapy and treatment is stopped if arrhythmia, prolonged QT interval or concave ST segments develop. Liver function tests should be monitored. Other toxic effects are myalgia and rarely pancreatitis
- Pentamidine is an antiprotozoal agent and acts by damaging the kinetoplast DNA–mitochondrial complex. The standard dose is 2 mg/kg IVI every other day, a total of seven injections producing good results in New World cutaneous leishmaniasis (Soto-Mancipe et al. 1993). The patient should be monitored for hypotension and hypoglycaemia. Liver function tests and white cell count should be monitored
- Amphotericin B is an antifungal agent that is selectively taken up by macrophages and attain high concentrations in the reticuloendothelial

system and binds firmly to the ergosterol in the cell membrane of the protozoa. It is used only for disseminated mucocutaneous leishmaniasis when other treatments fail. It is first administered as a test dose of 1 mg by slow IVI infusion and then increased to 0.25–1 mg/kg every other day for 8 weeks. The side-effects are fever, hypotension and arrhythmias including cardiac arrest, blood dyscrasias and liver failure. Liposomal amphotericin is less toxic

Oral medications

- Dapsone 1–2 mg/kg/day for 6 weeks is associated with a cure rate of 80%. Toxic effects are blood dyscrasia, arrhythmias, hepatocellular disturbances and allergic reactions
- Allopurinol is used in New World cutaneous leishmaniasis at a dose of 20 mg/kg/day for 15 days; however, its efficacy is doubtful
- Ketaconazole is used in Old World cutaneous leishmaniasis. Dose: 10 mg/kg in three divided doses a day for 4 weeks. The response is species-dependent. It was ineffective in South American leishmaniasis. Toxic effects are hepatocellular changes, gynaecomastia and allergic manifestations
- Levamisole is given as 150 mg/day on 2 successive days each week for 8 weeks producing a 100% cure rate in one study. Toxic effects are nausea, vomiting, abdominal pain, leukopenia, agranulocytosis and pruritis
- Rifampicin 10 mg/kg for 6–12 weeks. The mode of action is by strong binding to DNA-dependent RNA polymerase and inhibition of RNA synthesis. Toxic effects are confusion, drowsiness, headaches and muscle weakness. Body fluids are coloured red by the drug

Visceral leishmaniasis

Parenteral

- Pentavalent antimonial compounds are recommended for treatment of visceral leishmaniasis. Dosages are similar to those for cutaneous leishmaniasis given above
- Aminosidine (paromomycin) is used alone or in combination with other drugs and is effective in

all leishmania species (Scott *et al.* 1992). Dose: 14 mg/kg/day diluted in 250 ml normal saline given over 4 h (infusion pump) in single dose, for 20 days. Aminosidine is not hepatotoxic. It has been reported to be as efficacious as stibogluconate alone, and is more appropriate in patients with pre-existing liver disease and in visceral leishmaniasis. It has also been used in combination with sodium stibogluconate 20 mg/kg/day for 20 days when resistance develops. The toxic effects are disturbances of hearing, renal impairment, fever, myalgia, anaemia and headaches. Monitoring during infusion is essential

- Amphotericin B as with cutaneous leishmaniasis. Liposomal amphotericin B has been used in children with drug-resistant visceral leishmaniasis (Giacchino *et al.* 1993). Drug-resistant visceral leishmaniasis in children is treated with 3 mg/kg/day for 30 days, up to a total dose of 60 mg/kg. It is recommended for young children and patients in poor physical condition
- Pentamidine is used at 4 mg/kg on alternate days with a total of 20 injections producing cure rates of ~70%

Oral

- Allopurinol as a single drug is given in doses of 20 mg/kg/day for 14–70 days with a cure rates of 80% and used in cases showing resistance to antimonials
- Ketaconazole as in the treatment of cutaneous leishmaniasis
- A combination of ketaconazole and allopurinol at their normal dosage

Immunotherapy

During the active stage of visceral leishmaniasis there is a defect in interferon-γ production (Cook 1993), hence methods of stimulating cell-mediated immunity seem a rational therapeutic approach. However, this form of treatment is still in its infancy and more experience is required.

- Pentavalent antimony and interferon-γ. Dose of interferon-γ 100–400 μg/m^2 body surface/day

for 10–40 days, especially recommended for AIDS patients with visceral leishmaniasis. A short course (10 days) of high-dose IV meglumine antimonate 20 mg/kg plus interferon-γ has been reported to be effective in treating cutaneous leishmaniasis in Guatemala

- Intradermal human recombinant interferon-γ in cutaneous leishmaniasis has proved to be effective
- Heat-killed Leishmania promastigotes and bacillus Calmette-Guerin (BCG) to stimulate interferon-γ production. Three vaccinations over 32 weeks achieved a 94% cure rate in cutaneous leishmaniasis

VECTOR AND RESERVOIR CONTROL

The epidemiology of the disease in the specific geographical area should be considered when planning control of reservoir and vector. The reduction in rodents and the use of insecticides are difficult public health measures and mass treatment with a specific drug such as antimonials or pentamidine is not a proper solution as the parasite soon develops resistance, as in India (Russell 1993).

REFERENCES

Brandon-Filho S, Shaw J. *Leishmani*asis in Brazil. *Parasitology Today* 1994; **9**: 329–330

Cook GC. *Leishmani*asis – some recent development in chemotherapy. *Journal of Antimicrobial Chemotherapy* 1993; **31**: 327–330

El-On J, Livshin R, Evan-Paz ZE *et al.* Topical treatment of cutaneous leishmaniasis. *British Medical Journal* 1993; **291**: 1280–1281

Giacchino R, Giambartolomei G, Tasso L *et al.* Treatment with liposomal amphotericin B of a child affected with drug resistant visceral leishmaniasis [Short report]. *Transactions of the Royal Society of Tropical Medicine and Hygiene* 1993; **87**: 310–312

Gradoni L, Gramiccia M. *Leishmania infantum* tropism, strain genotype or best immune response. *Parasitology Today* 1994; **10**: 264–267

Navim TR, Aran FE, de Merida AM *et al.* Cutaneous leishmaniasis in Guatemala: comparison of diagnostic methods. *American Journal of Tropical Medicine and Hygiene* 1990; **42**: 36–42

Rossell RA de, de Duran R de J, Rossell O *et al.* Is leishmaniasis ever cured. *Transactions of the Royal Society of Tropical Medicine and Hygiene* 1992; **86**: 251–253

Russell RD. Vector-borne diseases and their control. *Australian Medical Journal* 1993; **158**: 681–690

Saravia NG, Weigle K, Segura I *et al.* Recurrent lesions in human *Leishmania braziliensis* infection or reinfection. *Lancet* 1990; **336**: 398–402

Scott JAG, Davidson RN, Moody AH *et al.* Aminosidine (paramomycin) in the treatment of Leishmania imported into UK. *Transactions of the Royal Society of Tropical Medicine and Hygiene* 1992; **86**: 617–619

Soto-Mancipe J, Ceroge M, Berman JD. Evaluation of pentamidine for the treatment of cutaneous leishmaniasis in Columbia. *Clinical Infectious Diseases* 1993; **16**: 417

World Health Organisation. *The Leishmaniasis.* Technical Report Series 702. Geneva: World Health Organisation, 1984

9

Trypanosomiasis

African Trypanosomiasis
Parasitology
Presentation
Pathology
Investigations
Trypanosoma cruzi (American

Trypanopsomiasis or Chagas' disease)
Parasitology
Presentation
Pathology
Investigations
Treatment
References

TRYPANOSOMIASIS

Haemoflagellated protozoa transmitted to man by an insect vector cause trypanosomiasis. Two types of trypanosomes recognized are sleeping sickness or African trypanosomiasis and Chagas' disease or American trypanosomiasis. Thirty-six African countries are affected by African trypanosomiasis, with 50 million people at risk and > 100 000 infected. American trypanosomiasis or Chagas' disease is a major public health problem with 400 000 new cases reported each year. According to the estimates of the World Health Organisation, 16–18 million people are actually infected, with 100 million at risk.

AFRICAN TRYPANOSOMIASIS

The two species responsible for African trypanosomiasis are *Trypanosoma brucei gambiense* and *rhodesiense*. The distribution of *T. brucei gambiense* is over a wide area of West Africa where infections are much higher compared with *T. brucei rhodesiense* (East African trypanosomiasis). Transmission of the infection is also different in the two infections. The gambiense trypanosomiasis is

transmitted by the tsetse fly from person to person, whereas *T. brucei rhodesiense* is a zoonosis where the vector feeds on animals and transmission can therefore be from person to person or animal to person. Gambiense trypanosomiasis is mainly found in the rural areas. Tourists are therefore rarely affected. Rhodesian trypanosomiasis occurs among tourists who live and/or as an occupational hazard among those who work for long periods in the game parks of East Africa. Five possible causes for sleeping sickness outbreaks have been suggested. These are variations in rainfall, in vectorial potential, host immunity, parasite virulence and the impact of explorers and colonizers on the environment.

PARASITOLOGY

In West Africa the vector is *Glossina palpalis* and *G. tachinoides,* whereas in East Africa it is *G. pallipedes* and *G. morsitans.* *T. brucei gambiense* has no documented animal reservoirs, although it can be transmitted to animals such as the bushbuck. The life cycle (Fig. 9.1) begins with the introduction of the infective stage to humans by the bite of a tsetse fly. Once the infective forms are introduced into the blood stream, the trypomastigote

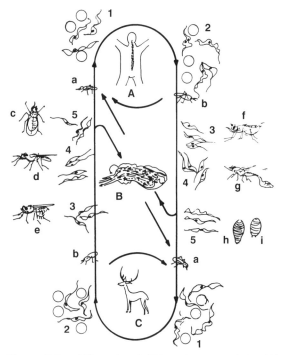

Figure 9.1 – Life cycle of African trypanosomiasis. (A) Development in man: trypanosomes in the peripheral blood: infection of the central nervous system; (1, 2) dividing trypanosomes. (B) Development in the tsetse fly; (3) trypanosomes from the stomach of the fly; (4) crithidial forms from the intestine of the fly (D); (5) metacyclic forms from the salivary glands (S); (a, b) blood-sucking Tsetse flies; (c) Glossina: resting position of the fly; (d) fasting fly; (e) fully engorged fly; (f) pregnant fly; (g) Glossina lays a larva; (h) larva; (i) pupa. Route of the migration of the trypanosomes in Glossina. (C) Development similar to (A) in the peripheral blood of the reservoir host (e.g. antelope, 'parasite reservoir'). Transmission by the species of Glossina can occur: (1) from man to man: A → B → A; (2) from animal to animal as reservoirs of the parasite: C → B → C; (3) from animal to man: C → B → A and the reverse: A → B → C.

forms develop and multiply and can be found in the blood, lymph nodes, cerebrospinal fluid and at the site of the bite. The morphology of the trypomastigote varies from the fully developed trypomastigote with a long flagellum, 30 μm in length, to short stumpy forms without a free flagellum, half the length of the flagellate type. The trypomastigote forms are 14–33 μm long and 1.5–3.5 μm wide. The stumpy forms are the infective forms that develop in the tsetse fly. The trypomastigotes develop by binary fission. They have a central nucleus that stains red with the Giemsa stain, granular cytoplasm and a kinetoplast that stains red at the posterior end. The flagellum and the undulating membrane arise from the kinetoplast and the flagellum runs along the edge of undulating membrane. The flagellum becomes free to extend beyond the anterior end of the body and undulating membrane.

When the tsetse fly bites an infected human, trypanosomal forms are ingested. They multiply in the lumen of the mid- and hindgut of the fly. From the gut, the organisms migrate to the salivary ducts, attach to the epithelial cells of the ducts and develop into the epimastigote forms. These are different from the trypomastigotes in that the kinetoplast is anterior to the nucleus. There is further development in the salivary gland for 3–5 days where transformation into the infective or metacyclic forms takes place.

PRESENTATION

In West African trypanosomiasis a painful chancre develops at the site of the bite; this heals quickly. Initially there is a low-grade parasitaemia with minimal symptoms that regress or develop further. In the early stage of the disease there is invasion of the lymph nodes with painless enlargement of posterior cervical nodes (Winterbottom's sign) as well as other nodes. The accompanying fever is irregular and remittent, with headaches. Experimental evidence suggests that Winterbottom's sign may indicate a cerebral infection, and trypanosomes may possibly enter the brain via lymphatics (Ormerod 1991). The liver and spleen may be palpable. Myocarditis, thrombocytopenia and anaemia may occur at this stage of the infection. Delayed sensation to pain (Kerandel's sign) is another feature.

The disease may progress as a gradual onset of daytime somnolence, insomnia and restlessness at night. Extrapyramidal signs develop with ataxia and Parkinson's disease. If untreated, there is progression to coma and death. Hypogonadism is a feature of African trypanosomiasis in both men, women and animals through its effects on hypothalamo-anterior-pituitary gonadal axis functions. This stage may last for years, the illness taking a chronic course. Tourists can therefore develop symptoms on returning to their home countries.

The incubation period of East African trypanosomiasis is only a few days. The preneurological state is similar to *T. gambiense* but is short, with a very acute course. Persistent tachycardia, myocarditis with arrhythmias and cardiac failure may cause death even in this stage of the illness. Late disease is very rapid in onset, producing the classical sleeping sickness, sleepy during daytime and restless and awake at night. Confusion and loss of coordination follow personality changes. Secondary infection and emaciation complicate this stage of the disease.

PATHOLOGY

Pathologic changes in both forms of trypanosomiasis are similar. The enlarged lymph glands contain macrophages filled with the trypanosomes. An inflammatory response with vascular congestion and oedema associated with perivascular endarteritis and obliteration of the small vessels is also seen. The glands later become fibrotic. In the central nervous system there is oedema of the brain and leptomeninges. Round cells with perivascular cuffing infiltrate blood vessels. The cerebral cortex contains granulomas with large numbers of trypanosomes surrounded by small glial cells. Scattered throughout the brain are the plasma cells, many engorged with immunoglobulin globules (Mott cells).

The surface of the trypomastigote has a variant surface glycoprotein (VSG). African trypanosomes have the ability to change the surface coat of this outer membrane probably every week. By this mechanism it can evade the host's humoral immune response (Barry and Turner 1991) thereby producing a wave of parasitaemia every week or fortnight. During the infection there is selective dysregulation of suprachiasmatic nucleus of the hypothalmus. This may be responsible for the disruption of endogenous rhythms in sleeping sickness (Bentivoglio *et al.* 1994).

INVESTIGATIONS

1. Trypomastigotes may be identified in the chancre in the case of West African trypanosomiasis and in blood, lymph nodes and cerebrospinal fluid in both forms of the disease. The stains used are Giemsa or Wrights. Trypomastigotes occur in the peripheral blood in large numbers during the spikes of fever (Fig. 9.2). Blood examination should be done to monitor response to treatment. The presence of Mott cells in cerebrospinal fluid is characteristic of African trypanosomiasis.
2. Parasite-specific DNA probes, non-radioactive probes and PCR methods are available (Eshita and Fukuma 1992).

Morphologic differentiation of *T. brucei gambiense* and *T. brucei rhodesiense* is not possible. Differentiation can

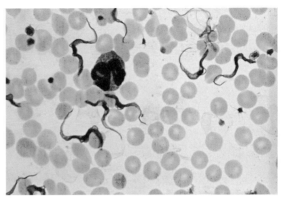

Figure 9.2 – Trypomastigotes in peripheral blood (Wright stain).

be made on different characteristics of isoenzymes, RNA and DNA methods.

TRYPANOSOMA CRUZI (AMERICAN TRYPANOSOMIASIS OR CHAGAS' DISEASE)

The disease was named after Carlos Chagas from Brazil who described the life cycle of the parasite at the beginning of this century. Chagas' disease is a zoonosis occurring in the American continent, transmitted by the reduviid bugs to humans through the faeces of the bug. Rarely transmission occurs transplacentally, by blood transfusions or accidental ingestion of the bug. The reservoirs are opossums, dogs, cats and rodents. With migration of South Americans to other countries, there is the possibility of encountering patients suffering from chronic Chagas' disease in non-endemic countries.

PARASITOLOGY

The life cycle (Fig. 9.3) begins when humans are infected by the metacyclic trypomastigotes released in the faeces when the reduviid bug takes a blood meal. The saliva causes an allergic reaction, resulting in scratching and entry of the trypomastigotes. These transform into amastigotes (non-flagellate form) that multiply in the host's cells. The amastigotes have a predilection for cardiac muscle, skeletal muscle, smooth muscle, ganglion cells and reticuloendothelial cells. The trypomastigotes are found as long or short forms with a central nucleus and a kinetoplast at the posterior end. The kinetoplast is different from the

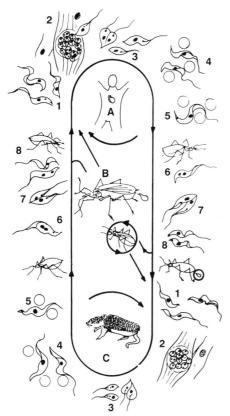

Figure 9.3 – Life cycle in Chagas' disease. (A) Development in man; (1) metacyclic trypanosomes enter man with the faeces of the bug (a); (2) intracellular multiplication in the Leishmania stage; (3) crithidia stage; (4, 5) trypanosoma forms from the peripheral blood. (B) development in the intestine of the triatoma bug; (6) freshly ingested trypanosomes in division; (7) change to the crithidia form; (8) metacyclic trypanosome forms from the faeces of the bug. (C) Development that occurs in man (A) also occurs in the reservoir hosts (armadillo, opossum, dog and other animals).

African forms as it has a small blepharoblast and a large oval parabasal body. The blepharoblast gives rise to a flagellum that extends beyond the anterior end with an undulating membrane medial to it. The nucleus and kinetoplast stains red with Giemsa stain.

On reaching the host tissue cell the parasite loses its flagellum, divides by binary fission and transforms into amastigotes. The amastigotes are 2–6 μm in diameter, have a large nucleus and kinetoplast. The infected cells eventually release both amastigote and trypomastigote forms. During a blood meal the reduviid bug ingests trypomastigotes which transform into epimastigotes in the midgut of the lung. After 7–10 days, the metacyclic trypomastigotes, which have developed from epimastigotes, are passed in the faeces of reduviid bug. Macrophages and muscle cells are the main targets of *T. cruzi*. These cells are invaded by endocytosis.

PRESENTATION

At the site of the bite a painful, subcutaneous nodule or chagoma may develop. It can persist from 10 to 12 weeks. If the infection is in the eyelid, oedema of conjunctiva and eyelids occurs (Romana's sign).

In the acute phase, the infection spreads to lymph nodes draining the site of the bite. The nodes become painful and tender. Trypomastigotes are found in blood ~7–10 days after the infection. Acute symptoms such as hepatosplenomegaly, lymphadenopathy, skin rashes and swelling of face and legs are more common in young children. An acute myocarditis may occur which can be fatal. The central nervous system may also be involved. Chagas' disease can present as an acute meningoencephalitis in children and in immuno-compromised patients.

HIV infected patients may show multifocal or diffuse meningoencephalitis with necrosis and large numbers of parasites (Rocha *et al.* 1994). These patients develop pseudotumours and show expanding lesions with a mass effect, causing intracranial hypertension, which may mimic a cerebral neoplasm. Acute myocarditis, which is fatal, can also manifest in HIV patients. HIV can also reactivate Chagas' disease.

The chronic phase may manifest after several years. The organs affected are myocardium, oesophagus and colon. Damage to the myocardium causes cardiomyopathy with its attendant complications such as arrhythmia, heart block, biventricular failure, thrombosis and embolism. ECG changes seen are sinus tachycardia, ventricular tachycardia, supraventricular tachycardia, premature beats, left anterior hemiblock and complete right bundle branch block. Chagas' disease of the oesophagus results in dilatation of the oesophagus and loss of contractibility resulting in dysphagia, regurgitation and aspiration. Colonic disease causes dilatation of the colon, with abdominal distension, discomfort and constipation.

Congenital Chagas' disease results from transplacental transmission and manifests as low birth weight, stillbirth or death soon after birth. Death occurs from myocarditis or central nervous system infection.

Children born to seropositive mothers should be monitored by periodic examination of their blood for parasites.

PATHOLOGY

Pseudocysts of intracellular aggregates of multiplying parasites are seen in infected tissue. Chagomas, seen mainly on the face, demonstrate intracellular parasites with lymphocyte infiltration and reactive hyperplasia in regional lymph nodes.

The heart is dilated, walls are thin with aneurysmal dilation at the apex and there is formation of mural thrombi. Histologically, fibrosis, atrophy of myocardial fibres and lymphocytic infiltration is seen. Myocardial damage and left ventricular dilatation precede cardiac parasympathetic nerve changes with an apparent correlation between the degree of left ventricular parasympathetic nerve changes. *T. cruzi* probably selectively destroys the postganglionic parasympathetic vagal nerve.

The oesophagus and colon are grossly dilated and hypertrophied. Microscopically, there is lymphocytic infiltration and reduction in the number of neurones in the myenteric plexus.

INVESTIGATIONS

1. Positive diagnosis depends on identifying trypomastigotes in the blood, in chagoma or lymph glands. Blood should be collected without anticoagulants for buffy coat preparations. The trypomastigotes should be differentiated from *T. rangeli*, which does not cause disease in humans and can occur in symptomatic individuals. However, morphologic differentiation may not be possible.
2. Serology – in chronic disease trypomastigotes are very few. Serologic tests are ELISA, indirect haemagglutination and complement fixation tests. Depending on antibodies, cross-reactivity can occur with leishmaniasis and schistosomiasis.
3. Polymerase chain reaction (PCR) is useful in chronic disease where organisms are very few and to distinguish *T. rangeli* from *T. cruzi*. PCR results corroborate with immunoperoxidase methods for detection of *T. cruzi* in cardiac biopsies (Wincker 1994). Monoclonal antibodies can be used for differentiation of *T. cruzi* and *T. rangeli*.

TREATMENT

The drugs currently available for treatment of African trypanosomiasis are: (1) suramin (Bayer 205) – a diamidine; (2) pentamidine isethionate – a diamidine derivative; (3) melarsoprol – trivalent arsenical; (4) deflornithine – a difluromethylornithine compound; and (5) nifurtimox – a nitrofuran. They are all toxic drugs.

- Before CNS involvement the drug of choice is suramin, given IV. It is contraindicated in renal disease. A test dose is recommended. Side-effects are hepatitis, CNS complications, shock, haemolysis and leucopenia. A 100–200 mg test dose should be given IV. For adults the maximum dose is 1 g on days 1, 3, 7, 14 and 21, for children it is 20 mg/kg on days 1, 3, 7, 14 and 21 (maximum 1 g) should be administered under monitoring conditions
- Alternative therapy is pentamidine isethionate. However, resistance to this drug is now known. Administration is by IM injection and flare-up of the disease (Herxheimer type reaction) may occur. A daily dose of 4 mg/kg for children and adults should be given IM or IV for 10 days monitoring for tachycardia and hypotension
- When there is CNS involvement melarsoprol is the drug of choice as it penetrates the blood–brain barrier. Toxic effects are encephalopathy and exfoliative dermatitis. A post-treatment reactive encephalopathy has been described during treatment of end-stage sleeping sickness. A 2–3.6 mg/kg dose IV in three divided doses for 3 days and 1 week later 3.6 mg/kg in three divided doses for 3 days is administered. The last course to be repeated in 10–21 days. The drug is very toxic and the patient should be monitored during its administration
- Alternative therapy is deflornithine in *T. gambiense* in early and late stages if resistant to melarsoprol. The development of deflornithine (DFMO) for treatment of Gambiense sleeping sickness has been a great advancement in treatment in view of its safety compared with other drugs and has been named the 'resurrection drug'. Dosage is 400 mg/kg/day in four divided doses for 2 weeks is given. This should be followed by 80 mg/kg/day for 3–4 weeks. DL-α-Difluromethylornithine (DFMO) inhibits ornithine decarboxylase and so lowers the levels

of spermine and spermidine, thereby inhibiting multiplication by parasites

- Nifurtimox (Lampit) can be used for *T. gambiense* infection is unresponsive to melarsoprol. The drug is toxic and the dosage should be increased gradually. The recommended doses are: children 15–20 mg/kg; adults 12–15 mg/kg for 30–60 days. Surveillance after treatment should be continued for up to 3 years. Relapses appear to be common

The drugs available for Chagas' disease are: nifurtimox, allopurinol; benznidazole and amphotericin B.

- In the acute stage, oral nifurtimox has been used successfully. It is very toxic and dosage should be gradually increased over 6–7 days. It is administered over long periods for up to 120 days. Resistance has developed. Recommended dose is 8–10 mg/kg/day in four divided doses for 120 days for adults. For children: 20 mg/kg in four divided doses for 15 days is recommended. It is not useful in chronic disease. Side-effects are neurological symptoms, paraesthesia, fits, disorientation and abdominal pain
- Benznidazole is the second line of drugs in acute Chagas' disease. Oral dosage is 5 mg/kg/day for 60 days. Side-effects are peripheral neuropathy and granulocytopenia. There is a correlation between the susceptibility of *T. cruzi* to benznidazole and to nifurtimox
- Purine analogues as chemotherapeutic agents are used in leishmaniasis and American trypanosomiasis. Parasites metabolize certain purine analogues to neucleotides and aminated to the analogue adenine neucleotide. These subsequently halt protein synthesis and RNA breakdown. Allopurinol at 5 mg/kg two to three times daily for 60 days has been reported to give high cure rates. Side-effects are uncommon, although hepatic toxicity, interstitial nephritis along with bone marrow depression and vasculitis has been reported
- Amphotericin B at a dosage of 1.5 mg/kg given by slow, IV injection for up to 90 days. Commencing with a test dose is recommended where other forms of treatment have failed

Drug treatment in chronic Chagas' disease is unsatisfactory. Limited studies have suggested that allopurinol may be useful in chronic Chagas' disease.

Prevention of African trypanosomiasis and Chagas' disease by vector control measures through the elimination of breeding grounds has not been very successful. The most effective methods are fly traps and insecticides. There should be regular screening of the population and attempts to eliminate the parasite to low levels although these methods too are not entirely satisfactory.

REFERENCES

Barry JD, Turner CMR. The dynamics of antigenic variation and growth of African trypanosomiasis. *Parasitology Today* 1991; **7**: 207–221

Bentivoglio M, Grassi-Zacconi, Kristensson K. From trypanosomiasis to the nervous system, from molecules to behaviour. A survey on the occasion of the 90th Anniversary of Castellani's discovery of the parasites in sleeping sickness [Review]. *Italian Journal of Neurological Sciences* 1994; **15**: 75–87

Eshita Y, Fukuma T. Diagnosis of trypanosomiasis with the parasite specific DNA probes – non-radioactive probes and PCR methods [Review]. *Nippon Rinsho, Japanese Journal of Clinical Medicine* 1992; **50 (suppl)**: 480–485

Ormerod WE. Hypothesis, the significance of Winterbottom's sign [Review]. *Journal of Tropical Medicine and Hygiene* 1991; **94**: 388–400

Rocha A, de Meneses AC, da Silva AM *et al.* Pathology of patients with Chagas' disease and acquired immunodeficiency syndrome [Review]. *American Journal of Tropical Medicine and Hygiene* 1994; **50**: 261–268

Wincker P. Use of a simplified polymerase chain reaction procedure to detect *Trypanosoma cruzi* in blood samples from chagasic patients in rural endemic areas. *American Journal of Tropical Medicine and Hygiene* 1994; **51**: 771–777

10

Cryptosporidiosis

Parasitology
Presentation
Pathology

Investigations
Treatment
References

Cryptosporidiosis is a diarrhoeal disease of vertebrates produced by protozoa of the genus Cryptosporidium, a zoonoses with a wide variety of hosts such as sheep, cattle, rodents, dogs, cats, poultry and primates, including man. Besides being a zoonoses, person-to-person transmission is now of importance. A survey in Victoria, Australia, revealed that Cryptosporidium was present in 4% of 884 hospital patients with gastroenteritis. Unknown as a human pathogen before 1976, cryptosporidia now rank as a major enteric pathogen of humans.

PARASITOLOGY

Most strains of this tiny parasite are morphologically similar in appearance. Cryptosporidia exhibit alternating cycles of sexual and asexual reproduction and are thereby classified as sporozoan protozoa. Both cycles are completed within the gastrointestinal tract of a single host. The infective forms of oocysts, 5 μm in diameter, are shed into the intestinal lumen of the parasitized animal. These hardy structures are resistant to most disinfectants including the chlorine concentrates generally present in municipal water supplies and survive in temperatures between –20 and 60°C. In cool, moist environments they may survive for months.

The oocysts are fully mature and immediately infective upon passage in the faeces. Following ingestion by another animal, sporozoites are released from the oocyst, attach to the epithelial surface and begin a series of developmental changes. Although excluded from the cytoplasm of the epithelial cell, trophozoites and all subsequent developmental stages are surrounded by a double membrane of host origin and are, by definition, intracellular parasites.

Domestic animals constitute an important reservoir of disease for humans. However, disease outbreaks in daycare centres, hospitals and urban family groups indicate that most human infections result from person-to-person transmission rather than zoonotic spread. Since oocysts are found almost exclusively in stools, the principal transmission route is undoubtedly faecal-oral. In daycare centres and among male homosexual groups the spread is probably direct. The recovery of oocysts from drinking water and the documentation of at least two waterborne outbreaks makes it likely that indirect transmission via water, and possibly food and fomites, is not uncommon.

The trophozoites divide asexually by a process of multiple fission (schizogony) to form meronts containing eight daughter cells known as type I merozoites. Upon release from the meront, each merozoite attaches itself to another epithelial cell, where it repeats the schizogony cycle, producing another generation of type I merozoites. Eventually, meronts containing only four daughter cells are seen. Incapable of continued asexual reproduction, these type II merozoites are transformed into male (microgamete) and female (macrogamete) sexual forms. Following fertilization, the resulting zygote develops into an oocyst (Figure 10.1). The majority possesses a thick, double-layered protective cell wall that ensures their intact passage in the faeces and survival in the external environment. About 20% of the oocysts, however, fail to develop such a wall. Their thin, single cell membrane ruptures, releasing infective sporozoites directly into the intestinal lumen and initiating a new 'auto-infective' cycle within the original host. In the normal host, the presence of innate or acquired immunity dampens both the cyclic production of type I merozoites and the formation of thin-walled oocysts, halting further parasite multiplication and terminating the acute infection. In the immunocompromised both merozoites and oocysts presumably continue, explaining why such individuals develop severe, persistent infections in the absence of repeated reinfections.

OOCYSTS

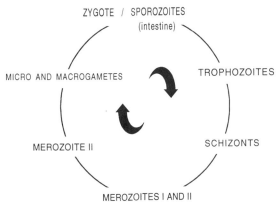

Figure 10.1 – Life cycle of Cryptosporidium in man.

PRESENTATION

The incubation period is 4–12 days. The severity of the infection depends on the host's immune status. The main symptom is watery diarrhoea that can vary in severity. Diarrhoea is associated with nausea, vomiting, anorexia, flatulence and colicky abdominal pain. Normal individuals have a self-limiting disease lasting up to 3–4 weeks. Cryptosporidial disease is a more severe illness in the immunocompromised patients resulting in marked volume depletion, loss of weight, malabsorption and electrolyte imbalance. The loss of fluids is comparable with cholera although no toxins have been isolated. Patients with AIDS often cannot clear the organism from the gastrointestinal tract and the cryptosporidia may persist for the remainder of their lives. In the USA, half the patients with AIDS and cryptosporidiosis survive for < 6 months. They may have cryptosporidiosis in the biliary tract, pharynx and large intestines. Biliary tract strictures have been reported in AIDS patients similar to sclerosing cholangitis. In patients with AIDS, Cryptosporidium has been found in sputum and in lung biopsy material.

PATHOLOGY

Although the jejunum is the most heavily infected organ, cryptosporidia have been found in the pharynx, bronchi, oesophagus, stomach, duodenum, gallbladder, ileum, appendix, colon and rectum of immunocompromised subjects. They appear as small, basophilic, spherical organisms measuring 2–4 μm in diameter arranged in rows or clusters along the brush border of the columnar epithelial cells, often mistaken for epithelial blebs (Figure. 10.2).

With haematoxylin and eosin staining, the parasite is either basophilic or golden brown in colour; with Giemsa it displays a bright red centre. It does not stain with either methenamine silver or PAS. As the parasite is very tiny, definitive diagnosis is best made by electron

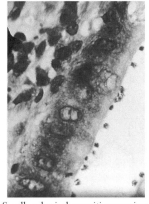

Figure 10.2 – Small, spherical parasitic organisms arranged in a row along the brush border of the small intestine in H&E.

microscopy where the trophozoite can be seen intimately attached to the microvillous membrane of the epithelial cell.

INVESTIGATIONS

The diagnosis of cryptosporidiosis must be pursued in any immunocompromised patient who develops diarrhoea. Before 1978, the diagnosis required small-bowel biopsy. The development of effective concentration and staining techniques, as well as the growing laboratory experience with this parasite, has made the recovery and identification of cryptosporidia oocysts from stool the diagnostic procedure of choice. Oocyst excretion is most intense during the first 4 or 5 days of illness, tapers during the second week and generally stops within 1 or 2 weeks of the cessation of diarrhoea. Oocysts are rarely recovered from solid stool.

1. Stool examination – specimens should be examined immediately after passage or preserved in 2.5% potassium dichromate or 10% buffered formalin. Initially, an iodine wet mount can be made from the unconcentrated specimen and examined microscopically. The spherical 5 μm oocysts are differentiated from yeasts, which they resemble in size and morphology, by their failure to take up the iodine. Also available are special methods of immersion of the specimen in sucrose solution, which allows the oocyst to float and examination by direct-phase contrast microscopy using acid-fast stains. Oocysts appear as highly refractile spherical bodies (4–5 μm). The Kinyoun acid-fast stain has a high sensitivity of 96.4% (Kehl et al. 1995). Accurate measurement of oocysts with an ocular micrometer is useful in the identification (González-Ruiz and Bendall 1991).
2. Small-bowel biopsy for the identification of the parasite in the form of schizonts containing merozoites and micro- and macrogametes.
3. Newer enzyme immunoassays and direct immunofluorescent assays are now available (Kehl et al. 1995).

A study of different methods for detection of Cryptosporidium species revealed that Kinyoun staining and direct immunofluorescent assays were sensitive tests.

Other tests to assess the secondary biochemical abnormalities include serum electrolytes and arterial blood gases, full blood count and haematocrit, and liver function tests.

TREATMENT

At present there is no drug that is 100% effective. In immunocompetent persons cryptosporidiosis is a self-limiting disease and supportive treatment is all that is essential. The treatments available currently are:

- Spiramycin 50–100 mg/kg in three divided doses for 12 days. Recent studies suggest that spiramycin is effective in hastening recovery and reduction of oocyst excretion in both immunocompetent and non-immunocompetent patients (Fafard and Lalonde 1990)
- Hyperimmune bovine colostrum – obtained from cows vaccinated with cryptosporidiosis antigen. There have been some successful reports using this treatment. (Ungar et al 1990).
- Paromomycin and azithromycin – Current trials are underway to determine the efficiency of these two drugs
- Supportive treatment including fluid and electrolyte replacement and parenteral nutrition

REFERENCES

Fafard J, Lalonde R. Long standing symptomatic cryptosporidiosis in normal man. Clinical responses to spiramycin. *Journal of Clinical Gastroenterology* 1990; **12**: 190–191

González-Ruiz A, Bendall RP. The use of the ocular micrometer in diagnostic parasitology. *Parasitology Today* 1995; **11**: 83

Kehl KSC, Cicirello H, Havens PL. Comparison of four different methods for detection of Cryptosporidium species. *Journal of Clinical Microbiology* 1995; **33**: 416–418

Ungar BL, Ward DJ, Fayer R *et al.* Cessation of Cryptosporidium-associated diarrhoea in an acquired immunodeficiency syndrome patient after treatment with hyperimmune bovine colostrum. *Gastroenterology* 1990; **98**: 486–489

11

Microsporidiosis

Parasitology
Presentation
Pathology

Investigations
Treatment
References

Microsporidiosis is an infection caused by protozoa of the Order Microsporidia, a group of obligate intracellular protozoa parasites. The organisms have only been recently identified and the number of diagnosed cases of microsporidiosis continues to increase because of HIV infection. In normal people the disease is self-limiting but in AIDS patients and other immunosuppressed patients microsporidiosis can produce severe intestinal infection. As with cryptosporidiosis, it has a variety of both vertebrate and invertebrate hosts. *Encephalitozoon hellem* is another form of disseminated microsporidiosis in AIDS patients.

PARASITOLOGY

More than 100 microsporidial genera and almost 1000 species have now been identified. Five species have been identified in AIDS patients as well as some unclassified Microsporidia.

The species identified in AIDS patients are *Enterocytozoon bineusi*, *Encephalitozoon cuniculi*, *E. hellem*, *Septata intestinalis*, *Pleistophora* spp. and other unidentified microsporidia. The method of transmission in humans is uncertain. Microsporidia have a nucleus, with a nuclear envelope, an intracytoplasmic membrane system and chromosome separation on mitotic spindles (Weber *et al.* 1994). They are

exclusively intracellular parasites and do not have active stages outside the host cell. The life cycle involves a spore stage proliferative merogenic stage followed by the sporogenic stage, which results in mature spores. The spores have a tubular extension apparatus for penetrating the host cell. Some microsporidia affect many organs, while others are limited to one organ.

The life cycle of microsporidia in humans is complete in the human host and there is no secondary host or a vector transmitting the development stages of microsporidia. However, more work needs to be done on the taxonomy of microsporidia infecting humans and some species have not been classified because the life cycle has not been properly worked out.

PRESENTATION

The commonest clinical manifestations of microsporidiosis are intestinal, ocular, muscular and cerebral. Systemic manifestations may also be seen. The presentation depends on the immune status of the host. In the immunocompetent host, it is a self-limiting disease with mainly gastrointestinal symptoms. Patients with HIV present with chronic diarrhoea and wasting syndrome. However, they may present with disseminated infection, depending on the infecting species.

Disseminated infection is generally caused by *E. hellem*, *E. cuniculi* or *S. intestinalis*. Keratoconjunctivitis is caused by species *E. hellem*. Jaundice secondary to infection in the biliary tree, referred to as 'AIDS cholangiopathy', may cause bile duct dilatation and acalculous cholecystitis. Hepatocellular necrosis has been described in patients infected with species *E. cuniculi* resulting in fulminant hepatic failure (Terada *et al.* 1987). Peritonitis has also been attributed to the same organism. Other presentations include nephritis, ureteritis, prostatitis, cystitis, encephalitis, myositis, respiratory tract infection and progressive respiratory failure.

PATHOLOGY

E. bineusi and *S. intestinalis* in humans affect the small intestines. Histological changes vary from none to severe epithelial degeneration, blunted villi, intra-epithelial lymphocytic infiltrates and lamina propria mononuclear cells, i.e. the changes of partial villus atrophy. *E. bineusi* has been identified in biliary epithelium, liver cells, pancreatic ducts epithelium and upper respiratory tract epithelium. Infections of the biliary tract can cause epithelial hyperplasia with bile duct obstruction, dilatation of bile ducts, acalculous cholecystitis and sclerosing cholangitis (Beaugerie *et al.* 1992). *S. intestinalis* affects not only the mucosa, but also the lamina propria to a greater extent than *E. bineusi* with infiltration of macrophages and fibroblasts. Histological changes have been found in kidneys in *S. intestinalis* infection such as granulomatous nephritis containing Langerhans' type multinucleated giant cells. Mode of transmission is likely to be through macrophages.

E. hellem is not found in the intestine. It affects the superficial epithelial layers of the cornea, conjunctiva, respiratory tract and urinary tract. Renal involvement may be extensive in AIDS patients with tubular necrosis, granulomatous lesions in ureters and ulcerative cystitis (Schwartz *et al.* 1992).

Myositis caused by the *Pleistophora* spp. has been reported in AIDS patients. There is atrophic degeneration of skeletal muscle without inflammatory cells contrasted with seronegative patients where the inflammatory reaction is very marked with lymphocytes, plasma cells and histiocytes.

INVESTIGATIONS

There are several diagnostic procedures available but the direct visualization of the organism is by far the most definitive.

1. Demonstration of the organism is done by light or electron microscopy. Initial detection can be achieved by light microscopy. Diagnostic specimens are stools, duodenal aspirates, sputum, urine, bronchoalveolar lavage, and smears or scrapings from conjunctiva. There are several staining methods available to highlight the organisms such as the trichrome or Giemsa stains (Weber *et al.* 1992). A coprodiagnostic staining technique developed improved the identification methods (Weber *et al.* 1994) and is routinely used in the USA for the examination of stools. This procedure involves removal of large faecal particles, fixation in gluteraldehyde followed by osmium tetroxide, embedded in an epoxy resin mixture, and finally stained with lead citrate and examined in the electron microscope. Others have found the Warthin Starry stain to be as good as electron microscopy for the detection of microsporidiosis (Field *et al.* 1993).

2. Chemofluorescent agents and examination under a fluorescence microscope is another method of identifying the spores. The chitinous wall of the microsporidia is brightened but staining is not very specific as other faecal elements may be highlighted.

3. Histologic examination is another diagnostic method where specific stains are necessary and diagnosis depends to a large extent on the expertise of the pathologist. The stains used are periodic acid-Schiff, methamine silver and acid-fast. The spore has a small PAS, positive posterior body, the spore coat will stain with silver and spores are acid-fast variables.

4. Electron microscopy helps in the identification of the species. Examination is done of tissue biopsies as well as stools and body fluids.

5. Serological tests are available for detecting antibodies to *E. cuniculi* in several species of animals. However, it is of little value in AIDS patients as detection of antibodies to any parasite is unreliable in immunocompromised patients.

Cell culture is unsuitable for routine diagnosis and it is difficult to culture some species of microsporidia.

TREATMENT

Symptomatic treatment such as fluid and electrolyte replacement and even parenteral nutrition for intestinal infection. There is no definitive chemotherapy available at present. However, albendazole and metronidazole has been tried in small uncontrolled series. *S. intestinalis* is supposed to be cured by albendazole (Weber *et al.* 1994). Dose of albendazole: 400 mg twice daily for 4 weeks or longer. It is not recommended in pregnancy. Topical ophthalmic application with intraconazole has been reported to be successful, but this has not been confirmed.

There are no definite good preventive measures because the modes of transmission are not fully known. Personal hygiene will prevent faecal-oral and urinary-oral route transmission. Transmission by aerosol method is extremely difficult to control.

REFERENCES

Beaugerie L, Teilhac MF, Debinol AM *et al.* Cholangiopathy associated with microsporidial infection of the common bile duct mucosa in a patient with HIV infection. *Annals of Internal Medicine* 1992; **117**: 401–402

Field AS, Hing MC, Milliken ST *et al.* Microsporidia in the small intestine of HIV infected patients a new diagnostic approach. *Medical Journal of Australia* 1993; **158**: 390–394

Schwartz DA, Bryan RT, Hewan-Lowe KO *et al.* Disseminated microsporidiosis (*Encephalitozoon hellem* and acquired immunodeficiency syndrome). *Archives of Pathology Laboratory Medicine* 1992; **116**: 660–668

Terada S, Reddy KR, Jerrers LJ *et al.* Microsporidian hepatitis in the acquired immunodeficiency syndrome. *Annals of Internal Medicine* 1987; **107**: 61–62

Weber R, Bryan RT, Owen RL *et al.* Improved light microscopic detection of microsporidia spores in stool and duodenal aspirates. *New England Journal of Medicine* 1992; **326**: 161–166

Weber R, Sauer B, Spycher AM *et al.* Detection of *Septa intestinalis* microsporidia in stool specimens and coprodiagnostic monitoring of successful treatment with albendazole. *Clinical Infectious Diseases* 1994; **19**: 342–345

12

Isosporiasis including Coccidian/Cyanobacterium-like Body Infection (CLB)

Isospora belli and coccidian/cyanobacterium-like body (CLB) are intestinal coccidian sporozoa. *I. belli* probably infects only humans. Recent outbreaks of diarrhoea have been attributed to CLB, which appears to be present worldwide.

ISOSPORA BELLI

PARASITOLOGY

This intestinal coccidian is endemic in South East Asia, Africa and South America. It is a cause of diarrhoea among travellers who are immunocompetent. The incidence of *I. belli* infection is even greater today because of immunocompromised patients, and is an important cause of diarrhoea in AIDS patients. In the USA ~0.2% of AIDS patients has this infection and the figure in developing countries is 3–20% (Pape and Johnson 1992). Isospora, like cryptosporidia, can also be found in animals. However, it has not been established that Isospora is acquired from animals.

Immature oocysts of Isospora are released from the intestinal wall and all stages of oocyst development occur in the stools. The oocysts are oval and long, 20–33 × 10–19 μm containing only one or two immature sporonts. In the stool, each oocyst contains two mature sporocysts, each containing four sporozoites. The sporulated oocyst is the infective stage which, when ingested, excyst in the small intestine, releasing the sporozoites which then penetrate the mucosa of the small intestine, particularly the distal duodenum and proximal jejunum, where they undergo the stages of trophozoites, schizonts, merozoites, gametocytes, gametes and oocysts. The schizogonic and sporogonic stages in the life cycle have been described from studies of human intestinal mucosal biopsies (Fig. 12.1).

PRESENTATION

The incubation period is 4–12 days. Patients present with profuse diarrhoea and there are muscular pains, fever, anorexia and weight loss. The diarrhoea may be very severe, up to 30–40 stools/day. Fatal cases of intractable diarrhoea have been reported (Liebmar *et al.* 1980). Malabsorption may occur if infection continues for a long time, especially in immunocompromised patients.

INVESTIGATIONS

Diagnosis is by identification of the organisms in direct or concentrated wet mounts of faeces. Iodine stains the oocyst and sporocyst. The oocyst may not be passed in faeces until symptoms of infection have cleared. Cysts of *Cyclospora cayetanensis* are larger (8–10 μm) and have a large, central morula with greenish refractile globules. There are no immunological tests for diagnosis and identification depends on morphology and accurate measurements using an ocular micrometer (González-Ruiz and Bendall 1995).

Duodenal aspirate or small bowel biopsy are other modes of identifying the oocyst. Biopsy may contain

the organisms despite negative stool examination due to small numbers of organisms (Liebmar *et al.* 1980).

TREATMENT

- Cotrimoxazole – trimethoprim 6 mg/kg sulphamethoxazole at 33 mg/kg/day, given for 21 days is the treatment of choice (Pape *et al.* 1989). A shorter course of 14 days would suffice for immunocompetent patients. In HIV patients, once infections are controlled, prophylactic treatment two or three times a week is recommended
- Pyrimethamine or metronidazole – an alternative treatment in cases of sulphonamide allergy. Metronidazole at 20–25 mg/kg/day for 5–10 days, and pyrimethamine 1.25 mg/kg for 28 days. Pyrimethamine can also be used in combination with sulphadiazine at dose of pyrimethamine 1.25 mg/kg with sulphadiazine 67 mg/kg for 28 days. Pyrimethamine is contraindicated in pregnancy and watch for blood dyscrasias. Metronidizole is contraindicated in pregnancy (Bozdech and Mason 1992)
- Supportive treatment including the patient's fluid resuscitation and correction of electrolyte imbalance.

COCCIDIAN/CYANOBACTERIUM-LIKE BODY INFECTION (CLB) (CYCLOSPORA)

PARASITOLOGY

Little is known about this organism named coccidian/cyanobacterium-like body infection (CLB). Originally CLB were considered a species of blue-green algae (Cyanobacteria); however, it is now considered to be a coccidian protozoan similar in structure to Isospora. Some of the evidence available indicates that it could be waterborne (Wurtz *et al.* 1991). CLB has been implicated as the cause in large outbreaks of diarrhoea in Chicago, USA, and Nepal. CLB-associated diarrhoea has been reported in travellers to the Caribbean, North and Central America, South America, South East and Eastern Europe. There is some evidence that CLB-associated diarrhoea may be seasonal increasing with rise in temperature and rainfall

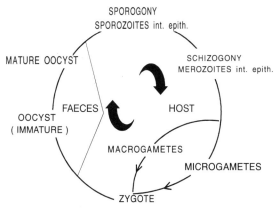

Figure 12.1 – Life cycle of *Isospora belli*.

(Shlim *et al.* 1991). It can affect both immunocompetent and immunocompromised hosts and has been associated with protracted diarrhoea in AIDS patients. The detection of CLB in faeces is very suggestive of a faecal/oral transmission.

Based on its ability to sporulate, the CLB have been assigned to Coccidian genus *Cyclospora*. Members of the genus *Cyclospora* have two sporocysts per oocyst and two sporozoites per sporocyst. During sporulation the oocyst produces two sporocysts, each containing two sporozoites. Oocysts are passed in the stools and are wrinkled spheres measuring 8–10 μm in diameter. The oocysts passed in fresh stools are not sporulated. The organisms fluoresce under UV illumination and are acid-fast. There are several questions that remain unanswered about the life cycle, epidemiology and clinical manifestation of *Cyclospora* (Wurtz 1994). Patients passing stools with oocysts produce antibodies against *Cyclospora*; however, immunity is not lasting as recurrent infections are common (Hoge *et al.* 1993).

Duodenal and jejunal aspirates have demonstrated *Cyclospora*. The organisms are also seen in biopsies of duodenum and jejunum where the changes of villous atrophy may be seen.

PRESENTATION

The incubation period is four to twelve days. There is severe intermittent watery diarrhoea and fatigue. Other less prominent symptoms include abdominal cramps, vomiting and weight loss. The illness is self-limiting. After 3–4 days there may be an improvement in the clinical condition, followed by a relapse. The duration of the symptoms in an outbreak in Nepal ranged from 4 to 107 days (Shlim *et al.* 1991). In immunocompromised, especially HIV, patients, diarrhoea may last several months (Wurtz *et al.* 1993).

INVESTIGATIONS

Diagnosis is made by the demonstration of CLB (oocysts) in faecal smears using either phase-contrast or bright-light microscopy and is confirmed by using UV microscopy and a modified Ziehl-Neelsen stain. The CLB are spherical cysts 8–10 μm in diameter. Accurate measurement of the size is important to distinguish from cryptosporidium oocysts, which are smaller, 4–6 μ (MMWR 1991).

TREATMENT

There is no specific chemotherapy available. There have been reported responses to trimethoprim-sulphamethoxazole. The mean duration of illness in 34 patients on antibiotics was 46 days, and in 14 untreated patients diarrhoea lasted on an average for 35 days (Shlim *et al.* 1991). The dose of trimethoprim-sulphamethoxazole is 5/25 mg/kg/day (Madico *et al.* 1993). Treatment is mainly symptomatic with rehydration and maintenance of electrolyte balance.

Travellers should avoid drinking unboiled water and consuming raw vegetables when travelling in endemic areas.

REFERENCES

Bozdech V, Mason P. *The Chemotherapy of Human Parasitic Disease.* Harare: Print Brokers, University of Zimbabwe, 1992, 31–32, 127–129, 150–151

González-Ruiz A, Bendall RP. The use of the ocular micrometer in diagnostic parasitology. *Parasitology Today* 1995; **11**: 83

Hoge CW, Shlim DR, Rajah R *et al.* Epidemiology of diarrhoea illness associated with Coccidian-like organism among travellers and foreign residents in Nepal. *Lancet* 1993; **341**: 1175–1179

Liebmar W, Thaller MA, Delonimer A *et al.* Intractable diarrhoea of infancy due to intestinal coccidiosis. *Gastroenterology* 1980; **78**: 579–584

Madico G, Gilman RH, Miranda E *et al.* Treatment of Cyclospora infections with cotrimoxazole [Letter]. *Lancet* 1993; **342**: 122–123

Outbreaks of diarrhoea illness associated with Cyanobacteria (blue-green) like bodies. Chicago and Nepal 1989 and 1990. *Morbid Mortal Weekly Report* 1991; **40**: 325–327

Pape JW, Johnson WD Jr. *Isospora belli* infections. *Prognostics of Clinical Parasitology* 1992; **2**: 119–127

Pape JW, Verdier RI, Johnson WD. Treatment and prophylaxis of *Isospora belli* infections in the acquired immunodeficiency syndrome. *New England Journal of Medicine* 1989; **320**: 1044–1047

Shlim DR, Cohen MT, Eaton M *et al.* An algae-like organism associated with an outbreak of prolonged diarrhoea among foreigners in Nepal. *American Journal of Tropical Medicine and Hygiene* 1991; **45**: 383–389

Wurtz R, Kocka FE, Kallick C *et al.* Blue green algae associated with a diarrhoea outbreak. In *Abstracts of the 91st General Meeting of American Society of Microbiology*, Dallas, Texas 1991, abst. C21, p. 345

Wurtz R. A newly identified intestinal pathogen of humans. *Clinical Infectious Diseases* 1994; **19**: 620–623

Wurtz RM, Kocka FE, Peters CS. Clinical characteristics of severe cases of diarrhoea associated with novel acid-fast organisms in the stool. *Clinical Infectious Diseases* 1993; **16**: 136–138

II

General Features of Nematodes

Nematodes are helminths which are multicellular organisms with three germ layers. The helminths are divided into two groups; the flat worms (Platyhelminthes) and round worms (Nemathelminthes), see Table II.1.

Those of medical importance are outlined in Table II.2.

Nematodes, commonly known as round worms are characterized by an elongated, cylindrical, unsegmented body and lack appendages (no suckers or rostellum). They have an alimentary canal that is complete (anus is present), Only nematodes contain a body cavity. There is no circulatory system. The body wall is covered by a cuticle with subcuticular cells and a muscular layer all of which help to identify some nematodes in tissue section. The nervous system consists of a nerve ring around the oesophagus and sensory papillae on the cuticle.

The digestive system is represented by a buccal cavity (mouth) may or may not contain teeth or cutting plates. Followed by muscular oesophagus, intestine (mid gut), terminating in rectum and anus.

The sexes are separate. The male reproductive system consists of single convoluted tubules differentiated into testis, vas deferens and seminal vesicle. The ejaculatory ducts open into a cloaca (a common passage for digestive and reproductive tubules). The accessory copulatory apparatus includes one or two spicules and a gubernaculum. Hookworms have a copulatory bursa which is umbrella-like.

The female reproductive system consists of a single, double or multiple group of tubules. The tubular ovary is followed by an oviduct, seminal receptacle, uterus, ovijector, vagina and vulva.

The nematodes that lay eggs are called oviparous (e.g. *A. lumbricoides*) and those that give birth directly to larvae are called viviparous (e.g. *T. spiralis*). Rarely larvae containing eggs hatch out immediately after deposition when they are known as ovoviviparous (e.g. *Strongyloides stercoralis*).

There are three modes of transmission. The first method is where eggs are ingested or inhaled as in *Enterobius vermicularis*; or larvae present in the intermediate host are ingested as in *Trichinella spiralis*.

The second method is by skin penetration where the filariform larvae penetrate the skin or mucosa directly (e.g. Hookworm).

The third method is by an insect bite where the larvae are transmitted into the host during a blood meal (e.g. Filarial nematodes).

The life cycle can be direct where ova are swallowed and mature in the intestine e.g. *Trichuris trichiura* or indirect through ingestion (e.g. Ascaris); skin penetration (Hookworm); or insect-bite (Filarial worms).

NOTE: Most nematodes (except filariae and *D. medinensis*) do not require an intermediate host.

Table II.1 – Classification of helminths

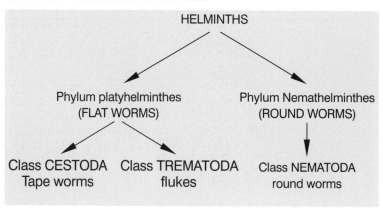

Table II.2 – Helminths of medical importance

Class	Common name	Principal human
Nematode	roundworm	*Enterobius*★
		Trichuris★
		Ascaris★
		Strongyloides★
		Necator
		Ancylostoma★
		Toxocara★
		Filariae
		(Dirofilaria)★
		Trichinella★
		Angiostrongylus★
Trematode	fluke	*Schistosomes*★
		Clonorchis
		Paragonimus
		Fasciola★
Cestode	tapeworm	*Taenia saginata*★
		Taenis solium
		Echinococcus★

★Infections encountered in Australia.

13

Strongyloidiasis

STRONGYLOIDES STERCORALIS

Parasitology

Strongyloidiasis is caused by *Strongyloides stercoralis*. Its distribution is worldwide with a higher prevalence in the tropics and Australia in the Aboriginal community. Its ability to cause auto-infection makes it the only helminth that causes opportunistic infection in debilitated and immunosuppressed persons. A higher prevalence is also seen in patients of mental institutions. A second species, *S. fuelleborni*, has been reported in adults in Africa and in infants in Papua New Guinea. *S. stercoralis* is a soil-transmitted nematode. The recent discovery of human T lymphocytic virus type (HTLV-1) infection in Northern Territory Aborigines in Australia is of particular interest in an endemic environment of *S. stercoralis* (Fisher *et al.* 1993). Fourteen communities with *Strongyloides* were reported in North Queensland over 5 years from 1985 of whom nine were aboriginal communities (Yiannkon *et al.* 1992). A survey of 122 communities, among Aboriginal and Torres Strait Islanders, revealed that 52 communities were infected (Porciv and Luke 1993). In Mornington Island the prevalence

rate fell from 26.2% to < 7% after treatment with the antihelminthic drug thiabendazole (Porciv and Luke 1993).

The incidence or prevalence increases in the wet season. Man is the most important host, while dogs and chimpanzees have been found to be infected. Expatriates can harbour the worm for many years because this is a parasite that causes auto-infection in man. Immunocompromised patients are at special risk and the disease is now prevalent in patients with HIV infection or on steroids and transplant patients.

The infective form of strongyloides is a filariform larva which penetrates skin or mucosa and gains access to the bloodstream (Fig. 13.1).

Under special circumstances, internal and external auto-infection occurs (rhabditiform larvae metamorphose into filariform larvae in the intestine or perianal skin). Occasionally, transmammary transmission occurs with infants being infected by larvae in breast milk. Instrument transmission has been reported from peptic ulcer patients infected with strongyloides via a contaminated gastroscope.

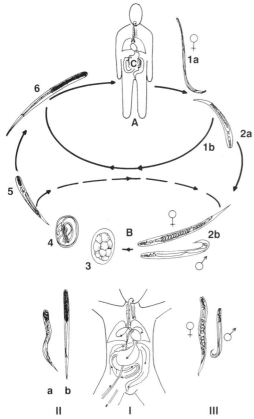

Figure 13.1 – Life cycle of strongyloides: (1a) parasitic female. (A) Direct development outside the host: (1b) rhabditiform larva from a fresh stool sample; (c) filariform larva (infective stage). (B) Indirect development outside the host: (2a) rhabditiform larva from a fresh stool sample; (b) unisexual generation: male-female; (3) egg of the unisexual generation; (4) egg containing a larva; (5) rhabditiform larva; (6) filariform larva. (C) Endo-auto-infection; (I) migration route of the *Strongyloides* larvae in man; (IIa) rhabditiform, (b) filariform larva (× about 100); (III) sexually mature forms of the free-living generation.

Presentation

On invading the skin, the filariform larvae produce petechial haemorrhages that are pruritic. The larvae invade pulmonary capillaries, break into the alveoli and invade the bronchial epithelium producing respiratory symptoms such as an irritating cough, shortness of breath and wheezing. The clinical picture is that of bronchopneumonia with pulmonary eosinophilia. In the intestinal phase, depending on the intensity of the infection, there can be watery mucous diarrhoea alternating with constipation, abdominal pain, nausea and vomiting. Abdominal symptoms may be associated with urticaria and eosinophilia. Patients may present with a sprue-like syndrome with malabsorption of iron and vitamin deficiency due to small intestinal mucosal dilatation of lymphatics from granulomatous lymphangitis.

Complications

Hepatic disease and jaundice is seen in immunocompromised patients due to disseminated strongyloidiasis. Disseminated strongyloidiasis is an acute and often fatal illness, with severe abdominal pain, diarrhoea, dehydration, fever and shock. This is the result of invasion of the small intestine by the larvae and intestinal organisms entering through the breached mucosa, produces septicaemia. Bacteraemic meningitis and endocarditis have been reported in *S. stercoralis*. This occurs when filariform larvae, in large numbers which carry bacteria from intestines as they penetrate the mucosa and enter the circulation. *Strongyloides* has been a cause of partial bowel obstruction in children (Walker *et al.* 1976). Strongyloidiasis colitis has been reported in non-immunocompromised patient resulting in aphthoid ulceration and intense tissue infiltrates (Al Samman *et al.* 1999).

Pathology

Pathologic changes seen are due to mechanical injury caused by adult worms, eggs and larvae. Lesions can occur anywhere between stomach and colon but are mostly found in the duodenum and proximal jejunum. Macroscopically, the wall of the small intestine is congested and oedematous. The mucosa may show petechiae and superficial ulceration. Microscopically, the lamina propria is infiltrated by neutrophils and eosinophils in the early stages and by mononuclear cells and eosinophils in the late stages. The cellular infiltrate may extend into the submucosa, muscularis and serosa inducing localized peritonitis. Patients with malabsorption show partial villous atrophy. In the chronic cases, degenerating larvae act as a nidus for causing granuloma formation and finally fibrosis. Definite diagnosis is made by identification of adult female worms, eggs, rhabditiform/filariform larvae in mucosa, submucosa and lumen in tissue sections (Fig. 13.2a and 13.2b). Mild-to-moderate eosinophilic infiltration with exudation and haemorrhage can be seen in the lungs. Worms and larvae can be seen in alveoli and sputum. In hyperinfection, filariform larvae can be seen in liver, heart, thyroid, parathyroid, adrenals, pancreas, lymph nodes, kidney, prostate, gall-

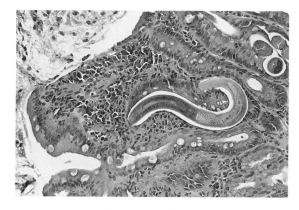

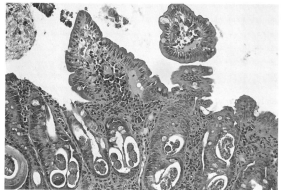

Figure 13.2 – Sections through small intestinal mucosa containing *S. stercoralis* larvae; (a) H&E × 100; (b) H&E × 100.

bladder, ovary and central nervous system. Cellular reaction and granulomata can be seen in these organs.

Investigations

1. Examination of stools for rhabditiform or filariform larvae should be carried out at least on three consecutive samples. The chance of missing the diagnosis is only 1.8% (Yiannakon *et al.* 1992). Stools should, if possible, be examined by concentrated larval techniques. In a study of clinically infected returned servicemen, a single stool examination detected 68% of cases, whereas repeated examination increased the yield to 84%. Duodenal aspirates yield a higher positive result (Yiannakon *et al.* 1992). In pulmonary infection, sputum may be examined for the larvae. Examination of urine may occasionally identify the larvae in the disseminated disease.

2. Serology can be particularly useful. An ELISA test developed in Perth, Western Australia, gives a sensitivity of 93% (Naguire *et al.* 1989).

3. White cell count – eosinophil counts of $> 0.45 \times 10^9$ are found in most patients. The haemoglobin level is usually normal (Yiannakon *et al.* 1992).

4. Blood cultures are recommended in febrile or immunosuppressed patients.

Treatment

- General supportive measures should be taken to resuscitate the patient with appropriate fluids and electrolytes. The drugs available are thiabendazole and albendazole

- Thiabendazole – recommended dose is 25 mg/kg twice a day for 2–3 days. Maximum dose is 3 g/day. Side-effects are common and include nausea, anorexia, vomiting, hypoglycaemia, bradycardia and disturbances of colour vision. Rarely, hypersensitivity reactions can occur such as fever, skin rashes, pruritus, conjunctival oedema and angio-oedema, erythema multiforme including Stevan-Johnson's syndrome. Cholestatic hepatitis has been ascribed to thiabendazole (Pungpak *et al.* 1987)

- Albendazole – overseas studies reveal a daily dose of 200 mg for children < 10 kg and 400 mg for those > 10 kg for 3 days as a successful replacement for mebendazole (Pungpak et al. 1987). Pregnancy is a contraindication. Adverse effects include gastrointestinal upset, headache, dizziness, pruritus, rash, rise of hepatic enzymes

- Ivermectin is less toxic and more effective. Dose of 200 μg/kg given in a single dose. Side-effects include gastrointestinal upset, dizziness and pruritis

- Appropriate IV antibiotics are indicated in cases of secondary infection. Once specific therapy has commenced, steroids are contraindicated at any stage as it will exacerbate auto-infection and may result in fatality. After treatment, patients must be followed up for successful eradication of the infection. The serology titres should diminish

Prevention

Improved sanitation, educational programmes should be targeted at susceptible groups. All clinicians should be aware of this condition and should rule out infection with Strongyloides before commencement of immunosuppressive drugs and transplantation, as these will cause a fatal infection.

STRONGYLOIDES FUELLEBORNI/FUELLEBORNI KELLYI

Parasitology

S. fuelleborni is a parasite of non-human primates in Africa, Asia and of humans in Africa (Ashford *et al.* 1992). A new subspecies named *S. fuelleborni kellyi* has been recently reported in Papua New Guinea in infants. Papua New Guinea is primate-free and how the infection reached the country is unsolved. Transmammary and transcutaneous transmission have been postulated for *S. fuelleborni*. *S. fuelleborni kellyi* is found where the annual rainfall is > 1500 mm (Ashford *et al.* 1992). The string bags ('bilums') with dried leaves or cloth that hold the infants and carried by mothers in Papua New Guinea are responsible for infection as these bags are often not cleaned for months.

The New Guinea Strongyloides is distinguishable from *S. fuelleborni* by the position of phasmidial pore and cuticle at the perivulval region. This species of Strongyloides pass eggs in the stools that hatch in 1 h and invade the skin. The egg counts are very high, up to 300 000 eggs/ml faeces (Ashford *et al.* 1992). They are 50 × 35 μm, embryonated and may resemble hookworm ova. Transmammary transmission to the infants has not been established in infants in New Guinea.

Presentation

Infected infants in New Guinea present with abdominal distension, diarrhoea, occasional vomiting and peripheral oedema due to hypoproteinaemia, features referred to as the distended belly syndrome. They may present with respiratory distress due to the distended belly. If the condition is undiagnosed and untreated mortality rate is high. The infants are anaemic and have reduced serum proteins. Diagnosis is established by finding large number of eggs in the faeces and moderate eosinophilia.

Treatment

- Thiabendazole 25 mg/kg twice daily for 3 days
- Plasma transfusion if indicated 40 ml/kg with frusemide 0.1 ml/kg IM
- Antibiotics if there is secondary bacterial infection

REFERENCES

Al Samman M, Haghe S, Long JD. Strongyloidiasis colitis: a case report and review of literature. *Journal of Clinical Gastroenterology* 1999; **28**: 77–80

Ashford RW, Barnish G, Viney ME. *Strongyloides fuelleborni kellyi*: infection and disease in Papua New Guinea. *Parasitology Today* 1992; **8**: 314–318

Fisher D, McCarry F, Currie B. *Strongyloides* in the Northern Territory. Underrecognized and undertreated? *Medical Journal of Australia* 1993; **159**: 88–90

Naguire C, Jimeriez G, Guessa JG *et al.* Ivermectin for human strongyloides and other helminths. *American Journal of Tropical Medicine and Hygiene* 1989; **40**: 304–309

Porciv P, Luke R. Observations on strongyloides in Queensland Aboriginal communities. *Medical Journal of Australia* 1993; **158**: 160–163

Pungpak S, Bunnag D, Chindanond D *et al.* Albendazole in the treatment of strongyloides. *South Asian Journal of Tropical Medical Public Health* 1987; 207–210

Walker AC, Blake G, Downing D. A syndrome of partial intestinal obstruction due to *Strongyloides stercoralis. Medical Journal of Australia* 1976; **1**: 47–48

Yiannakon J, Croese J, Ashdown LR *et al.* Strongyloides in North Queensland. Re-emergence of a forgotten risk group. *Medical Journal of Australia* 1992; **156**: 24–27

14

Enterobiasis (Oxyuriasis)

Parasitology
Presentation
Pathology
Investigations

Treatment
Prevention
References

PARASITOLOGY

This nematode worm infestation is caused by *Enterobius vermicularis* (syn. *Oxyuris vermicularis*) commonly known as pinworm or threadworm.

The mode of transmission is by ingestion of eggs from soiled clothes and inhalation or swallowing of airborne dust containing the eggs from contaminated bedclothes. The female worms migrate from the anus at night to deposit eggs in the peri-anal region (Fig. 14.1).

The adult female worm measures 6–12 × 0.3–0.5 mm; the male worm is 2–5 × 0.1–0.2 mm. The adult worm is characterized by the presence of a pair of cephalic, wing-like alae and a prominent muscular oesophageal bulb. The bilateral thorn-like cuticular crests seen in cross-sections are a reliable marker for its identification (Figure 14.2). Both female and male contain a single reproductive tube. In the gravid female, the egg-filled uterus occupies most of the body cavity.

The eggs measure 50 × 30 × 30 μm and are asymmetric, one side flattened with a transparent shell. A fully developed larva is seen inside when detected in stools. Eggs are infective at body temperature ~6 h after deposition. Man is the only natural definitive host.

PRESENTATION

Most infected persons are asymptomatic. In heavy infections there may be a mild peripheral eosinophilia. The main clinical symptom is pruritus ani. Worms and eggs are found in the anal canal. This can lead to eczema and secondary pyogenic infection in the peri-anal region. Infected persons have restless sleep due to the pruritus. Fig. 14.3 illustrates numerous pinworms in the peri-anal region in a child with pruritus ani.

Complications are vaginal enterobiasis (Chung *et al.* 1997), intense enterobiasis with peri-anal abscess or granuloma (Aviolo *et al.* 1998) and appendicular enterobiasis (Ajao *et al.* 1997).

PATHOLOGY

In non-endemic areas, pinworms are an incidental finding in the appendix; hardly causing a tissue reaction (Figure 14.4). In endemic regions high worm loads of 50 000–100 000 eggs are seen.

Lesions are found in the caecum and appendix with superficial ulceration, petechial haemorrhages including secondary bacterial infection with mucosal and submucosal abscesses.

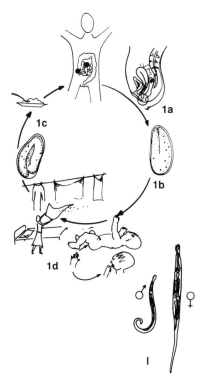

Figure 14.1 – Life cycle of *Enterobius vermicularis* – man as the only host of *E. vermicularis* (pinworm); (1a) eggs of the pinworm are laid outside the anus; (b) freshly laid egg of the pinworm; (c) an infective egg ~6 h old; (d) when scratching of the perineum allows hand to mouth transmission; in adults chiefly through eggs in dust arising from the bed or ingestion of air-borne eggs.

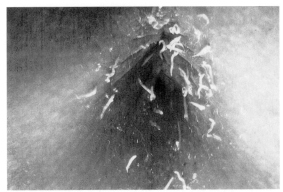

Figure 14.3 – Numerous pinworms in the peri-anal region in a child with pruritus ani.

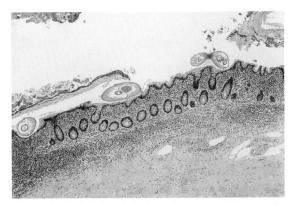

Figure 14.4 – Incidental finding of worms in the appendix (H&E × 40).

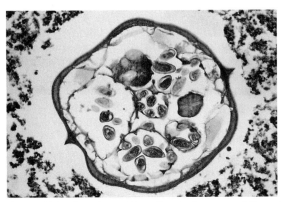

Figure 14.2 – Prominent, bilateral, cuticular crests of *E. vermicularis* in cross-section (H&E × 200).

Superficial mucosal invasion causes granulomatous inflammation characterized by abundant eosinophils or the 'oxyuris nodule'. These are also seen in the pelvic peritoneum, inguinal ligament, greater omentum and mesocolon. The centre of the nodule is necrotic with the adult worm or ova, surrounded by a rim of granulation tissue enclosed by a fibrous capsule infiltrated by eosinophils, lymphocytes and giant cells. The Splendore-Hoeppli phenomenon may be seen. These nodules later fibrose and hyalinize.

INVESTIGATIONS

1. Ova are found in the faeces in < 10% of cases.
2. Definitive diagnosis is made by recovery of the eggs from the peri-anal region by adhesive cellophane swabs or direct swabs.

TREATMENT

- Albendazole as a single dose of 7 mg/kg is considered to be very effective in up to 100% of cases (Amato-Neto *et al.* 1985)
- Pyrantel embonate is an alternative drug if albendazole is not available. It is a broad-spectrum antihelminthic. It produces a depolarizing block

on neuromuscular transmission and causes paralysis of the worm, which is then expelled from the gastrointestinal tract. Side-effects are very minimal. Nausea, vomiting, rash, fever and abdominal pain have been known to occur. The standard dose is 11 mg/kg base; maximum 1 g given with or without food, repeated in 2–4 weeks

- Mebendazole for adults and children > 2 years: one 100 mg dose; repeat in 2 weeks.

Albendazole, pyrantel and mebendazole are not recommended in pregnancy.

PREVENTION

1. This parasitic disease is well known for auto-infection. Therefore, attention to personal hygiene during treatment such as washing the peri-anal region regularly, trimming of finger nails and changing into fresh night clothes is strongly recommended.

Washing of clothing and bedding is also recommended, as is regular vacuuming of bedrooms. If one member of the family is infected, the whole family needs to be treated.

2. In pregnancy due to teratogenic effects, antihelminthic drugs should be avoided. Improved hygiene is recommended.

REFERENCES

Ajao OG, Jastaniah S, Malatani TS et al. Enterobius vermicularis (pinworm) causing symptoms of appendicitis. Tropical Doctor 1997; **27**: 182–183

Amato-Neto V, Castillo VLP, Moreira AA et al. Efficacy of albendazole treatment in enterobius. Revista de Instituto de Medicina Tropical De Sao Paulo 1985; **27**: 143–144

Aviolo L, Avoltini V, Ceffa. Peri-anal granuloma caused by Enterobius vermicularis, report of a new observation and review of the literature. Journal of Paediatrics 1998; **132**: 1055–1056

Chung DI, Kong HH, Yu HS et al. Live female Enterobius vermicularis in the posterior fornix of the vagina of a Korean woman. Korean Journal of Parasitology 1997; **35**: 67–69

15

Ascaris lumbricoides (Round Worm)

Parasitology
Presentation
Pathology

Investigations
Treatment
References

PARASITOLOGY

Ascariasis is caused by *Ascaris lumbricoides*. It is the most prevalent helminthic infection in the world with ~25% of the world population infected.

Infection is transmitted from person to person by the faecal-oral route by eggs passed in the faeces and found in the soil or on contaminated hands (Fig. 15.1). Transplacental transmission has rarely been reported.

A. lumbricoides is a large human nematode, the female worm measuring 220–350 mm in length and 3–6 mm in diameter; the adult male worm measures 150–310 mm in length and 2–4 mm in diameter. Sexes can be identified grossly by the presence of a coiled tail and two copulatory spicules in the male, and a constricting area known as vulva waist or genital girdle at the junction of anterior and middle third in females. The human species can be distinguished from animal species by the presence of lips. The female worm has ovaries, oviducts, seminal receptacles and uteri in the posterior two-thirds of the body. The male has a single tube composed of testis, vas deferens and ejaculatory ducts situated in the posterior half of the body. In a cross-section of the adult worm, the typical polymyarian musculature is seen with many muscles projecting into the body cavity. There are lateral, ventral and dorsal cords that divide the body cavity into quarters. Tall columnar cells and reproductive organs line the intestines. The fertile eggs which consist of an outer albuminous coat and a thick inner shell, are ovoid in shape and measure 60–40 μm (Sun 1979) (Fig. 15.2). They are golden brown in colour due to bile staining. The infertile eggs, however, are longer and measure 90–40 μm and are irregular in shape. The decorticated ovum (when it loses the outer albuminous coat) resembles hookworm eggs and needs to be separated from them. The eggs are highly resistant to acid, alkaline, dehydration, toxic salts and even formalin. They can resist temperatures up to 39–40°C and are destroyed by desiccation, temperatures > 65°C, freezing at < –20°C, direct sunlight and organic solvents. The eggs are infective in soil in 3–4 weeks. For the life cycle, see Fig. 15.1.

PRESENTATION

During the phase of larval migration from the small intestine to the liver and lungs, there may be mild fever, asthma and eosinophilia. Urticarial rash may appear. In severe infections there could be a significant

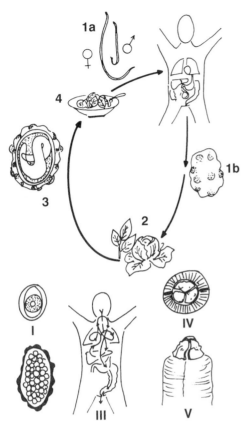

Figure 15.1 – Life cycle of *Ascaris lumbricoides*; (1a) sexually mature worms: male and female; (b) typical egg from the faeces; (2) manuring with the faeces of worm carriers brings the worm eggs to fresh vegetables; (3) egg containing an infective larva; (4) the eating of the leaves of salad plants, to which the eggs containing larvae adhere, leads to infection. (I) Fertilized egg without its outer wall: optical section; (II) unfertilized worm egg; (III) migration route of the worm larvae after eggs containing larvae have been taken in through the mouth; (IV) anterior end ('mouth opening') seen from above; (V) anterior end of the female, ventrolateral view.

pneumonitis resulting in bronchial irritation and haemoptysis.

When the adult worms establish in the small intestine, the symptoms depend on the worm load. Most infected persons remain asymptomatic (Fig. 15.3), others have non-specific abdominal symptoms such as abdominal discomfort and flatulence. Ascarides may be found to pass out of the anus resembling earth worms. Fig. 15.4 illustrates a large worm load passed by a woman. A large worm load in children could lead to intestinal obstruction and sometimes intestinal perforation. Rarely a roundworm can obstruct the duodenal papilla resulting in obstructive jaundice and pancreatitis. Invasion of the appendix can lead to acute appendicitis. *A. lumbricoides* has migrated from intestine to lodge itself in pleural cavity (Sen *et al.* 1998) and Reiters syndrome has been reported (Carballada *et al.* 1998).

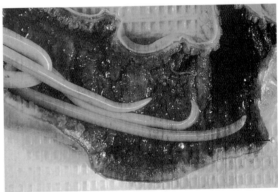

Figure 15.3 – Ascaris in the small intestine an incidental finding in an Australian Aboriginal woman (Courtesy Professor R Cook, Brisbane).

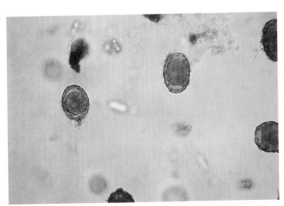

Figure 15.2 – Eggs of Ascaris, oval in shape with outer albuminous coat and thick inner shell.

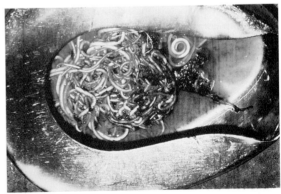

Figure 15.4 – Large worm load passed by a woman from Harare (Courtesy Professor Clement Kiire, Zimbabwe).

PATHOLOGY

In the liver Ascaris larvae produce a granulomatous reaction with epithelioid cells, multinucleated giant cells and also the Splendore-Hoeppli's phenomenon where, at the edge of the granulomas, amorphous eosinophilic material (presumed to be immune complexes) is seen together with eosinophils, neutrophils and histiocytes. The larvae that migrate to the lungs may be seen in the alveolar walls, alveoli, bronchioles and bronchi. Eosinophils, macrophages and a fibrinous exudate surround them. Granuloma formation may also be seen at a later stage. Features of broncho-pneumonia have also been seen. In the intestines, heavy worm load produces intestinal obstruction, intussusception and volvulus with local circulatory disturbances, and resultant infarcts or gangrene of intestines. Granulomas may also develop around worms or ova in the peritoneal cavity. These can be frequently misdiagnosed as tuberculous peritonitis (Crompton *et al.* 1989). Fistulae have also been reported in extra-intestinal lesions.

INVESTIGATIONS

1. The most common method of diagnosing intestinal ascariasis is by examination of a direct stool smear. As the female worm lays 200 000–250 000 eggs/day, the equivalent of 2925 eggs/1 g faeces, eggs are easily detected in the faeces. Stools should be examined at least on three occasions.

2. Radiological examinations – adult worms may sometimes be detected by barium meal, when the ascarides outline is clearly seen.

3. Real-time sonography presents an efficient, reliable and non-invasive diagnostic approach for hepatobiliary enteric and pancreatic ascariasis (Carballada 1998, Ferreyra *et al.* 1998).

4. Identification of worm – if cross-sections of the adult worms are seen, they can easily be identified by their typical musculature. Their bilateral alae, intestine and the two excretory columns identify the larvae.

TREATMENT

The benzimidazoles are very effective drugs for ascariasis.

- Albendazole (7 mg/kg) – a single dose for adults and children > 2 years gives up to 100% cure (Pamba *et al.* 1989). The safety of albendazole has not been established in children < 2 years. It should not be used in pregnancy. Adverse effects such as nausea, dizziness, lassitude, epigastric discomfort and headaches are mild

- Levamisole (2.5 mg/kg) may be used as an alternative. 2.5 mg/kg in a single dose has a reported cure rate of ~90% (Asaolu *et al.* 1991). It is not used in pregnancy. Adverse drug reactions are flu-like syndrome, dermatitis, myalgia, peripheral neuropathy and agranulocytosis

- Pyrantel embonate – one single dose 10 mg/kg. It is available in liquid and tablet form. It may be repeated if eggs are still found after a fortnight. Adverse effects such as nausea, vomiting, rash, fever and abdominal pain are minimal. To be used with caution in patients with liver disease and during pregnancy.

- Mebendazole – for adults and children > 2 years, 100 mg twice a day for 3 days. This should not be used in pregnancy

REFERENCES

Asaolu SO, Holland CV, Compton DWT. Community control of *Ascaris lumbricoides* in rural Ogo State, Nigeria. Mass targeted and selective treatment with levamisole. *Parasitology* 1991; **103**: 291–298

Carballada RC, Amenciros LE, Gonzalez MJ *et al. Review Clinical Espania* 1998; **198**: 714

Crompton DWT, Neisheim MC, Pawlowski ZS (eds). *Ascariasis and its Public Health Significance*. London: Taylor & Francis, 1989, 289

Ferreyra NP, Cerri GG. Ascariasis of the alimentary tract, liver, pancreas and biliary system: its diagnosis by ultrasonography. *Hepatogastroenterology* 1998; **45**: 932–937

Pamba HO, Buibo NO, Chunge CN *et al.* A study of the efficacy and safety of albendazole in the treatment of intestinal helminthiasis in Kenyan children less than 2 years of age. *East African Medical Journal* 1989; **66**: 197–202

Sen MK, Chakrabarti S, Ojha UC *et al.* Ectopic ascariasis: an unusual case of pyopneumothorax. *Indian Journal of Chest Disease Allied Science* 1998; **40**: 131–133

Sun T. Intestinal parasitic infections: Part 2. Diagnostic criteria. *Laboratory Medicine* 1979; **10**: 277–287

16

Hookworm Infestation

Ancylostoma duodenale and Necator americanus
 Parasitology
 Presentation
 Pathology
 Investigations
 Treatment

Trichostrongyliasis
 Parasitology
 Investigations
 Treatment
 Prevention
 References

ANCYLOSTOMA DUODENALE AND NECATOR AMERICANUS

Parasitology

Hookworm infestations are caused by *Ancylostoma duodenale* and *Necator americanus*. Several other species of *Ancylostoma* such as *A. braziliense* and *A. ceylonicum* do not cause hookworm disease but creeping eruption in humans.

About 20% of the world population is infected with ancylostomiasis (Carrole *et al.* 1990). The filariform larvae remain viable for weeks in the appropriate environment such as damp and loose soil. *A. duodenale* is prevalent in temperate climates such as in Southern Europe, North Africa, Japan and China. *N. americanus* is prevalent in the tropics, most parts of Africa, North America, Panama and South America. Man acquires the infection when the filariform larva in the soil penetrates the bare foot. Agricultural labourers and gardeners may acquire the infection through the skin of the hand. The infective larva may also be swallowed in infected water. Man is the only important definitive host. *A. duodenale* is the only species found in Australia

(Porciv and Luke 1995) and in the Northern Territory. The dog hookworm *A. caninum* has been implicated in eosinophilic enteritis in non-aboriginals (Currie 1994).

The adult female of *A. duodenale* measures 10–30 × 0.6 mm while *N. americanus* measures 9–11 × 0.35 mm. The male is smaller in both species and measures 8–11 × 0.45 mm in Ancylostoma and 5–9 × 0.3 mm in Necator. The buccal capsule in *A. duodenale* has four ventral teeth and two dorsal rudimentary teeth, whereas the Necator has two ventral and two dorsal cutting plates. The male has a copulatory bursa and the position of the vulva and the presence or absence of a caudal spine in the female are used for differentiation of the different species of hookworms. The ova and larva are indistinguishable among the species. *N. americanus* produces 6000–11 000 eggs/day and *A. duodenale* has a daily production of 15 000–20 000 eggs. The eggs measure 60 × 40 μm with a thin and transparent eggshell. A clear space separates the shell from the yolk cells that vary from two to eight when the eggs are deposited in stools. The eggs have rounded ends that distinguish them from those of *Trichostrongylus* spp., which have one or both ends tapered.

The eggs hatch in 24 h after reaching warm or moist soil. The first stage larvae are the rhabditidiform larvae which moult in 3 days and become the second stage larvae. The second moult, which takes place in ~6–7 days, results in the third stage infective filariform larvae. The filariform larvae penetrate the skin of man and enter the lymphatics or capillaries. They may also penetrate the oral mucosa if contaminated vegetables or fruits are ingested. Some larvae may become entrapped in the regional lymph nodes while the remaining migrate to the lungs where they rupture the pulmonary capillaries and escape into the alveolar spaces and travel up the bronchial tree. They can be coughed up and swallowed into the small intestine where they moult once more to become adult worms that remain mainly in this site but may be found anywhere from the stomach to the colon. Prenatal or transmammary infection has also been reported in infants of few weeks old and occasionally larvae have been found in breast milk. The time from skin penetration to egg deposition is ~1–3 months, depending on the species and the extent of infection (Fig. 16.1).

Presentation

At the site of entry, the filariform larva produces an itchy papular or vesicular eruption. During the passage through the lungs the symptoms are a dry cough and sore throat. This may be associated with infiltrates in the lung with peripheral eosinophilia. The principal clinical features are in the small intestine and depend on the adult worm load. The worms cause injury to the mucosa and absorb blood, resulting in secondary hypochromic microcytic anaemia. Ancylostomes can remove > 0.5 ml blood per worm/day. In the acute stages there may be abdominal pain and bloody diarrhoea but these tend to disappear in the anaemic stage. Heavy infection in children leads to mental retardation and they develop a characteristic pot belly appearance.

Pathology

The intestinal lesions vary from inconspicuous to marked alterations like those seen in tropical sprue. There may be petaechial haemorrhages, superficial erosions, congestion and oedema of the mucosa. The mucosal and submucosa contain eosinophils, lymphocytes and plasma cells. The parasite can sometimes be seen with its mouth cavity grasping the intestinal

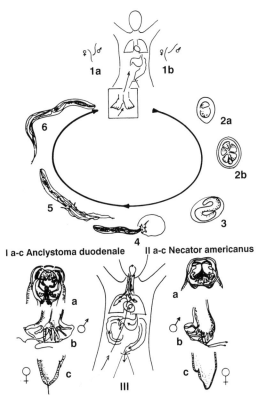

Figure 16.1 – Life cycle of hookworm; (1a) *Ancylostoma duodenale* (characteristic copulations); (b) *Necator americanus* (position and natural size). Development outside the host; (2a) freshly laid egg, two-celled stage; (b) egg in the six-celled stage; (3) egg containing a larva; (4) rhabditiform larva after emerging from the egg; (5) first ecdysis; (6) filariform larva after the second ecdysis; the larva remains inside the old larval skin ('sheathed larva'). Species differences; (I) *Ancylostoma duodenale*. (II) *Necator americanus*; (a) buccal capsule with mouth apparatus; (b) bursa copulatrix of the male; (c) posterior end of the female. (III) Migration route of the hookworm larvae.

mucosa. This should be distinguished from other nematodes that invade the intestinal mucosa such as *Capillaria philippinensis* and *Strongyloides stercoralis*, which are much smaller and readily distinguishable. In a cross-section of the worm the typical meromyarian type of musculature with three to four muscle cells in each quarter is seen; the quarters divided by two lateral, one ventral and one dorsal cord help to identify hookworm.

Peripheral eosinophilia is seen in the early stages of infection. In the later stages, due to blood loss, iron deficiency anaemia is the major finding. A definite diagnosis is established only by identifying the typical eggs in stool specimens often together with Charcot-Leyden crystals. If the stool specimens are stored at room temperature for > 1 day, rhabditidiform larvae may be hatched and can be definitely identified and distinguished from strongyloides larvae. The rhabditidiform larva of hookworm has a longer buccal cavity than strongyloides.

Investigations

1. Stool examination – definitive diagnosis is made by repeated examination of stools, either by direct smear or by concentration methods for ova, and have to be differentiated from other ova. The number of ova in the stool gives a rough indication of the worm load. Each female worm passes ~50 eggs/g faeces.
2. Blood examination – a full blood count with examination of red cell morphology gives an indication of the severity of anaemia.
3. Endoscopy – if diagnosis is suspected with negative stools examination, an upper gastrointestinal endoscopy with biopsies of duodenum is recommended (Kato *et al*. 1997).
4. Polymerase chain reaction has been used recently to confirm the identity of eggs from faeces and larvae from environment and identifying species (Monti *et al*. 1998).

Treatment

- The drug of choice in ancylostomiasis is a benzimidazole called albendazole. This drug blocks glucose uptake by the parasite and depletes glycogen stores, causing paralysis followed by death. A single dose of 7 mg/kg albendazole gives a cure rate of 89–100% (Pugh *et al*. 1986). As it is teratogenic in animals, albendazole is not recommended in pregnancy. Albendazole cleared hookworm infections when pyrantel failed (Reynoldson *et al*. 1997)
- Levamisole – as a single dose of 2.5 mg/kg gives a high cure rate and prolonged administration of 5 mg/kg/day for 5 days improves efficiency (Sinniah and Sinniah 1981). It is contraindicated in chronic hepatic or renal disease. Side-effects such as headaches, nausea and vomiting are infrequent. Hypotension has been reported but occurs infrequently
- Pyrantel (embonate) – dose 10 mg/kg as a single dose. Preparations are available in tablet and liquid

form. The adverse reactions are gastrointestinal upsets, headache, drowsiness and skin rash. Contraindications are acute hepatic disease. It is not indicated in pregnancy. Pyrantel had no significant effect against hookworm in 29 individuals treated in the Kimberley region of North West Australia (Reynoldson *et al*. 1997)
- Mebendazole (Vermox) – recommended for adults and children > 2 years age. Dose one tablet (100 mg) in the morning and one in the evening for 3 days; for children 3 mg/kg not exceeding adult dose, twice daily for 3 days. Available in tablet form and as suspension. Adverse reactions are gastrointestinal upsets. It is not indicated in pregnancy, children < 2 years age and lactation
- Anaemia should be treated with oral iron preparations
- Control of hookworm disease is only possible with proper sanitation and by mass treatment. Individual prophylaxis is carried out by the wearing of shoes.

TRICHOSTRONGYLIASIS

Parasitology

The ova of the hookworm resemble the ova of human trichostrongyliasis. Human trichostrongyliasis is caused by *Trichostrongylus* spp., which are zoonotic nematodes. Five cases were reported in 1992 in Queensland, Australia (Boreham 1995). It has been described in humans who have had contact with herbivores such as sheep, goats and cattle. The species that infect man are *T. orientalis* and *T. colubriformis* in addition to a few others (Ghadirian and Arfaa 1975). Man is an incidental host and is infected by ingestion of raw plants contaminated with infective larvae. The larvae develop from eggs passed in the faeces of herbivores. Once swallowed by humans, the larvae attach to the intestinal mucosa and mature sexually in 25 days. The life span of the adult worm is long, up to 18 years. The life cycle differs from hookworm larvae in that the portal of entry is not the skin and there is no migration through the lungs for completion of life cycle (Wolfe 1978). Clinical symptoms are non-specific and generally absent. However, heavy infections can cause abdominal pain, diarrhoea, fatigue, anorexia and anaemia with eosinophilia. The latter may be the only feature (Miyazaki 1991).

Investigations

1. Diagnosis is by examination of stools. The eggs have pointed ends and are smaller than the eggs of the hookworm.
2. Faecal culture may help identify the species.

Treatment

- Pyrantel embonate 600 mg given as a single dose. It is not indicated in pregnancy. Repeat stool examination after a few weeks

PREVENTION

Prophylaxis is the avoidance of used animal manure as a fertilizer, proper washing and cooking of vegetables before consumption especially in endemic areas.

REFERENCES

Boreham RE, McCowan MJ, Ryan AE *et al*. Human tricho-strongyliasis in Queensland. *Pathology* 1995; **27**: 182–185

Carrole SM, Walker JC. Hookworm infection in South East Asia, Oceania and Australia. In Schad GA, Warren KS (eds), *Hookworm Disease: Current Status and New Directions*. London: Taylor & Francis, 1990, 33–47

Currie B. *Northern Territory Communicable Diseases Bulletin* 1994; **4**: 1–17

Ghadirian E, Arfaa F. Present status of trichostrongyliasis in Iran. *American Journal of Tropical Medicine and Hygiene* 1975; **24**: 935–941

Kato T, Kaomi R, Iida M *et al*. Endoscopic diagnosis of hookworm disease of the duodenum. *Journal of Clinical Gastroenterology* 1997; **24**: 100–102

Miller TA. Hookworm infection in man. *Advances in Parasitology* 1979; **17**: 315–384

Miyazaki I. *An Illustrated Book of Helminths Zoonoses*. Fukuoka: International Medical Foundation of Japan with Shukosha, 1991

Monti JR, Chilton NB, Qian BZ *et al*. Specific amplification of *Necator americanus* or *Ancylostoma duodenale* DNA by PCR using markers in ITS-1. DNA and its implications. *Molecular Cell Probes* 1998; **12**: 71–78

Porciv P, Luke RA. The changing epidemiology of human hookworm in Australia. *Medical Journal of Australia* 1995; **162**: 150–152

Pugh RNH, Teesdale CH, Burnham GM. Albendazole in children with hookworm infection. *Annals of Tropical Medicine and Parasitology* 1986; **80**: 565–567

Reynoldson JA, Bechnke JM, Pallant IJ et al. Failure of pyrantel in treatment of human hookworm infections (*Ancylostoma duodenale*) in the Kimberley region of Northwest Australia. *Acta Tropica* 1997; **68**: 301–312

Sinniah B, Sinniah D. The antihelminthic effects of pyrantel pamoate, oxanthel pamoate, levamisole and mebendazole in the treatment of intestinal nematodes. *Annals of Tropical Medicine and Parasitology* 1981; **75**: 315–321

Wolfe MS. Oxyuris, trichostrongylus and trichuris. *Clinics in Gastroenterology* 1978; **7**: 201–217

17

Trichuriasis (Whipworm Infection)

Parasitology	**Treatment**
Presentation	**Prevention**
Pathology	**References**
Investigations	

PARASITOLOGY

Trichuriasis caused by *Trichuris trichiura* is of world-wide distribution most prevalent in tropical and subtropical regions where there is heavy rain. In Australia these worm infestations are found mainly in the north east among the aboriginal population (Grove 1993). Man gets infected by the faecal/oral route where the Trichuris ova in faecal contaminated food or water are ingested (Fig. 17.1). Hence, the mode of transmission depends to a large extent upon the socio-economic state of the area. The eggs may be dormant in the soil but may remain infective for several months.

The greyish-white adult worm is characterized by two distinct body parts, a slender thread-like anterior portion (whip) and a thick posterior portion (handle). The worm measures 30–45 mm in length with the male containing a cellular oesophagus in the attenuated anterior portion and a tail curved through 360° containing a single spicule in the sheath, which is studded with spines. The female has the posterior half occupied by a short uterus filled with eggs. The barrel-shaped egg measures 50×22 μm, is brown and has a single shell with a plug at either end and an embryo within.

The worms inhabit the caecum and large intestine and lie in the mucus in the intestinal crypts. The eggs are unembryonated. It takes 3 weeks for embryonation to take place. The eggs hatch in the intestine, the larvae penetrate the intestinal villi and develop for 1 week until they re-emerge and pass to the caecum and large intestine where they develop into adults.

PRESENTATION

The majority of infected persons are asymptomatic in light infections. In medium infections there may be abdominal pain and diarrhoea, which may mimic bloody dysentery. Anaemia may be severe. Severe infections may present with matted masses of worms in the rectum. Worms may obstruct the appendix. Whipworms may perforate the intestine rarely causing peritonitis. In heavy infections, rectal prolapse, appendicitis, volvulus and sessile polyps of colon could occur (Pampiglione *et al.* 1997).

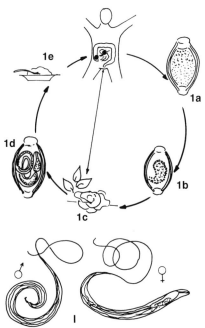

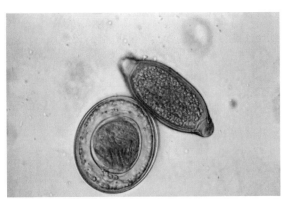

Figure 17.2 – Egg of trichuris barrel-shaped, single shell with bipolar knobs. Egg of hookworm for comparison.

Figure 17.1 – Life cycle of *T. trichiura*; man as the only host of *T. trichiura* (Whipworm). (1) Site of the worm in the lower small intestine, caecum and large intestine; (1a) whipworm egg soon after it has been laid; (b) commencing development of the embryo; (c) salad plants contaminated with eggs by the use of the faeces of worm carriers as manure; (d) infective egg containing a larva; (e) man can ingest the infective eggs, which are very resistant, by, for example, eating fresh salads. (I) Sexually mature whipworms, and male and female.

PATHOLOGY

A few worms do not cause damage. A heavy load causes damage to intestinal mucosa with mucopurulent stools, haemorrhage and symptoms of dysentery with rectal prolapse. Trichuris can be associated with *Ascaris lumbricoides*, hookworms and even *E. histolytica*, which can in addition cause ulceration.

INVESTIGATIONS

1. Specific diagnosis depends on the identification of the characteristic eggs in the faeces by direct smear or by concentration methods (Fig. 17.2). More than 30 000 eggs/g stool are considered a heavy infection.
2. Proctoscopy will show the worms attached to the reddened and sometimes ulcerated mucosa.
3. Colonoscopy can directly diagnose trichuriasis, confirming that the thread-like form of worms with an attenuated end provided colon preparation is satisfactory (Joo *et al.* 1998).

TREATMENT

- Benzimidazoles are used in the treatment, with the aim of reducing the worm load and thereby reducing the bloody diarrhoea. Mebendazole given to children > 2 years of age at 2 mg/kg twice daily for 3 days and adults at 100 mg twice a day for 3 days gives a 100% cure rate (Holzer and Frey 1987, Grove 1993). The drug kills the worms. Treatment can be repeated after 2 or 3 weeks. Low dose mebendazole is free of major side-effects. It is especially contraindicated in the first trimester of pregnancy. In children, a single dose therapy of 500 mg mebendazole had an 85% reduction in egg count and 400 mg albendazole had a reduction of 75% in egg count (Jackson *et al.* 1998)
- Ivermectin (200 µg/kg) repeated after 12 h gives 85% cure rates (Naquira *et al.* 1989). Ivermectin paralyses the nematodes by intensifying Gamma-aminobutyric acid (GABA) transmission of signals in peripheral nerves of the nematode. GABA causes mostly inhibitory responses in the central nervous system. The drug is well tolerated and side-effects are rare
- Pyrantel pamoate (Embonate) – dose 15 mg/kg twice daily – a 3-day regimen (Cabrera and Cruz 1980). Effectiveness is controversial (Kale 1981)

PREVENTION

Soil-transmitted nematode infections such as trichuriasis, ascariasis, hookworm disease and strongyloidiasis can all be controlled by improved sanitation and the prevention of faecal soil contamination.

REFERENCES

Cabrera BD, Cruz AC. Clinical trial of oxantel-pyrantel (quantrel) against trichuriasis. *Acta Medica Philippina* 1980; **16**: 95–102

Grove DI. Worms in Australia. *Medical Journal of Australia* 1993; **159**: 464–466

Holzer BR, Frey FJ. Differential efficacy of mebendazole and albendazole against *Necator americanus* but not for *Trichuris trichiura* infestations. *European Journal of Clinical Pharmacology* 1987; **32**: 635–637

Jackson TF, Epstein SR, Gouws E *et al.* A comparison of mebendazole and albendazole in treating children with *Trichuris trichiura* infection in Durban, South Africa. *South African Medical Journal* 1998; **88**: 880–883

Joo JH, Ryu KH, Lee YH *et al.* Colonoscopic diagnosis of whipworm infection. *Hepatogastroenterology* 1998; **45**: 2105–2109

Kale OO. Controlled comparative study of the efficacy of pyrantel pamoate and a combined regimen of piperazine citrate, bephenium hydroxynaphthoate in the treatment of intestinal nemathelminthiasis. *African Journal of Medicine and Medical Sciences* 1981; **10**: 63–67

Pampiglione S, Rivasi F, Rubbiani C. Cryptic infection by whipworm mimicking a sessile polyp of the colon. *Italian Journal of Gastroenterology and Hepatology* 1997; **29**: 365–366

Toxocariasis (Visceral Larva Migrans)

Toxocara worms cause Toxocariasis. It is a common disease in animals. *Toxocara canis* and to a lesser extent the cat ascarid *T. cati* are the aetiological agents of visceral larva migrans. Human toxocariasis is universal and has been reported in many parts of the world including Australia.

PARASITOLOGY

The adult worm lives in the small intestines. Man becomes infected by swallowing infective eggs from dog faeces and food contaminated with eggs or transferred by flies. The infection is transmitted from puppies to children through intimate contact. In the USA, 100% of puppies < 6 months of age are infected. Of children up to the age of 11 years, 7.3% are seropositive; it is 30% in socially disabled people (Hope 1993). Infected dogs and puppies shed ~200 000 eggs/day, which survive for many years (Kerr-Muir 1994). Puppies can get infected by transplacental transmission and can pass infective larvae in their stools. Hence, it is a difficult disease to eradicate from the public health point of view. Other non-definitive hosts are cattle and sheep and transmission to man by uncooked meat is therefore possible. Humans serve as a paratenic host for toxocara, which means that the parasite arrests its development in the new host at larval stage. The larvae can remain in humans for 4–5 years (Figure 18.1).

Adults of Toxocara spp. are large, ~6–18 cm in length and 2–3 mm in breadth. *T. canis* larva is 357–445 × 18–21 μm; *T. cati* larva is 357–445 × 15–17 μm. The larvae of the two species are similar, differing only in their diameter. The larva has an oesophagus in the anterior region, an intestine in the middle region with two excretory canals. The intestines are also in the posterior region. In cross-sections of the larvae bilateral alae can be identified. The life cycle of the parasite is similar to the human *Ascaris lumbricoides*. The dog ascarid can directly invade organs from the lungs. They may bypass the liver and lung and also migrate directly from the intestine. The larvae remain in the host till they are pregnant and become active, pass in through the placenta to infect puppies. In puppies < 5 weeks, the larvae complete a migratory cycle and mature into adults. In older puppies or adult dogs the larvae cannot complete the cycle.

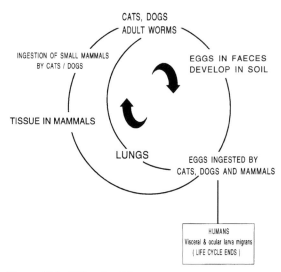

Figure 18.1 – Life cycle of Toxocara.

PRESENTATION

Toxocara can infect any organ. The infection is often subclinical. The clinical manifestations may be considered under subclinical or overt toxocariasis, visceral larva migrans and ocular larva migrans.

Subclinical or overt infection – the serum is positive for antibodies. Clinical presentation is bizarre with transient fevers in childhood, sleep disturbance, cough and wheeze. There is also a significant eosinophilia.

Visceral larva migrans

The patients present with fever, malaise, cough, failure to thrive in babies, lymphadenopathy and hepatomegaly. They may present with severe pulmonary symptoms such as asthma (Nesme *et al.* 1998) and pneumonitis, or rarely with allergic symptoms such as urticaria and rhinitis. Liver involvement may mimic hepatitis. Neurological manifestations such as seizures (tonic or clonic), encephalopathy, meningo-encephalitis and transverse myelitis may occur. Larvae invade the brain but they do not encapsulate. Infection with *Toxocara* species has been considered a cause of epilepsy in the absence of other identifiable causes. Meningoencephalitis is associated with eosinophilic pleocytosis in toxocariasis (Bouchard *et al.* 1998). Myocarditis is found in severe infections. Oesophageal muscular hypertrophy with eosinophil infiltration is a rare complication (D'Alteroche *et al.* 1998).

Ocular toxocariasis

Hemispherical, solitary lesions in the retina were often misdiagnosed for retinoblastoma in the past. Of 47 eyes enucleated for retinoblastoma, 23 had larvae or hyaline remnants and eosinophilic granulomatous lesions, which were positively identified as *T. canis* (Wilder 1952). There is a broad spectrum of ocular lesions found in *Toxocara* infection (Sakai *et al.* 1998). The symptoms are red eye, impaired vision, leukor-rhoea and strabismus. There may be peri-orbital infection, intra-ocular granulomas, chorioretinitis, papillitis uveitis or endophthalmitis and unilateral blindness if the macula is affected. A single worm can cause unilateral blindness. Chronic ocular involvement may lead to retinal fibrosis and detachment.

The clinical features depend on the larval load and host immune response, the latter directed to the larval outer coat. The two clinical syndromes visceral larva migrans and ocular larva migrans do not seem to overlap. A possible explanation is that the larval load in ocular larva migrans is very minute.

PATHOLOGY

The liver is enlarged with scattered greyish-white or tan nodules. Sometimes they are umbilicated, ranging from 1 to 10 mm in diameter and can be seen on the liver surface, resembling metastatic tumour or miliary tuberculosis. On microscopic examination, the lesions are granulomatous sometimes with central eosinophilic necrosis. On serial sectioning larvae can sometimes be detected especially with the PAS stain, which stains the parasite a brilliant blue colour. The cellular infiltrate in the granulomas not only is predominantly composed of eosinophils, but also includes epithelioid cells, multinucleated giant cells, lymphocytes and plasma cells. With time, the cellular infiltrate is gradually replaced by fibrosis and in the late stages the entire lesion can be fibrosed and calcified. Eosinophils, lymphocytes and plasma cells infiltrate portal tracts. The hepatocytes are generally not involved. In the lungs, early lesions show diffuse eosinophilic infiltration, oedema and widening of the alveolar septa. In the late stages, granuloma formation is seen. The central nervous system may show gliosis with perivascular cuffing by eosinophils, lymphocytes and macrophages and occasionally granulomas. Similar pathology can be seen in the heart, eyes and other organs. Histological examination of myotomy biopsy showed an eosinophilic infiltration of the oesophageal muscle layer (D'Alteroche *et al.* 1998).

INVESTIGATIONS

1. Histology – a definitive diagnosis can only be made by detecting larvae in tissue sections.
2. Serology – investigations show that the ELISA test is superior to other tests such as indirect haemagglutination, bentonite flocculation and the Ouchterlony double diffusion technique. Elevated antibody titres can be detected in the aqueous humour in the ocular forms of the infection. The serum antibody in toxocara is directed against antigens (outer coat) and excretory-secretory products released from *T. canis* larvae. ELISA can assess this. Sensitivity is 78%; specificity 92%. Sensitivity and specificity are low for ocular larva migrans. The immunodiagnostic tests are positive in 45% of cases with ocular lesions. However, a higher positivity can be found by using vitreous or aqueous humour.
3. IgG, IgM and IgE hypergammaglobulinaemia is observed in visceral toxocara.
4. Anti-striational antibodies (sStrAbs) were positive in 44 of 66 patients with anti-toxacara antibodies (Macura-Biegun *et al.* 1998).
5. In the systemic forms, eosinophilia is a consistent finding. Leukocyte counts can be as high as 30 000/ml with 80% eosinophils. Eosinophilia is mild or absent in the ocular forms.
6. Liver biopsy for granulomas is helpful in establishing the diagnosis. Biopsies of other organs are seldom contributory.

TREATMENT

Visceral larva migrans

- The successful use of mebendazole in an adult has been reported. Dose of mebendazole: 50 mg/kg/day for 21 days
- Albendazole 10 mg/kg in divided dose, daily for 5 days has given slightly better cure rates than thiabendazole (Bekhti 1984, Sturcher *et al.* 1989). Stevens-Johnson syndrome has been reported after albendazole (Dewerdt *et al.* 1997)

- Dose of thiabendazole is 50 mg/kg in divided doses for 7 days. This drug is contraindicated in pregnancy
- Myotomy for eosinophilic oesophagitis with oesophageal motor disorder (D'Alteroche *et al.* 1998)
- Anticonvulsants, bronchodilators, steroids when indicated

Ocular toxocariasis

- Management depends on the extent of damage. Vitriectomy and membrane peeling for macular detachment may improve the vision. Ocular larvae close to the macula require photocoagulation
- Thiabendazole has been shown to enter to a large extent the aqueous and vitreous humour in minimally inflamed eye (Maguire *et al.* 1990)

PREVENTION

Antihelminths can be used to kill worms in dogs. Strict laws should be in place to prevent pollution by dogs in public places, especially where children play. Proper personal hygiene is a preventive measure.

REFERENCES

Bekhti A. Mebendazole in toxocariasis. *Annals of Internal Medicine* 1984; **100**: 463

Bouchard O, Bosseray A, Leclercq P *et al.* Meningoencephalitis caused by *Toxocara canis*. *Annals of Internal Medicine* 1998; **149**: 391–392

D'Alteroche L, Bourlier P, Picon L *et al.* Myotomy for oesophageal muscular hypertrophy with eosinophil infiltration of the oesophagus associated with toxocariasis revealed by oesophageal motor disorder. *Gastroenterology Clinical Biology* 1998; **22**: 541–545

Dewerdt S, Machet L, Jan-Lamy V *et al.* Stevens-Johnson syndrome after albendazole. *Acta Dermatology and Venereology* 1997; **77**: 411

Hope PJ. Visceral and ocular larva migrans. *Seminars in Neurology* 1993; **13**: 175–179

Kerr-Muir MG. *Toxocara canis* and human health. *British Medical Journal* 1994; **309**: 5–6

Macura-Biegun A, Pituch-Noworolska A, Rewicka M *et al.* Antistriational antibodies during *Toxocara canis* and *Trichinella spiralis* infections. *Comprehensive Immunology, Microbiology and Infectious Diseases* 1998; **21**: 101–106

Maguire AM, Zarbin MA, Conor TB *et al.* Ocular penetration of thiabendazole. *Archives of Ophthalmology* 1990; **108**: 1675

Nesme P, Deniaud F, Perol M *et al.* Larva migrans syndrome: a rare differential asthma diagnosis. *Review of Pneumonary Clinics* 1998; **54**: 225–227

Sakai R, Kawashima H, Shibui H *et al. Toxocara cati*-induced ocular toxocariasis. *Archives of Ophthalmology* 1998; **116**: 1686–1687

Sturcher D, Schubarth P, Gualzata M *et al.* Thiabendazole vs albendazole in treatment of toxocariasis: a clinical trial. *Annals of Tropical Medicine and Parasitology* 1989; **83**: 473–478

Wilder HC. Nematode endophthalmitis. *Transactions of the American Academy of Ophthalmology and Otolaryngology* 1952; **55**: 99–109

19

Trichinosis

Parasitology	**Treatment**
Presentation	**Prevention**
Pathology	**References**
Investigations	

PARASITOLOGY

This is an infection caused by the nematode *Trichinella spiralis*. It is of cosmopolitan distribution and most prevalent where undercooked pork or meat containing encysted larvae is consumed.

The highest incidence of trichinosis is reported from China. It is also common in Spain, Italy and France. The US Center for Disease Control, Atlanta, GA, reported 52 cases during 1987–90 with two large outbreaks in 1990 (McAuley *et al.* 1991). Trichinosis has been reported in Eastern Europe, Germany, Poland, Yugoslavia and Thailand. To date, the only documented cases of human trichinosis from infected herbivores were from horsemeat in Italy and France (Murell 1994). The common source of infection of man is through the domestic cycle, mainly the pig. Three distinct sylvatic cycles exist. One in the temperate zone involving pigs and rats, with strains of low infectivity such as *Trichinella spiralis nativa*, unlike the highly infectious *T. spiralis*. They are resistant to freezing. The strain in the sylvatic cycle of African tropics, called *T. spiralis nelsoni*, is of low infectivity to pigs but high infectivity for carnivores and humans. From the public health point of view, feeding pigs with uncooked meat scraps is the main cause of transmission of trichinosis.

The adult worms are small, thread-like, with a slightly thickened posterior end. The female is 3–4 mm long and 60 μm wide; the male is 1.4–1.6 mm long and 40 μm wide. A series of large glandular cells (stichocytes) surround the oesophagus in the anterior portion. The female has a single reproductive tube composed of a vulva, vagina, uterus, seminal receptacle, oviduct and ovary. The male reproductive tube consists of a testis, vas deferens, seminal vesicle and ejaculatory duct, the latter joining the intestine to form the cloaca.

As soon as the worms mature, mating takes place and larvae are produced 3 days after fertilization. Larvae mature within 5 days and larval deposition takes place as long as the adult female remains in the intestine. The larvae enter the lymphatics in the mucosa and gain access to the general circulation. The larvae measure 80–160 × 5–7 μm. When they encyst in muscles they measure 800–1300 × 30–40 μm. The larvae in cross-section show the oesophagus, stichocytes, intestine and the immature reproductive tube. From the capillaries they penetrate the muscle fibres and reach their full size in ~4 weeks. The larvae become coiled and lie in a spiral surrounded by a sheath derived from the muscle. When fully developed, they measure 1 mm in length. They can remain encysted and viable for many years, even after the capsule has calcified.

More than 100 different animals are infected by this nematode. The cysts are digested by host gastric juices allowing the larvae to encyst, penetrate the mucosa and moult four times before developing into adults in 30–40 h (Fig. 19.1).

PRESENTATION

The clinical features may be considered under the intestinal phase of parasite and phase of muscle invasion which may overlap.

During the intestinal phase there may be no symptoms, or patients may present within 24 h of infection with abdominal cramps, general malaise, diarrhoea and nausea, simulating food poisoning. This phase lasts ~1 week. However, in infection with the Arctic strain *T. spiralis nativa*, the gastrointestinal symptoms may be more severe and prolonged. This has followed eating walrus meat by Eskimos. Diagnosis is seldom made at this stage; however, gastroenteritis in a group of individuals, 2–7 days after ingestion of uncooked

pork products should be suspected of being due to trichinosis.

In the phase of muscle invasion, the symptoms depend on the intensity of the infection. Fever and eosinophilia are prominent. Muscle pain and characteristic circumorbital oedema may be present. Muscle damage causes difficulty in chewing, breathing, swallowing and movement (Garcia and Bruckner 1993). The severity of muscle pain extends up to ~3 weeks, and they are tender. Splinter and subconjunctival haemorrhages are features in a large percentage of patients. Trichinosis can affect the central nervous system in ~10–20% of patients. If untreated, the mortality rate may reach 50%. The neurological features can mimic acute psychosis, space occupying lesions, meningoencephalitis, cerebrovascular accident, polyneuritis or acute anterior poliomyelitis. With moderate infections, symptoms begin to abate during the fifth or sixth week after ingestion and in fulminant infection, death may occur in 4–6 weeks. The most common cause of death is myocarditis.

Complications are neurotrichinosis with symptoms of meningitis, encephalitis, polyradiculoneuritis, poliomyelitis, myasthenia gravis and paralysis.

PATHOLOGY

The most frequently infected tissues are the skeletal muscles of limbs and diaphragm. Tongue, masseters, intercostal, extensor ocular, laryngeal and paravertebral muscles have all been involved. Larvae migrate and invade muscle 8 days after ingestion (Fig. 19.2). The muscle fibres degenerate with surrounding inflammation and atrophy of adjacent muscle fibres. Within 2 months a hyaline layer surrounds the cyst containing the parasite, which is ovoid, refractile, has sharp ends and varies in size. The size of the cyst varies with the number of larvae contained, from commonly one to seven. Occasionally, a histiocytic and giant cell reaction may surround the cyst. In the late stages, these cysts undergo calcification. If only the cyst wall calcifies, the larvae remain viable and infective. Larvae in cardiac muscle cause myocarditis characterized by focal eosinophilic, neutrophilic and lymphocytic infiltration. Although encystment of larvae is not seen, myocardial changes regress without scarring. Peripheral eosinophilia is common. Polycythaemia and hypochromic anaemia has also

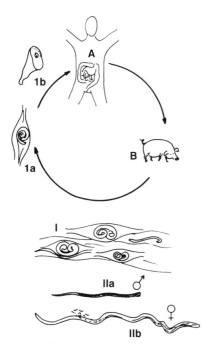

Figure 19.1 – Life cycle. (A) Man: infection with trichinae results from eating uncooked meat containing muscle trichinae (trichina larvae; 1a, b); (B) domesticated and wild pigs, the chief sources of human infection. (I) 'Muscle trichinae' – microscopical preparation: muscle fibres containing Trichina larvae, some of them encapsulated; (II) 'Intestinal trichinae'; (a) male; (b) female expelling larvae (× ~30:1).

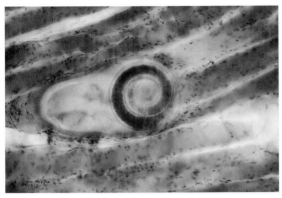

Figure 19.2 – Cyst in muscle (Masson's trichrome stain × 100).

been described. There is marked hyperplasia of bone marrow with eosinophilia. Larvae cysts or granulomas cause obstruction of blood vessels with toxic vasculitis, secondary thrombosis and haemorrhages. Immune complex deposits may be found in kidney causing mesangial proliferation. These are reversible with treatment of trichinosis.

INVESTIGATIONS

1. Full blood count – eosinophilia is consistently seen during invasion of muscle and varies from 10 to 90%. It increases very rapidly and returns to normal after ~1 month.
2. Examination of the suspected meat by laboratory digestion procedure may reveal larvae. A biopsy from the gastrocnemius, biceps or deltoid muscle of ~1 g, squashed between two slides and examined under a low-power microscope, may reveal larvae. A rough estimation of the larval load will predict the severity of disease. A level of 50–100 larvae/g is considered moderate infection and 1–10 larvae/g is usually asymptomatic. The muscle may also be examined after digestion performed between two glass slides.
3. Radiographs will not demonstrate calcified cysts in the acute stage. They may be seen by xeno-radiography.
4. Serology is very useful. Bentonite flocculation test is the standard test and recommended as the test of choice for trichinosis (Nikobi 1998). A dot enzyme-linked immunosorbent assay (ELISA), using purified antigens, has been developed for detecting *T. spiralis* in swine (Su and Prestwood 1991).

5. Muscle breakdown enzymes such as lactate dehydrogenase, aldolase and creatinine phosphokinase are often elevated.
6. Computerized tomography (CT) for neurotrichinosis (Nikolic *et al.* 1998).
7. Magnetic resonance imaging for neurotrichinosis (Nikolic *et al.* 1998).
8. Antibodies against *T. spiralis* in cerebrospinal fluid in neurotrichinosis (Nikolic *et al.* 1998).
9. Dissociated enhanced lanthamide fluoro-immunoassay (DELFIA) is highly sensitive in detecting circulating antigens (Ko 1997).
10. Presence of antistriational antibodies for *Toxocara canis*, *T. spiralis* infections (Macura-Biegun 1998). All sera with active trichinellosis showed positive anti-striatal antibodies, which suggest the occurrence of anti-muscle anti-immune response.

TREATMENT

- Most patients with trichinosis have minimal symptoms. They require analgesics and rest. There is no specific therapy for trichinosis
- Thiabendazole (tiabendazole) at 25 mg/kg twice daily for 5–7 days (maximum 3 g/day) has given beneficial effects. However, it has toxic effects such as dermatitis, drug fever and abdominal discomfort
- Mebendazole is active against the adult and larval stage, used in dose of 400 mg, three times a day for 2 weeks. It is contraindicated in children and in pregnancy
- Prednisolone is indicated in allergic manifestations at an initial dose of 20–60 mg/day and taper within a few days to a minimal dose. The disadvantage of steroids is it tends to increase the duration of larval stage and antihelmintics should be used
- Patients with severe allergic reactions, cardiac involvement should be monitored in hospital

PREVENTION

Refrigerate uncooked pork at –15°C for > 20 days or deep-freeze at –37°C. Microwave cooking might not kill the larvae. All parts of pork muscle tissue must be heated to 60°C. Avoid feeding pigs with uncooked meats.

REFERENCES

Garcia LS, Bruckner DA. *Diagnostic Medical Parasitology*, 2nd edn. Washington, DC: American Society of Microbiology, 1993, 217

Kagan IG, Normal L. Serodiagnosis of parasitic diseases. In Rose NR, Friedman H (eds), *Manual of Clinical Immunology*. Washington, DC: American Society for Microbiology, 1976, **70**: 10

Ko RC. A brief update on diagnosis of trichinellosis. *South East Asian Journal of Tropical Medical Public Health* 1997; **1**: 91–98

Macura-Biegun A, Pituch-Noworolska A, Rewicka M. Anti-striational antibodies during *Toxocara canis* and *Trichinella spiralis* infections. *Comprehensive Immunological Microbiological Infectious Diseases* 1998; **21**: 101–106

McAuley JB, Michelson MK, Schantz PM. *Morbidity and Mortality Weekly Report*. Center for Disease Control, 1991

Murell KD. Beef as a source of trichinellosis. *Parasitology Today* 1994; **10**: 434

Nikolic S, Vujosevic M, Sasis M *et al.* Neurological manifestations in trichinosis. *Serbian Archives Celok Lek* 1998; **126**: 209–213

Su X, Prestwood AK. Western blot test for the detection of swine trichinellosis. *Journal of Parasitology* 1991; **77**: 76–82

20

Angiostrongyliasis

Two known species cause angiostrongyliasis, *Angiostrongylus cantonensis*, the rat lung worm that causes cerebral angiostrongyliasis, which can also cause eye and lung lesions in humans, and abdominal angiostrongyliasis caused by *A. costaricensis*, which has been present in Costa Rica since 1952.

ANGIOSTRONGYLUS CANTONENSIS (CEREBRAL ANGIOSTRONGYLIASIS)

Parasitology

Angiostrongyloides, a parasitic nematode belonging to the family mestrongylidae, a rat lungworm, has been found to be endemic in Australia, at least in Queensland (Heaton and Gutteridge 1980). It is also found in the tropical Pacific region (Porciv and Brindles 1984), Thailand, Taiwan, Philippines and Sumatra. The parasite is confined to the brain. Human cases have been reported in which the parasites were found in the lung as well.

The female adult worm measures 21–25 mm in length and 0.30–0.36 mm in diameter; the male worm measures 16–19 mm in length and 0.26 mm in diameter. Both have an intestine, but the female has two reproductive tubes, with the male having only one. The adult worms live in the pulmonary arteries and the right heart of rodents. Eggs are laid in blood vessels and the larvae hatch and break through the pulmonary capillaries to enter the alveoli. The first stage larva then migrates to the bronchus and trachea and is coughed up and swallowed where they enter the gastrointestinal tract and finally exit in the faeces.

Further development takes place if the intermediate host swallows it, which are either slugs or land or water snails. The larvae, which invade these hosts, moult twice to become the infective third stage larvae. To continue the life cycle, these molluscan hosts have to be eaten by rats where the third stage larvae are found. These penetrate the rat intestinal wall and enter the systemic circulation where they can be carried to the brain. In the brain, the larvae moult twice and become young adult worms. From there they enter the subarachnoid space and the cerebral veins, finally entering the pulmonary circulation where they become mature adults (Fig. 20.1).

Presentation

Human infection occurs when molluscs containing larvae of *A. cantonensis* or parentic hosts such as fresh water prawns, land crabs or frogs are ingested. The parasite is believed to be the commonest cause of the clinical syndrome, which includes eosinophilic meningitis, although only rarely the parasite is identified in human tissue. Patients may present with fever, headache, stiff neck, nausea, vomiting, arthralgia and non-specific abdominal symptoms. They can present with bizarre mental symptoms, sometimes with psychotic features, incoherence, disorientation, impairment of memory and coma. Some patients develop cranial nerve palsies, local hyperaesthesia, which can be a very distressing and persistent symptom, have signs of raised intracranial pressure with papilloedema. However, most patients show almost complete recovery. The meningeal symptoms are secondary to the immunological response to the dead parasite whose life cycle terminates in the human. There is no inflammatory response to the live parasite. Ocular symptoms may be secondary to eosinophilic meningitis or secondary to the presence of the parasite in the anterior or posterior chamber of the eye with painless loss of vision or iridocyclitis or keratitis. Examination may rarely reveal the worms in the eyes in cases of ocular involvement. Few patients may become comatose. Infestation is rarely fatal. There is no immunity to this disease and second and third attacks have been described.

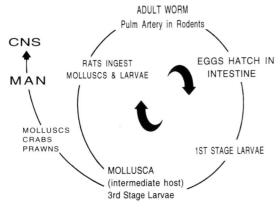

ADULT WORM
Pulm Artery in Rodents

CNS

MAN

RATS INGEST
MOLLUSCS & LARVAE

EGGS HATCH IN
INTESTINE

MOLLUSCS
CRABS
PRAWNS

1ST STAGE LARVAE

MOLLUSCA
(intermediate host)
3rd Stage Larvae

Figure 20.1 – Life cycle of *A. cantonensis*.

Pathology

In most cases no lesions are identifiable on macroscopic examination of the brain but occasionally opacity or thickening of the leptomeninges and mild subdural and subarachnoid haemorrhages are seen. The parasite can be seen on microscopic examination in sections of the brain or spinal cord.

There is eosinophilic infiltration together with lymphocytes, monocytes and plasma cells with occasional foreign body giant cells in the subarachnoid space. Sometimes small canals or microcavities in the cerebral tissue, representing the tract taken by the parasite may be seen lined by necrotic debris and gitter cells with surrounding tissue showing a cellular infiltrate, degenerating neurons and areas of demyelination. With time these lesions end up as glial scars with eosinophils, Charcot Laden crystals and haemosiderin pigment. A granulomatous response is also seen around the dead parasite. The living worm only provokes a mild cellular response. Sometimes the degenerating worm can be identified in cross-sections as they possess the transversely striated cuticle and the polymyarian type of musculature with prominent lateral cords, the immature reproductive tube (no sperms or eggs) and a relatively thick walled intestine. Vascular tissue changes vary from congestion to perivascular cuffing by eosinophils to damaged blood vessels with thrombosis and surrounding cerebral haemorrhage.

Investigations

1. If the cerebrospinal fluid (CSF) examination shows > 10% eosinophils, a diagnosis of cerebral angiostrongyliasis can be suspected. The eosinophilic count of the CSF varies from 10 to 90%. The glucose level is usually normal.
2. For a definitive diagnosis of cerebral angiostrongyliasis, identification of the parasite in the CSF or tissue is necessary, although this is a rare event. Examination of fresh teased specimens obtained from tissue or CSF under a dissecting microscope provides a higher positive rate than examination of histologic sections alone. This technique also preserves the parasite for further identification.
3. Serologic test – serology (EIA) may be used on serum and CSF to assist in diagnosis. Enzyme immunoassay detecting antibodies to *A. cantonensis* is being trialled.

4. ELISA (enzyme-linked immunosorbent assay) is used in the detection of circulating antigens in cerebrospinal fluid levels of which are markedly higher than in the serum (Chye *et al.* 1997).

5. A specific monoclonal antibody (Aw-3CZ) as revealed by ELISA was produced against the adult worm antigens, e.g. *Parastrongylus cantonensis*. The specificity of the assay was 100% and sensitivity 50% (Eamsobhana *et al.* 1997).

Treatment

- In the past, thiabendazole was used to shorten the duration of symptoms. However, the beneficial effect is probably due to its anti-inflammatory effects rather than antihelminthic effects
- Ivermectin 200 µg/kg has been used on animals and is effective, but clinical trials on humans have not been conducted (Ishii *et al.* 1985)
- There has been no definite evidence to support the use of corticosteroids (Beaver *et al.* 1984)
- Spinal fluid drainage 10 ml (repeated if necessary) has been done by some to relieve symptoms and may confirm the diagnosis (Beaver *et al.* 1984). However, this may not prevent long-term, permanent disability

Illustrative case

A 33-year-old Australian male army sergeant who had spent 6 weeks in Vanuatu presented with a 5-day history of fever, malaise, generalized headache, lower back pain and arthralgia. He developed nausea, vomiting, photophobia, bilateral pain over his tibiae and pain in both lumbar regions. He had taken oral doxycycline (100 mg/day) for malaria prophylaxis. The patient had consumed local foods while in Vanuatu including crustaceans and salads. A medical practitioner in Port Vila prescribed chloroquine and maloprim with no effect. He was evacuated to Australia.

On examination, the patient did not look unwell. He had a mild fever (37.5°C). There was no clinical evidence of meningism. Marked hyperaesthesia over the left tibia and both flanks was noted. The remainder of the examination was normal.

Full blood count revealed a white cell count of 10×10^9/litre with an eosinophilia (0.9×10^9/litre). Cerebral CT revealed old postoperative changes in skull only. Two unsuccessful attempts were made at lumbar puncture.

A clinical diagnosis of *A. cantonensis* meningitis was made on the history of residence in an endemic area and compatible clinical features with cutaneous pain and hyperaesthesia and peripheral blood eosinophilia. Symptoms resolved gradually without specific therapy (slight paraesthesia was present at discharge on day 8).

Diagnosis was confirmed by seroconversion to *A. cantonensis* demonstrated using an enzyme immunoassay (ICPMR, Westmead, NSW, Australia). Acute phase serum on day 10 of symptoms was negative; convalescent serum on day 27 was borderline and on day 47 was positive.

ANGIOSTRONGYLUS COSTARICENSIS (ABDOMINAL ANGIOSTRONGYLIASIS)

Parasitology

A. costaricensis causes abdominal angiostrongyliasis and is similar to *A. cantonensis* but the habitat of the adult worm is different in that they live in the mesenteric arteries of rodents and lay eggs in the intestinal wall. The first stage larvae migrate into the intestine and are excreted in the faeces. Humans acquire infection by accidentally ingesting food or drink contaminated by snails or slug mucus rather than by eating the intermediate host directly. The wall of the intestine of the host is penetrated by the infective larvae and mature in lymph nodes or lymphatic vessels. The young adults migrate to the mesenteric arteries but as humans are unsuitable or incidental hosts, eggs do not hatch out.

Presentation

Clinical features are abdominal pain mainly in the right iliac fossa. It may simulate acute appendicitis. There may be low-grade fever, vomiting, diarrhoea or constipation. On examination, there may be a mass in the right iliac region with guarding and tenderness. Eosinophilia with abdominal symptoms gives a clue to the differential diagnosis. Perforation of the bowel may occur with generalized peritonitis. No eggs or larvae are seen in the stools. Look for eggs or larvae in tissue sections under microscope.

Pathology

Eosinophilic micro-abscesses and granulomata with giant cells, eosinophils and mononuclear cells are found in the subserosa of small intestines, which may be oedematous and rigid (Loria-Cortes and Lobo-Sanakuja 1980). The lumen of the intestines can become partially or totally obstructed by this inflammatory mass. Lesions are mostly found in the appendix but the caecum, colon, ileum, lymph nodes of the mesentery, omentum and liver may also be involved. Sometimes adult worms are seen obstructing the mesenteric or intestinal arteries causing arteriolitis with thrombosis with degenerating eggs or dead worms forming the focus for granulomas (Wu 1997).

Treatment

There is no specific treatment available. Treatment is symptomatic. It is a self-limiting disease with a low mortality rate.

REFERENCES

Beaver PC, Jung RC, Cupp EW. *Clinical Parasitology*, 9th edn. Philadelphia: Lea & Febiger, 1984, 292–294

Chye SM, Yen CM, Chen ER. Detection of circulating antigen by monoclonal antibodies for immunodiagnosis of angiostrongyliasis. *American Journal of Tropical Medicine and Hygiene* 1997; **56**: 408–412

Eamsobhana P, Mak JW, Yong HS. Detection of circulating antigens of *Parastrongylus cantonensis* in human sera by sandwich ELISA with specific monoclonal antibody. *Southeast Asian Journal of Tropical Medicine and Public Health* 1997; **28**: 139–142

Heaton DC, Gutteridge BH. Angiostrongyliasis in Australia. *Australian and New Zealand Journal of Medicine* 1980; **10**: 255–256

Ishii AI, Terada M, Sano M. Studies on chemotherapy of parasitic helminths (XXII). Effects of ivermectin on *Angiostrongylus cantonensis* in rats. *Japanese Journal of Parasitology* 1985; **34**: 411–417

Loria-Cortes R, Lobo-Sanakuja JF. Clinical abdominal angiostrongyliasis. A study of 116 children with intestinal eosinophilic granuloma caused by *Angiostrongylus costaricensis*. *American Journal of Tropical Medicine and Hygiene* 1980; **29**: 538–544

Porciv P, Brindles PJ. Eosinophilic meningitis. *Medical Journal of Australia* 1984; **141**: 319

Wu SS, French SW, Turner JA. Eosinophilic ileitis with perforation caused by *Angiostrongylus* (parastrongylus) *costaricensis*. A case study and review. *Archives of Pathology and Laboratory Medicine* 1997; **121**: 989–991

21

Anisakiasis

Parasitology
Presentation
Pathology

Investigations
Treatment
References

PARASITOLOGY

Anisakiasis is caused by a larval nematode of the family Anisakidae, man being infected commonly by eating inadequately cooked salt-water fish. Three types of Anisakiasis are recognized in causing infection in man, Anisakis being the commonest.

The Anisakidae family infects large sea mammals, seals, dolphins, whales and porpoises. The larval stage is found in several fish such as herrings, mackerel and various rockfishes. It is also found in squid. Human infection has only recently been recognized. Humans get infected by eating fish, which are sometimes salted, containing the third stage larvae. A study of New Zealand fish showed that 57 species were infected with Anisakis such as Trevally, Snapper, John Dory, but were not found in Rainbow trout or Quinnat salmon. The larvae are killed at 60°C but not by common methods of food preservation. Cooking and freezing may not protect against allergenic reactions to ingested *Anisakis simplex* (Andicana *et al.* 1997).

The adult nematode worms found in the intestinal tract of sea mammals are large, stout ascarids with a mouth surrounded by three lips, an oesophagus with an oblong to cylindrical posterior ventriculus and an asymmetrical excretory system. Eggs are passed in the faeces and hatch out as first stage larvae in seawater.

These are swallowed by crustaceans in which they moult and become second stage larvae. These measure > 18 mm. When fish ingest the crustaceans the larvae penetrate the gastrointestinal tract and migrate to the body cavity and muscle. They are the third stage larvae. They can be transmitted to other fish or squids. When seawater mammals ingest fish or squid containing these third stage infective larvae, the latter develop into adults, thus completing the life cycle (Fig. 21.1). To date, only the larval forms have caused human infections. These larvae are 50 mm long and 1 mm wide and in the third stage of development. They have a thick multilayered cuticle, large lateral chords and general muscle cells in each quarter of worm. The intestine has plentiful columnar cells. There is a large excretory gland cell in the anterior portion of the worm. The reproductive organs are either absent or immature.

PRESENTATION

The infection may be symptomless or may present with gastric or intestinal symptoms. Gastric Anisakiasis resembles acute gastritis and presents with vomiting and abdominal pain ~5–6 h after ingestion of seafood. This may follow a chronic course with symptoms lasting for several weeks or months. Intestinal anisakiasis may mimic an acute abdomen, or

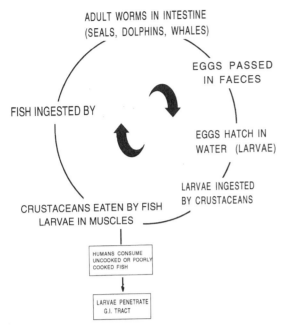

Figure 21.1 – Life cycle of Anisakidae sp.

be mistaken for carcinoma due to eosinophilic granuloma formation or regional ileitis.

Intestinal anisakiasis can occur up to 7 days after ingestion of infected seafood. Complications of swelling in the intestinal mucosa and bowel wall can lead to acute or subacute bowel obstruction. Peritonitis can occur due to perforation. Patients may also present as acute appendicitis (Ruschovich *et al.* 1983).

Acute urticaria and angio-oedema in sensitized patients occurs when parasitized by Anisakiasis. Allergic symptoms disappear in 24 h in most cases (Armentia *et al.* 1998). Asthma due to inhalation of antigens from Anisakis (Daschner *et al.* 1998) is another complication. Occupational conjunctivitis has been reported (Anibarro and Seoane 1998). Arthralgia or arthritis has been reported by rheumatologists in Spain (Cuende *et al.* 1998).

PATHOLOGY

There are no characteristic macroscopic features in resected specimens. The walls of the gastrointestinal tract may be oedematous and thickened in the segment where the parasites are lodged, with local ulceration and inflammation of the peri-intestinal fat. On microscopy, the early lesions show interstitial oedema with an inflammatory infiltrate consisting predominantly of eosinophils with lesser numbers of neutrophils, lymphocytes and plasma cells. Later lesions show granuloma formation sometimes with fragments of the degenerated larvae. Occasionally well-preserved larvae may be seen in the early lesions.

Diagnosis is made with confidence only if larvae are seen in tissue sections. Sometimes larvae are expelled from the mouth.

INVESTIGATIONS

1. Diagnosis can be very difficult. Peripheral eosinophilia is not always found. Stools examination is of no value as the larvae do not mature in humans or produce eggs. Gastric aspirates may demonstrate the larvae. Gastroscopy may show larvae penetrating the mucosa.
2. Abdominal X-rays may show fluid levels, dilated bowel loops suggestive of intestinal obstruction, or bowel loops with gas levels consistent with gastroenteritis. Sonographic abdominal X-rays may show small bowel dilatation, and focal oedema of mucosa (Ido *et al.* 1998).
3. Diagnosis is often made at laparoscopy when complications arise. Often the symptoms subside on their own and diagnosis is never made.
4. Cutaneous prick test with commercial extract of *A. simplex* and specific immunoblot serum IgE (Gomez *et al.* 1998).

TREATMENT

1 Treatment is symptomatic. There is no specific chemotherapy for the infection.
2 Rehydration with IV fluids and surgical intervention may be required if complications develop.

REFERENCES

Andicana L, Andicana MT, Fernande Z de Corres. Cooking and freezing may not protect against allergenic reactions to ingested *Anisakis simplex* antigens in humans. *Veterinary Records* 1997; **140**: 235

Anibarro B, Seoane FJ. Occupational conjunctivitis caused by sensitisation to *Anisakis simplex. Journal of Allergy and Clinical Immunology* 1998; **102**: 331–332

Armentia A, Lombardero M, Callejo A *et al.* Occupational asthma by *Anisakis simplex. Journal of Allergy and Clinical Immunology* 1998; **102**: 831–834

Cuende E, Audicana MT, Garcia M *et al.* Rheumatic manifestations in the course of anaphylaxis caused by *Anisakis simplex. Clinical and Experimental Rheumatology* 1998; **16**: 303–304

Daschner A, Alonso-Gomez A, Caballero T *et al.* Gastric anisakiasis: an underestimated cause of acute urticaria and angio-oedema? *British Journal of Dermatology* 1998; **139**: 822–828

Gomez B, Tabar AI, Tunon T *et al.* Eosinophilic gastroenteritis and anisakis. *Allergy* 1998; **53**: 1148–1154

Ido K, Yuasa H, Ide M *et al.* Sonographic diagnosis of small intestinal anisakiasis. *Journal of Clinical Ultrasound* 1998; **26**: 125–130

Ruschovich GO, Randall EL, Caprini JA *et al.* Omental anisakiasis. A rare mimic of acute appendicitis. *American Journal of Pathology* 1983; **80**: 517–520

22

Gnathostomiasis

Parasitology
Presentation
Pathology

Investigations
Treatment
References

PARASITOLOGY

Gnathostomiasis in humans is caused by a nematode *Gnathostoma spinigerum*. It is a form of larva migrans. The definitive hosts of this remarkable parasite are a variety of mammals including cats, dogs, lions and racoons. Infestation in humans has been reported in Thailand, Vietnam, the Philippines, Malaysia, Cambodia, Mynamar, Indonesia, Israel and Mexico. Man is an unsuitable host for the parasite, as it cannot mature so that the life cycle ends. The larvae can survive for > 10 years. More recently it has been shown that icthyophagus birds on dams and dykes near the city of Culiacar, Mexico were found to harbour Gnathostomiasis larvae identical to larvae found in humans (Diaz-Camacho *et al.* 1998).

Man acquires the infection by eating undercooked, infected fish, pork, chicken or any other intermediate host including frogs and snails. In Japan, raw fish consumption as 'Sushimi' and 'Smofak', a fermented fish in Thailand have been incriminated.

There are several species, *G. spinigerum* being the most common to infect man. The life cycle of *G. spinigerum* has been fully worked out (Fig. 22.1).

The adult females are 25–50 mm whereas the males measure 10–25 mm. The third-stage larva and the adult has a head bulb with four rows of hooklets and cuticular spines in the body, which are poorly developed in the third stage larva which measures ~1 cm in length. The male adult has paired papillae with no spines around the cloaca that differentiates it from the female. In the primary host, the third stage larvae migrate from the stomach, and in 3 months time re-enters the stomach. The life cycle is completed in a year.

PRESENTATION

Incubation is for 24–48 h. The larva causes both cutaneous and visceral migrans. In man, Gnathostoma produces superficial lesions in the subcutaneous tissue or in the muscles. The lesions may develop by migration of larvae to any peripheral part of the body including breasts, uterus, eye and central nervous system. They may present as abscesses with larvae emerging from the abscesses. If the lesion is accessible it should be surgically removed. The patient may have non-specific symptoms such as nausea, vomiting, urticaria and upper abdominal pain or discomfort. During the migratory phase the eosinophil count is high, the symptoms depending on the migratory path. Invasion of the thorax may produce pleuritic chest pain, cough with bloodstained sputum, pneumothorax and pneumonia (Priyanouda *et al.* 1995). The disease is generally self-limiting. Fatal cases have

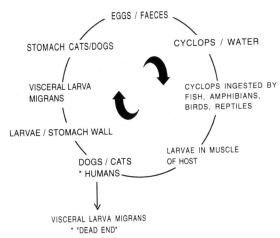

Figure 22.1 – Life cycle of Gnathostoma.

been reported following meningoencephalitis. The skin lesions would be difficult to distinguish from Calabar swelling, myasis, cutaneous paragonimiasis and a spargonosis. Cerebral symptoms can mimic *Angiostrongylus cantonensis*, sparganosis and toxocariasis.

Complications

Intracranial involvement with headaches, peri-orbital oedema, cranial nerve palsies and seizures. Many patients have impairment of memory. The mortality is ~13% following massive subarachnoid or intraventricular haemorrhage which are common causes (Punyagupta *et al.* 1968). Pulmonary infection has been reported (Charoentratanakul 1997). Ocular involvement causes iritis and palpebral oedema.

PATHOLOGY

In humans, the commonest lesions are found in the skin. The histological changes are secondary to mechanical causes, response to parasitic antigens and noxious secretions from larva such as an acetylcholine like substance, hyaluronidase, proteases and haemolysins. Compressive changes are seen around an advancing parasite followed by oedema, small haemorrhages with a cellular infiltrate of eosinophils, plasma cells and lymphocytes. Fibrogranulomatous reaction develops around the periphery of stationary parasites with inflammation and eosinophils in the centre. The parasite can be identified by its spinose cuticle, a muscular oesophagus and polymyarian

musculature. The larvae enter the central nervous system through the foramen magnum and cranial nerve foramina, resulting in an eosinophilic myeloencephalitis. The cerebrospinal fluid shows eosinophilic pleocytosis and xanthochromia. The brain shows features of encephalitis.

INVESTIGATIONS

1. Examination of the cerebral spinal fluid shows raised pressure, high protein, normal glucose, high eosinophil count and xanthochromia.
2. A full blood count shows increased eosinophils as high as 90%.
3. A CT scan needs to be carried out to exclude space-occupying lesions.
4. A chest X-ray should be done to exclude pulmonary pathology caused by the parasite during migration.
5. An enzyme-linked immunosorbent assay (ELISA) using a crude somatic extract of adult *Gnathostoma doloresi* worms showed 93% of clinically diagnosed patients with sero-positivity (Diaz-Camacho *et al.* 1998).

TREATMENT

- Administration of albendazole together with steroids for cerebral gnathostomiasis may be worthwhile. Albendazole tends to cause *G. spinigerum* larvae to migrate outward and can be removed by excision (Suntherasmi *et al.* 1992). Albendazole is not recommended in pregnancy. Changes of liver functions after albendazole has been reported (Inkatanuvar *et al.* 1998)
- Mebendazole given frequently has been reported to achieve results in ocular and skin lesions (Markell *et al.* 1992). Mebendazole 200 mg every 3 h for 6 days with glucocorticoids is administered in CNS disease. This drug is not recommended in pregnancy

REFERENCES

Charoentratanakul S. Tropical infection and the lung. *Monaldi Archives of Chest Diseases* 1997; **52**: 376–379

Diaz-Camacho SP, Zazneta-Ramos M, Pouce-Torrcillas E *et al.* Clinical manifestations and immunodiagnosis of gnathostomiasis in Culiacar, Mexico. *American Journal of Tropical Medicine and Hygiene* 1998; **59**: 908–915

Inkatanuvar S. Changes of liver function after albendazole treatment in human gnathostomiasis. *Journal of Medical Association of Thailand* 1998; **81**: 735–740

Markell EK, Voge M, John DT. *Medical Parasitology*, 7th edn. Philadelphia: WB Saunders, 1992, 339

Priyanouda B, Pradatsundarasar A, Viranuvatti V. Pulmonary gnathostomiasis. A case report from Thailand. *Annals of Tropical Medical Parasitology* 1995; **49**: 121–122

Punyagupta S, Juttijudata P, Bunnag T *et al.* Two cases of eosinophilic meningoencephalitis. A newly recognized disease caused by *Gnathostoma spinigerum*. *Transactions of the Royal Society Medical Hygiene* 1968; **62**: 801–809

Suntherasmi P, Riganti M, Chittamas S *et al.* Albendazole stimulates outward migration of *Gnathostoma spinigerum* to the dermis in man. *Southeast Asian Journal of Tropical Medical Public Health* 1992; **223**: 716–722

23

General Features of Filarial Nematodes

Filariasis is a debilitating and often disfiguring disease caused by filarial nematode worms. Mosquitoes in both rural and urban areas in the tropics transmit the disease.

Adult filariae (super family Filarioidea) live in the tissues or body cavities of vertebrate hosts including man where they parasitize the lymphatics, causing incompetence, lymph stasis and vulnerability to opportunistic infection. Symptoms of filariasis include painful attacks of lymphadenitis and obstructive lesions such as hydroceles and elephantiasis in which reaction to the worm is compounded by secondary infection. Filarial worms do not replicate in the human host. The disease appears similar to leprosy, with the spectrum represented by microfilaria carriers at one end and by patients with elephantiasis or other chronic lesions at the other.

Although there are more than 200 species of filarial nematodes, only a few infect humans. The females produce microfilariae that are less differentiated than the first-stage larvae of other nematodes. These are highly motile, threadlike prelarval forms that in some species retain the sheath (egg membrane), while in others the sheath ruptures and, therefore, are called unsheathed forms. Fig. 23.1 shows distinguishing features of microfilariae.

The microfilariae enter the blood stream or lymphatic vessels and can also enter the subcutaneous tissue where they may be ingested by bloodsucking arthropods. These microfilariae, which may survive for 1–2 years, are not capable of infecting other vertebrate hosts until they undergo further development. The microfilariae in the arthropod migrates through the wall of the digestive tract into the body cavity and in a suitable location (usually the thoracic muscles, malpighian tubules or fat bodies), develop through two distinct larval stages before reaching the infective or third stage larva.

When the arthropod takes its next blood meal, the infective stage larvae migrate to the arthropod mouthparts and escape into or onto vertebrate host skin.

Depending on the species, microfilariae exhibit periodicity in the blood circulation. If the highest number of microfilariae in the blood occurs at night, it is called nocturnal periodicity. Some species may be non-periodic or diurnal, in which case the microfilariae circulate both day and night. When microfilariae are not in the peripheral blood, they are found primarily in the capillaries and blood vessels of the lung. The basis for the filarial periodicity is not known. For species that exhibit nocturnal periodicity, it has been found that the insect vector also bites primarily at night, whereas in areas with non-periodic disease the vector feeds mainly during the day. Fig. 23.2 shows the life cycle of common filarial species parasitizing man.

In individuals who have resided or migrated from areas where filariasis is endemic and have a history of an insect bite, filariasis should be considered. A definitive diagnosis is based on the detection of microfilariae of

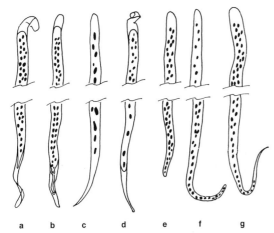

Figure 23.1 – Distinguishing features of the microfilariae. (a) *Wuchereria bancrofti*; (b) *Brugia malayi*; (c) *Onchocerca volvulus*; (d) *Loa loa*; (e) *Mansonella perstans*; (f) *Mansonella streptocerca*; (g) *Mansonella ozzardi*.

Wuchereria bancrofti, *Brugia malayi*, *Loa loa* and *Acanthocheilonema perstans* in the blood. For *Onchocerca volvulus*, microfilariae are detected in the skin although, occasionally, they may be seen in blood. Microfilariae may also be in the hydrocele fluid and urine of patients with a very high microfilaraemia or those who have been treated with dyethercarbamazine (DEC). In dirofilaria species, microfilariae are not produced; only adult worms are seen in tissue sections in humans. Therefore, the clinical history helps to determine the nature of the diagnostic specimen and the time of collection. For example, the best time for detection of *W. bancrofti* and *B. malayi* is between 22:00 and 04:00 hours. For *Loa loa*, blood should be taken between 10:00 and 14:00 hours, whereas blood for *Mansonella* can be taken at any time. Either finger prick or ear lobe blood may be taken for direct wet thin and thick blood smears. Blood films may be stained with Giemsa.

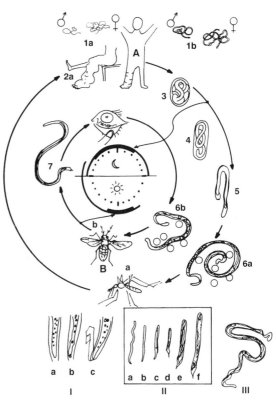

Figure 23.2 – Life cycle of Bancroftian, Malayan filariasis and Loiasis. (A) Final host: man. Sexually mature stages and (a) *Wuchereria bancrofti*; and (b) *Loa loa*. (2a) Characteristic symptom of an infection with *W. bancrofti*: elephantiasis and (b) *Loa loa* during its passage over the conjunctiva. Development of the microfilariae in the uterus: egg containing a microfilaria; commencing elongation of the egg; 'sheathed' microfilaria. (6a) *Microfilaria bancrofti* (*M. nocturna*); (b) *Microfilaria loa* (*M. diurna*). (B) Intermediate host and vector: Diptera. (a) Species of Aedes and Culex; (b) species of Chrysops. (7) Metacyclis, infective microfilaria. (I) Tail end of a sheathed Microfilaria of: (a) *Wuchereria bancrofti*; (b) *Wuchereria malayi*; and (c) *Loa loa*. (II) Development of the microfilaria in the vector to the metacyclic form: (a) microfilaria from the blood; (b–e) developmental period as far as the first ecdysis; and (f) growth by elongation until the second ecdysis. (III) Microfilaria malayi.

24

Dirofilariasis

Parasitology
Presentation
Pathology
Investigations

Treatment
Illustrative Case
References

PARASITOLOGY

Dirofilaria is a zoonosis transmitted by mosquitoes from animals to humans. Six species cause infection in humans. *Dirofilaria immitis*, known as the dog heartworm, causes lesions in the lung and heart. *D. immitis* is found in dogs in temperate, tropical and subtropical parts of the world. The other five species, *D. tenuis*, *D. subdermata*, *D. repens*, *D. striata* and *D. uris*, cause subcutaneous or conjunctival nodules in humans. *D. immitis* is also found in cats, foxes, muskrats, wolves, otters and sea lions. The vector is a mosquito of the genus Aedes, Anopheles and Culex.

Human *D. immitis* infection causes solitary pulmonary nodules that present as asymptomatic coin lesions (Wockel 1993, Green *et al.* 1994). The worm can lodge in the right ventricle and could be carried into the lungs and dies as man is an unsuitable host.

Subcutaneous lesions caused by *D. repens* have been documented in Spain, Italy and Czechoslovakia. On an island in Puerto Rico, where the incidence of canine heartworm is high, a sero-epidemiologic study was carried out on humans revealed antibodies in 2.66% (Villianveva and Rodriguez-Perez 1993).

In Australia, reports of cases in humans are few and occur mainly in the tropical north and Western Australia.

The larvae of *D. immitis* further migrate through the muscle sheaths or peritoneum into the veins and to the right heart where they mature within 180 days. In the dog, the adult worms are found in the chambers and large vessels of the right heart. The female measures 25–30 cm in length and 1 mm in width. The male is smaller, measuring 12–18 cm in length. *D. immitis* adult worm is characterized by cuticle of three to four layers thick (male 5–15 μm; female 5–25 μm) with transverse striations and bilateral internal cuticular ridge, abundant musculature – frequently retracted away from the cuticle during tissue processing and double uteri – not filling the body cavity, 300–350 μm in maximum diameter. The microfilariae are sheathless, measuring 300–325 × 7 μm. The microfilariaemia is subperiodic and nocturnal with levels higher in summer than in winter. Microfilariae cannot be found in blood or tissues.

PRESENTATION

The pulmonary type is of greater significance than the subcutaneous filaria. It is not because of the severity of the pathologic changes, but the radiologic findings are so alarming that unnecessary thoracotomy has been done (Yamazaki *et al.* 1998). Most patients are asymptomatic with 'coin' lesions in lung. The lesion is 1–3 cm in diameter (at times two or more coin lesions and bilateral). Symptomatic patients complain of pleuritic pain, cough and haemoptysis. Constitutional symptoms include fever, chills and malaise.

Subcutaneous dirofilariasis involves conjunctiva, eye lids orbit (Stianese *et al.* 1998), face, extremities, breast, upper part of chest, scrotum, penis and perianal region (Dissanaiyke *et al.* 1997). The nodules are erythematous, tender and painful, are moderately firm, and 1–6 cm in diameter. Occasionally, patients feel a crawling sensation in the skin.

PATHOLOGY

Pulmonary infarction is caused by a thrombus with the parasite as a nidus. The infarct is not typical end-artery type. It is rounded rather than wedge-shaped. Allergic reaction to the diffusion of parasite antigen is said to contribute to the necrosis. The pulmonary nodule is separated by surrounding atelectatic lung by a layer of cellular infiltrate composed of eosinophils, lymphocytes and plasma cells. When eosinophils are prominent the condition is known as eosinophilic pneumonitis. The layers forming the nodule include a hyaline fibrous capsule, a row of palisading histiocytes or a granulomatous layer containing multinucleated giant cells and a necrotic centre with the degenerate remains of the parasite. Worms may also be seen in adjacent arteries which show marked intimal hyperplasia and plasma cell infiltration of its entire wall. The composite histologic features of encapsulation of infarction, palisading histiocytes and plasma cell arteritis are diagnostic even if the parasite cannot be seen. In subcutaneous dirofilariasis a single parasite is seen in a small cavity containing fibrinous exudate or in an abscess. The inflammatory cells are neutrophils and eosinophils and the histology can also be similar to the lung lesions.

INVESTIGATIONS

1. The adult worm can be extracted from subcutaneous tissue as a thread-like opalescent structure and identified microscopically or the parasite is identified at biopsy.
2. Identification of a 44 kD antigen recognized by IgM against *D. immitis*. Human sera are analysed by an enzyme-linked immunosorbent assay (ELISA) for detection of anti-*D. immitis* IgM seropositive

individuals. Enzyme-linked immunoelectro-transfer blot (EITB) is also performed for the detection of polypeptides that specifically react with IgM anti-*D. immitis*. The 44 kD protein is a marker of recent *D. immitis* infection (Perera *et al.* 1994).

3. Non-specific fluorescence stains for the rapid recognition of pulmonary dirofilariasis employ Tinopal CBS-X (TBCS-X) and Calcofluor White (CFW) and are rapid and inexpensive. Deparaffinized rehydrated sections are stained for 1 min in 1% W/V aqueous solution of (CBS-X) or CFW. They are counterstained and examined under fluorescence microscope. The worm fragments are stained (Green *et al.* 1994).
4. ELISA using antigen β-galactosidase-*D. immitis* recombinant fusion protein (FP) using recombinant DNA technique is a useful diagnostic tool for human dirofilariasis. ELISA using (FP) is highly sensitive and specific compared with the use of crude somatic antigen (Sun and Sugane 1992).
5. Immunoblot technique using excretory-secretory (AS) antigen proteins with molecular weights 20–19.5, 17.5–17 and 14 derived from *D. immitis*. This has much less reactivity compared with adult worm extracts, with non-filarial parasite infection (Akao *et al.* 1991).
6. Histologic examination of lung lesion.

TREATMENT

The only treatment available is surgical excision of the nodules.

ILLUSTRATIVE CASE

A 55-year-old male, a heavy smoker, presented to his general practitioner with bronchitis. A chest X-ray showed a 20 mm diameter coin lesion in the periphery of the left mid-zone (Fig. 24.1), clinically suspected to be a carcinoma. A wedge resection of the apical segment of left lower lobe was done.

On microscopic examination a rounded area of infarction was seen. The nodule was separated from surrounding atelectatic lung by a layer of cellular infiltrate (Fig. 24.2) composed of eosinophils, lymphocytes and plasma cells. The typical granuloma was contained in its centre with degenerating parasite with bilateral internal cuticular ridge, and abundant musculature retracted from the cuticle (Fig. 24.4). At the periphery were palisading histiocytes and plasma cell arteritis.

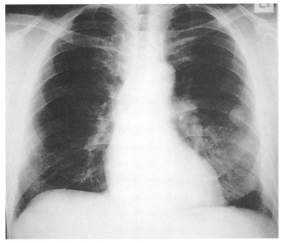

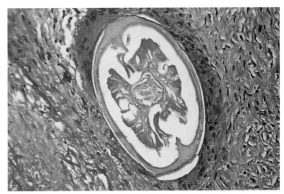

Figure 24.4 – Typical dirofilarial granuloma with degenerated parasite showing bilateral internal cuticular ridge and abundant musculature, retracted from the cuticle during tissue processing (H&E × 100).

Figure 24.1 – Chest X-ray from a 55-year-old man showing a 20 mm diameter coin lesion in the periphery of the left mid-zone.

REFERENCES

Akao N, Kondo K, Fujitak. Immunoblot analysis of *Dirofilaria immitis* recognized by infected humans. *Annals of Tropical Medical Parasitology* 1991; **85**: 453–460

Dissanaiyke AS, Abeywickreme W, Wijesundera MD *et al.* Human dirofilariasis caused by *Dirofilaria* (Nochtiella) *repens* in Sri Lanka. *Parasitologia* 1997; **39**: 375–382

Green LK, Ausari MQ, Schwartz MR *et al.* Non-specific fluorescent whitener stains in the rapid recognition of pulmonary dirofilariasis: a report of 20 cases. *Thorax* 1994; **49**: 590–593

Perera L, Muro A, Munoz I *et al.* Human dirofilariasis: identification of a 44 kD antigen recognized by IgM against *Dirofilaria immitis*. *Enfermedades Infecciosas y Microbiological Clinica* 1994; **12**: 193–196

Stianese D, Martini A, Molfino G *et al.* Orbital dirofilariasis. *European Journal of Ophthalmology* 1998; **8**: 258–262

Sun S, Sugane K. Immunodiagnosis of human dirofilariasis by enzyme-linked immunosorbent assay using recombinant DNA-derived fusion protein. *Journal of Helminthology* 1992; **66**: 220–226

Villianveva EJ, Rodriguez-Perez J. Immunodiagnosis of human dirofilariasis in Puerto Rico. *American Journal of Tropical Medicine and Hygiene* 1993; **48**: 536–541

Wockel W, Eckert J, Loscher T *et al.* Authochonus european dirofilaria of the lung. *Pneumologie* 1993; **47**: 227–231

Yamazaki A, Kubota K, Shimota H. Three cases of pulmonary dirofilariasis suspected of lung cancer. *Kyobu Geka* 1998; **51**: 457–460

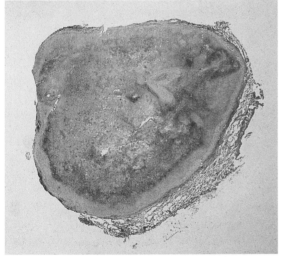

Figure 24.2 – Rounded area of infarction (H&E × 20).

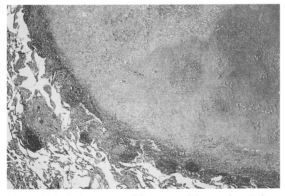

Figure 24.3 – Pulmonary nodule separated from atelectatic lung by a layer of cellular infiltrate (H&E × 40).

25

Lymphatic Filariasis

Parasitology
Presentation
Pathology
Investigations

Treatment
Prevention
References

PARASITOLOGY

Lymphatic filariasis is caused by the nematodes *Wuchereria bancrofti* and *Brugia malayi*, the adults of which inhabit lymphatic tissues. The clinical manifestations can vary from the very extreme, such as elephantiasis or none at all.

World incidence of lymphatic filariasis is 118 million, *W. bancrofti* 105 million and *B. malayi* 13 million. Disease prevalence is 43 million for overt lymphatic disease and 74 million microfilariae positive but asymptomatic.

W. bancrofti is found in Asia, Africa, Southern Europe, South and Central America. *B. malayi* is restricted to South and South East Asia. In some of these regions *B. malayi* occurs alone; in others it overlaps with *W. bancrofti*. Bancroftian filariasis is transmitted by several species of mosquitoes such as *Culex* (*C. fatigans* being the common example), *Aedes* and *Anopheles*. Malayan filariasis is transmitted by the vector Mansonia, which breeds in water-containing plants such as water lettuce and pistia. The Anopheles is found in more rural areas. Man gets infected with the bite of vector and is the usual reservoir, but certain species of Mansonia can transmit the parasite to cats and dogs. The incubation period in man is ~8 months–1 year. Continued re-infection is essential to develop the full clinical picture.

W. bancrofti adults are threadlike white worms with the male measuring 2.5–4 cm long; the female is 5–10 cm. *B. malayi* measures 2.5 cm long. The worms are present in lymph nodes or lymphatics. When the adult worms mate they produce microfilariae. Filariae are viviparous nematodes that release the first stage larvae into the tissue of the host where it can remain for months. Wuchereria and Brugia have very thin and delicate microfilarial sheaths surrounding the embryo as it circulates in the blood. The sheath is lost when it gets digested in the stomach of the mosquito. It is likely that the sheath antigens are not recognized by the host's immune system resulting in their survival. When the mosquito bites an infected person, microfilariae are ingested and enter the body cavity of the insect and the thoracic musculature where they grow and moult in the next 10 days to become infective-stage larvae, measuring from 244 to 296 μm. The infective larvae enter the proboscis and with the next blood meal of mosquito they escape into the skin. From the skin the microfilariae enter the peripheral lymphatics, the regional lymph nodes and larger lymph vessels, then after moulting twice, mature into adult worms. Sexual maturity is attained in probably several months. Adult worms are known to live for several years.

In blood films the microfilariae measure 245–300 μm and contain large numbers of nuclei. There is no alimentary canal and the body is cylindrical with a rounded anterior end and tail that tapers to a point where no nuclei are present, a feature which distinguishes this species from other sheathed microfilariae (Fig. 25.1a and b).

PRESENTATION

Although visitors to endemic areas may be infected, only a few develop symptoms. When the fully mature worms release microfilaria into the blood stream, a flu-like illness ensues with myalgia, lymphangitis, lymphadenopathy, epididymo-orchitis fever and mild eosinophilia. The clinical manifestations are probably secondary to an allergic response to the microfilaria. Acute attacks can recur periodically.

After several years there is lymphoedema, after repeated episodes of lymphangitis and lymphadenopathy. This is secondary to tissue response to the dead or live adult worm. The chronic lymphoedema of legs, scrotum, anus is referred to as elephantiasis, and is a

non-pitting oedema (Fig. 25.2). The early stage of elephantiasis is considered to be due to a hypersensitivity reaction and is reversible. Subsequently, there is an obstructing fibrous reaction in the lymphatic system and the chronic oedema results in a warty or verrucose skin. It can produce a hanging scrotum, which can weigh several kilograms. Hydrocele is a manifestation of filariasis. The skin can be secondarily infected by streptococcal or staphylococcal organisms causing acute adenolymphangitis. Exfoliative dermatitis is a manifestation of acute lymphatic filariasis. When lymphatic obstruction occurs in the urinary tract, the patient presents with chyluria. Lymphatic fibrosis in the abdomen causes chylous ascites. Obstruction to the thoracic duct can lead to a chylous pleural effusion. Weight loss is often the result of repeated bouts of fever, and the filarial worms acquire certain nutrients directly from their host including vitamin A, iodine, thiamine and pyridoxine (Storey 1993). Elephantiasis

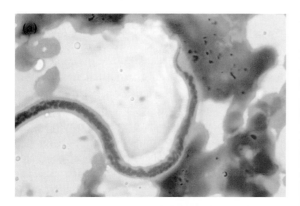

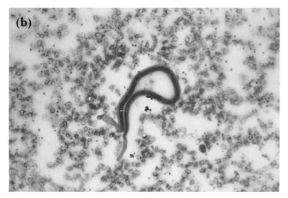

Figure 25.1 – Sheathed microfilariae in peripheral blood. (a) Large numbers of nuclei in the body; (b) rounded anterior end and tapering tail with no nuclei.

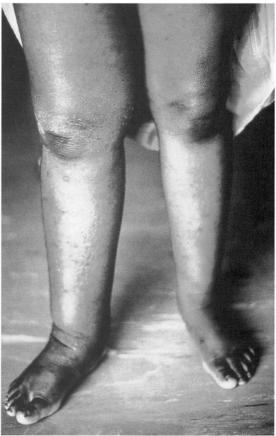

Figure 25.2 – Chronic lymphoedema of the legs in an African woman.

of the breast or breast lumps has been described (Chandrasoma 1978). Renal disease appears a common event in *B. malayi* filariasis, involving both the tubular and glomerular compartment of the organ and its pathogenesis is complex (Langhammer *et al.* 1997).

Tropical pulmonary eosinophilia is a clinical entity associated with microfilaria lodged in the pulmonary capillaries and resulting in a granulomatous reaction. The clinical features are fever, widespread crepitations and rhonchi, mimicking bronchial asthma. X-rays show marked reticular markings throughout the lung fields and small, nodular shadows of 2–3 mm in diameter. The criteria for diagnosis of tropical eosinophilia are an irritating cough, which becomes paroxysmal with asthmatiform dyspnoea and an eosinophilic count of > 2000/μl (Donough 1963). Pulmonary eosinophilia can also be caused by strongyloidiasis, toxocariasis and ascariasis. The pulmonary opacities in all these infections are transient. Complete immunity to any helminth infection is rare. However, some degree of acquired immunity to filarial parasites builds up over the years. The method of eliminating larval filarial parasites by the immune system is not clearly defined. Filarial infection has two phases. In active infection, a phase of hyporesponsiveness occurs with low T-cell proliferation.

Microfilariae are an uncommon finding in migrants reflecting an intense immunological reaction to the parasite (Chodakewitz 1995).

PATHOLOGY

Persistent lymphoedema of the scrotum, penis, vulva, leg, breast and arm is seen in chronic filariasis. Hydrocele, lymph node enlargement or rupture of a lymphatic varix with chyluria may also occur. Inflammatory nodular lesions or sterile abscesses of the epididymis or around the external genitalia may also occur. Elephantoid skin shows dilatation of the dermal lymphatics with widespread lymphocytic infiltrates and focal deposition of cholesterol. The epidermis is hyperkeratotic and hypertrophic.

Microscopically, filarial worms may be found in lymphatics or nodes. These may be alive or dead and calcified. It is associated with lymphangiectasia. In recurrent filarial funiculoepididymitis, an intense eosinophil inflammation is seen, which is probably immunologically mediated. Granulomatous inflam-

mation around the cuticular remnants of the parasite is sometimes recognized. Polypoid infoldings of the lymphatic vessel with persisting eosinophils and lymphocytes are features that are highly suggestive of lymphatic filariasis. Microfilariae are difficult to find in histological sections. Exudative glomerulonephritis referred to as acute eosinophilic nephritis has been described in *W. bancrofti*.

INVESTIGATIONS

1. Examination of peripheral blood – blood smears for microfilariae between 22:00 and 02:00 hours is the most reliable method of diagnosis. Some strains are not periodic and blood may be taken during daytime. Fresh blood can be examined on a direct smear or the centrifuge sediment may be used. The specimen can also be pumped through a millipore or nucleopore filter and the sediment examined (Denham and McGreevy 1977).

2. Serological assays – in the chronic phase, microfilariae will not be detected in the blood and serological assays are useful. Circulating antigens of *W. bancrofti* can readily be screened (Forsyth *et al.* 1985). In Brugian filariasis an IgG_4 antibody test appears to give the best result (Forsyth *et al.* 1985). ELISA is a diagnostic test for active infection in 'normal' individuals and in patients with elephantiasis when the parasite is not detected by other methods. The method is also used to assay the response to diethylcarbamazepine. A reduction of IgG_4 by 70% occurs in 8 weeks and by 90% in 2 weeks (Maizels *et al.* 1995). Trop-Ag *W. bancrofti* lymphatic filariasis detection kit is now available from James Cook University of North Queensland, Australia, which is specific and does not cross-react with other filarial worms. The assay configured as an antigen capture (Sandwich) ELISA and detects parasite antigen only.

3. Polymerase chain reaction – a PCR assay based on ELISA has been developed to detect *B. malayi* infection. PCR-ELISA detected 12 times as many *B. malayi* infections as did thick blood film examination (Rahman *et al.* 1998).

4. Antistreptolysin O (ASO) and anti-DNAase B (ADAB) are elevated in acute-convalescent stage due to streptococcal invasion of the lymphatics which triggers or amplifies lymphoedema and elephantiasis in patients with chronic filariasis (Vincent *et al.* 1998).

5. Lymphoscintigraphy – even in asymptomatic individuals, grossly abnormal lymphatic damage may be seen, emphasizing the urgency of treating patients.

6. Ultrasonography – a living adult worm in the lymphatics may be visualized using a 3.5-MHz transducer (Dreyer *et al.* 1998).

7. Monoclonal antibodies – circulating filarial antigen (CFA) in finger prick blood specimen can be detected by monoclonal antibodies rather than using blood to detect microfilariae. It has been shown that treatment of lymphatic filaria with ivermectin or diethylcarbamazine, the filarial antigen-specific reactivity was significantly increased over baseline level at 9 months.

8. Magnetic resonance imaging – filarial serotum imaging by MRI showed the pathological description of the three muscular layers (Atreaga *et al.* 1997).

TREATMENT

- Ivermectin is a semisynthetic product with antiparasitic activity. Ivermectin 400 µg/kg in a single dose reduces the microfilaria load within 4 days. At this dosage it has no action on the adult worm

- Albendazole 600 mg in combination with ivermectin 400 µg/kg in single dose was safe and effective regimen for suppression of microfilariae in bancroftian filariasis and has significant effect on adult worm (Ismail *et al.* 1998)

- Diethylcarbamazine 5 mg/kg in three divided doses for 21 days. It is also a macrofilaricidal but its action is slow. With heavy infection, a test dose of 25–50 µg diethylcarbamazapine should be given. This drug is also used for tropical pulmonary eosinophilia. It is contraindicated in pregnancy. Allergic reactions to released filarial antigens (Herxheimer reaction) such as hypotension, tachycardia, collapse and a higher incidence of inflammatory nodules or lymphadenitis can occur. Antihistamines are not indicated as they aggravate drowsiness. In multicentre trials using ivermectin 420 µg/kg and diethylcarbamazine 6 µg/kg for *W. bancrofti* infection, the microfilarial level was the same for patients receiving either drug. Treatment should be repeated yearly receiving either drug (Chodakewitz 1995). Elephantiasis of legs, scrotum, vulva or breasts may be surgically managed. A single dose treatment for *W. bancrofti*, 6 µg/kg, resulted in 89–97% success rate with 19–28% cure rate and 74–80% reduction in microfilarial density (Weerasooriya *et al.* 1998). Local hygiene, topical antibiotics or antifungal to prevent lymphangitis and arrest progression to elephantiasis.

PREVENTION

Treatment with single dose of diethylcarbamazine and ivermectin for those at risk in the community is recommended once yearly. Combined diethylcarbamazine and ivermectin reduces microfilaria by 99%. Use diethylcarbamazine fortified salt substitute for normal cooking. Salt also eliminates the infection for 9–12 months. Vector control by eliminating breeding sites. Toxin-producing *Bacillus sphaericus* has been used in some areas. Measures to prevent mosquito bites should be undertaken.

REFERENCES

Atreaga C, Salamand P, Mianne D *et al.* MRI aspects of Filaria scrotal elephantiasis. MRI-anatomopathological correlations. *Journal of Radiology* 1997; **78**: 1285–1287

Chandrasoma PT, Mendis KN. Filarial infection of the breast. *American Journal of Tropical Medicine and Hygiene* 1978; **27**: 770–773

Chodakewitz J. Ivermectin and lymphatic filariasis: a clinical update. *Parasitology Today* 1995; **11**: 233–235

Denham DA, McGreevy PB. Brugian filariasis epidemiological and experimental studies. *Advances in Parasitology* 1977; **15**: 244–311

Dreyer G, Santos A, Noroes J *et al.* Ultrasonographic detection of living adult *Wuchereria bancrofti* using a 3.5-MHz transducer. *American Journal of Tropical Medicine and Hygiene* 1998; **59**: 399–403

Donough DL. Tropical eosinophilia and lung injury. *New England Journal of Medicine* 1963; **269**: 1357–1364

Dunyo SK, Nkrumah FK, Ahorlu CK *et al.* Exfoliative skin manifestations in acute lymphatic filariasis. *Transactions of the Royal Society of Tropical Medicine and Hygiene* 1998; **92**: 539–540

Forsyth KP, Spark R, Kazura J *et al.* A monoclonal antibody-based immunoradiometric assay for detection of circulating antigen in bancroftian filariasis. *Journal of Immunology* 1985; **134**: 1172–1177

Ismail MM, Jayakody RL, Weil GJ *et al.* Efficacy of single dose combinations of albendazole, ivermectin and diethylcarbamazine for the treatment of bancroftian filariasis. *Transactions of the Royal Society of Tropical Medicine and Hygiene* 1998; **92**: 94–97

Langhammer J, Birk HW, Zahner H. Renal disease in lymphatic filariasis: evidence for tubular and glomerular disorders at various stages of the infection. *Tropical Medicine International Health* 1997; **2**: 875–884

Maizels RM, Sartono E, Kurniawan A. T-cell activation and the balance of antibody isotypes in human filariasis. *Parasitology Today* 1995; **11**: 50–56

Rahman N, Ashikin AN, Anwar AK *et al.* PCR-ELISA for the detection of *Brugia malayi* infection using finger-prick blood. *Transactions of the Royal Society of Tropical Medicine and Hygiene* 1998; **92**: 404–406

Storey DM. Nutritional interaction in human and animal host. *Parasitology* 1993; **107 (suppl.)**: 5147–5158

Vincent AL, Urena Rojas CA, Ayoub EM *et al.* Filariasis and erisipela in Santo Domingo. *Journal of Parasitology* 1998; **84**: 557–561

Weerasooriya MV, Kimura E, Dayaratne DA *et al.* Efficacy of a single dose treatment of *Wuchereria bancrofti* microfilaria carriers with diethylcarbamazine in Matara, Sri Lanka. *Ceylon Medical Journal* 1998; **43**: 151–155

26

Non-lymphatic Filariasis

Parasitology
  Loiasis
  Mansonella perstans
  Onchocerciasis
Presentation
  Loiasis
  Mansonella perstans
  Onchocerciasis
Pathology
  Loiasis
  Mansonella perstans
  Onchocerciasis

Investigations
  Loiasis
  Mansonella perstans
  Onchocerciasis
Treatment
  Loiasis and *Mansonella perstans*
  Onchocerciasis
Prevention
  Onchocerciasis
References

PARASITOLOGY: LOIASIS, *MANSONELLA PERSTANS* AND ONCHOCERCIASIS

Loa loa (the native name), the African eye worm, was first noted in the eye of a Negro girl in the West Indies in 1770. *Mansonella perstans*, until recently known as *Dipetalonema perstans*, is a common parasite of humans and apes in large areas of Africa. Both parasites cause swellings in residents of old Calabar in West Africa and hence the name 'Calabar swellings'. Onchocerciasis is caused by *Onchocerca volvulus*, the largest of the human filariae. It is also known as river blindness and is a major health problem as the infection is a leading cause of blindness in the world.

Loiasis

The vector for *Loa loa* is the blood-sucking female Mango fly of the genus Chrysops, Silacia and Dimidiata. The endemic areas are the rain forests and Savannas of West and Central Africa. The vector for *M. perstans* is midges of the genus Culicoides. The adult males of *Loa loa* are 2–3.5 cm long and 0.35–0.4 mm wide; females are 5–7 cm long and 0.45–0.6 mm wide. The microfilariae are sheathed and measure 185–300 × 5–10 μm. They differ from the other sheathed microfilariae such as Wucheraria and Brugia in that the body nuclei continue to the tip of the tail. The adult worms migrate in the subcutaneous and deep connective tissues of man and enter the blood stream where they cause a diurnal periodicity. When the Mango fly takes them they undergo a developmental cycle similar to the other microfilariae in the thoracic musculature. After ~10–12 days become infective larvae and are introduced to the host by the bite of a Chrysops.

Mansonella perstans

The vectors for *M. perstans* are the midges of the genus culicoides. The adult worms of *Mansonella perstans* are found in the body cavities of man, i.e. the peritoneal and pleural cavities, and are similar in size to the other filarial worms. The microfilariae measure 190–200 μm in length and 4–5 μm in diameter, and are unsheathed with the body nuclei extending to the tip of the tail. The insect vector, Culicoides species (midges), ingests the microfilariae that circulate in the blood.

Onchocerciasis

Onchocerciasis is one of the great public health problems in the world. About 40 million people in 34 countries are affected and nearly 2 million of these go blind (WHO 1987). The disease is mainly found in West Africa and South America. Man gets infected by the bite of a Simulium fly, the vector, which is a small black fly that requires a hot and moist, shady environment for breeding. The breeding is heaviest in the wet season and occurs near running streams. Man is usually the true reservoir host.

The adult female worm measures 50 cm in length and is white wire-like and lies coiled within fibrous tissue capsules. The males are much shorter and measure 5 cm. The microfilariae emerge from these nodules and are unsheathed larvae measuring 150–350 μm in length and 5–9 μm in width. The intermediate host and vector of *O. volvulus*, the black fly Simulium, ingests microfilariae which develops in the insect in a manner similar to other filarial larvae. The infective forms enter a new host and migrate in the subcutaneous tissue some becoming encapsulated in this site (Fig. 26.1). Nodules of adult worms in a fibrous tissue tumour-like mass are formed ~1 year after onset of infection. These range from a few millimetres to several centimetres in diameter and may be numerous.

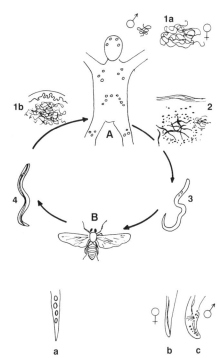

Figure 26.1 – Life cycle of Onchocerca. (A) Final host: man; (1a) male and female sexually mature worms; (1b) section through an Onchocerca nodule, about natural size; (2) microfilariae migrating in the subcutaneous connective tissue; (3) microfilaria. (B) Intermediate host: *Simulium damnosum*; (2) metacyclic microfilaria from the biting proboscis of the intermediate host; (a–c) tail ends of the microfilariae of various species; (a) *Onchocerca reticulata* from horse; (b) *O. volvulus* from man; (c) *O. gutturosa* from cattle.

PRESENTATION

Loiasis

The infection may be asymptomatic for years. When symptoms set in they are due to migration of the worm, causing local reactions. The worms are generally found in subcutaneous tissue and, if the tissue is loose, there is hardly any pain. However, if they are in tight skin or over joints, the swellings can be very painful. Systemic manifestations include fever, myalgia, urticarial rashes and marked peripheral eosinophilia. Some of the symptoms are due to the location of the adult worm. Infection in the central nervous system produces seizures. In the eye it causes pain and retinopathy. The swellings can appear in any part of the body but are more common in sites predisposed to trauma. The size of each swelling is 6–7 cm, and appears ~3 months after the onset of infection. They can reappear from time to time over many years. The skin lesions are itchy.

Adult worms may be seen periodically, moving in the eyelids, conjunctiva, scrotum, penis, tongue and buccal mucosa. The spleen may be palpable as the microfilariae are destroyed in the spleen. *Loa loa* may be associated with nephrotic syndrome, microhaematurea and renal failure (Pakasa *et al.* 1997). Thrombosis of veins is a rare complication (Petersen *et al.* 1998).

Mansonella perstans

The two species that affect man are *M. perstans* and *M. streptocerca* but they differ in clinical manifestations. In *M. perstans* infection the symptoms and signs are poorly defined. Infection causes cutaneous itching, Calabar swellings and vague abdominal symptoms. The liver, gallbladder and heart may be affected. *M. streptocerca* causes a chronic itching dermatitis, dermal thickening, lymphadenopathy and hypopigmented macules in the pigmented skin.

Onchocerciasis

The nodular changes in the skin, called onchocercomas, are subcutaneous, especially near bony prominences. They consist of adult worms entangled in a mass of fibrous tissue. The microfilariae cause more extensive lesions as millions of microfilariae migrate into the skin, lymph nodes, eyes and deeper organs. The skin lesions are acute papular onchodermatitis due to acute reaction, chronic papular onchodermatitis or lichenified onchodermatitis (Brieger 1998). The skin manifestations in chronic cases are pruritus, hypo- and hyperpigmentation. There may be loss of elastic fibres of the skin leading to a 'hanging groin' and other skin manifestations referred to as lizard skin or elephant skin. The skin nodules are non-tender unless over a joint and movable. Ocular lesions can present in many ways. The damage is caused by the microfilariae directly infiltrating the cornea producing a sclerosing keratitis, anterior uveitis, secondary glaucoma, optic atrophy and severe chorioretinal changes (Narita and Taylor 1993). The lymph glands are enlarged, with regional lymphoedema and elephantiasis of the scrotum. Hydroceles teeming with microfilariae is often seen. Cachexia is a common feature of longstanding onchocerciasis. Onchocerciasis is a progressive condition and the main impact is on the eye, resulting in blindness called 'river blindness'.

PATHOLOGY

Loiasis

Microfilariae are found in the capillaries around the sweat glands of the skin. Focal inflammatory cells are found in the dermis and fibrotic lesions may be seen. Reaction to living adult worms is mild. The dying adult worms cause suppurative inflammation. This subsequently leads to a granulomatous reaction with fibrosis. The granulomatous reactions can affect adjacent structures such as major nerves to cause paraesthesia or focal paralysis. Focal inflammatory lesions or microfilarial granulomas have been found in organs such as spleen, heart, brain and spinal cord, all of which contain microfilariae. Lymphocytes, histiocytes and foreign body giant cells surround these microfilariae. Membranous nephropathy has been described in *Loa loa* infection. Focal segmental glomerulosclerosis with microfilariae in renal microvasculature has been documented (Pakasa *et al.* 1997).

Mansonella perstans

The adult worms are found in the peritoneal, pericardial and pleural cavities including inguinal hernial sacs. Microfilariae are found mainly in the peripheral blood, rarely in the urine or cerebrospinal fluid. Pathological reactions to live adult worms have not been described with other filarial worms. The dying or the dead worms cause an inflammatory reaction. The dead worms are surrounded by inflammatory infiltrates comprising histiocytes, lymphocytes and plasma cells. The serous lining, as in inguinal hernia, may be thickened and fibrotic.

Onchocerciasis

Severe infections cause a chronic dermatitis with focal darkening or loss of pigment and scaling. Subsequently, atrophy of epidermis, subcutaneous oedema, redundancy and thickening of the dermis occurs. The skin is called 'leopard', 'lizard' or 'elephant' skin. There is depletion of lymphocytes in lymph nodes in the groin. There is fibrosis and loss of elastic fibres in the skin called 'hanging' groin. The initial reaction to the adult worms is an exudative reaction progressing to a granulomatous and finally fibrotic reaction with calcification. The eye lesions begin as punctate keratitis with fluffy opacities of cornea caused by degenerative microfilariae that elicit an eosinophilic infiltration. The sclerosing keratitis follows with the corneal opacity beginning at the limbus. In addition, iridocyclitis is caused by microfilariae in the anterior chamber resulting in glaucoma. The choroid and retina is involved with atrophy and irreversible loss of vision. The inflammation sometimes affects the optic nerve. Renal complications could occur in *O. volvulus* with immune complexes causing minimal change, mesangioproliferative, mesangio-capillary and chronic sclerosing glomerulonephritis.

INVESTIGATIONS

Loiasis

1. The microfilaria can be identified in the peripheral blood, in wet preparations, where they are mobile or by staining thick films. Blood should be drawn around midday. However, it is not always possible to demonstrate microfilaria in the blood.
2. Biopsies of cutaneous swellings may or may not contain adult worms or microfilaria.
3. Skin tests and compliment fixation tests using dirofilarial antigens may be positive but cross-react with other dirofilarial infections.
4. Full blood count for peripheral eosinophilia.
5. Detection of *Loa loa* specific DNA in the blood by using the polymerase chain reaction (PCR) with a sensitivity of 95% and for *M. perstans* 100% (Toure *et al.* 1997).

Mansonella perstans

1. Detection of microfilaria *M. perstans* in peripheral blood and occasionally in CSF or urine. Blood should be taken during midday.
2. Rarely, adult worms may be identified in tissue sections.
3. Peripheral eosinophilia is present.
4. *M. streptocerca microfilaria* is generally absent from the peripheral blood. Skin snips may detect microfilaria in the tissues.

Onchocerciasis

1. Skin biopsies, excision of subcutaneous nodules or sclerocorneal punch biopsies are used for the detection of microfilariae or adult worms (Figs. 26.2a and 26.2b).

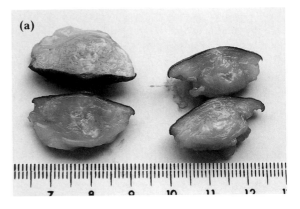

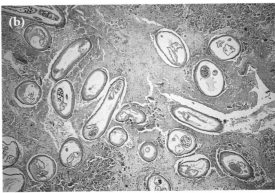

Figure 26.2 – Subcutaneous nodules (onchocercoma); (a) skin slices showing a conglomerate of nodules; (b) sections of several adult worms of Onchocerca (H&E × 200).

2. Slit lamp examination of the eye may reveal movement of microfilariae.
3. If microfilariae cannot be found, a small dose of diethyl carbamazine 50 mg can reactivate the microfilariae (Mazzotti test) and a skin snip will then be positive for microfilariae. Microfilariae of *O. volvulus* are rarely detected in the blood.

TREATMENT

Loiasis and *Mansonella perstans*

- Ivermectin 200 μg/kg as a single dose reduce the microfilaria load by 80–90%. It has no action on the adult worm (Richard-Lenoble *et al.* 1988) Since 1991 several cases with neurological manifestations including coma have been reported after ivermectin treatment of persons infected with *O. volvulus* who also had high microfilaria of *Loa loa* (Boussinesq *et al.* 1998).

- Diethylcarbamazine has been used in a test dose of 0.5–1 mg/kg on days 1 and 2, maximum dose 50 mg, then 2 mg/kg up to 100 mg twice daily on days 3–8. This drug is microfilaricidal; however, side-effects include fatal encephalitis (Carme *et al.* 1991). It crosses the blood–brain barrier and is toxic and contraindicated in renal disease. It can occasionally cause shock, collapse and exfoliative dermatitis. Diethylcarbamazine initially mobilizes and later kills microfilariae. Co-administration of prednisolone and use of cytapheresis to reduce microfilaraemia may reduce side-effects.

Onchocerciasis

The aim in management is to reduce the incidence of blindness by diminishing the quantity of microfilaria.

- Ivermectin (Mectizan) 150 mcg/kg is the drug of choice with a very high rate of reducing the microfilariae. It has only shown action against the adult worm and should be repeated at yearly and twice yearly intervals to suppress the microfilariae. Ivermectin acts as a GABA agonist and causes spastic paralysis of microfilariae and death. Other drugs with similar effects such as barbiturates and benzodiazepines should not be used together. The adult worm lives up to 15 years of which 30% die every year. Hence, the necessity to continue yearly doses. The use of Ivermectin has brought great benefit to patients infected with onchocerciasis and has brought this public health problem under control. It has been used on a large scale in Guatemala, under the auspices of the World Health Organisation. Ivermectin has the following actions: immediate killing of cutaneous microfilaria (Duke *et al.* 1992), prevents release of microfilariae from the uterus of adult females (Schulz-Key 1986), reduces the number of infective larvae stage available for the vector and reduction of both male and female adult worms in the nodules. When Ivermectin is used in multiple doses it acts as a macrofilaricidal.

Twice yearly treatment has been carried out on volunteers and 6 months after the second dose. Even highly infectious individuals were no longer able to serve as microfilarial donors to the vector *S. ochraceum*, the primary vector in Guatemala (Cupp 1992). During a 2-year study, there were significant reductions in eosinophils, IgG and IgE antibodies. The drug is contraindicated in pregnant women and in children < 5 years of age. Ivermectin given every 6 months controls troublesome itching (Ogbuagu and Eneanya 1998). Ivermectin treatment has a beneficial effect on onchocercal optic nerve disease and visual-field loss and reduction in blindness in endemic areas (Abiose 1998).

- Diethyl carbamazine has been used in the past but has side-effects such as hypotension and encephalopathy. Furthermore, it crosses the blood–brain barrier and exacerbates the eye lesions resulting in blindness (Mazzotti reaction). It is an effective microfilaricidal drug but has no effect on the adult worm.
- Surgical – nodule may be surgically excised from the head, particularly in children, reducing the risk and severity of ocular complication.

PREVENTION

Onchocerciasis

The WHO undertook to spray insecticides in 11 West African countries successfully preventing the breeding of the Simulium fly. The flies are usually found near rivers and streams. Different larvicides can be used when there is resistance to one particular larvicide.

REFERENCES

Abiose A. Onchocercal eye disease and the impact of mectizan treatment. *Annals Tropical Medical Parasitology* 1998; **(suppl.)**: S11–22

Boussinesq M, Gordon J, Gordon-Wendel N *et al.* Three probable cases of Loa loa encephalopathy following ivermectin treatment for onchocerciasis. *American Journal of Tropical Medicine and Hygiene* 1998; **58**: 461–469

Brieger WR, Awedoba AK, Eneanya CL *et al.* The effects of ivermectin on onchocercal skin disease and severe itching: results of a multicentre trial. *Tropical Medical International Health* 1998; **3**: 951–961

Carme B, Boulesteix J, Bento H. Five cases of encephalitis during treatment of loiasis with DEC. *American Journal of Tropical Medicine and Hygiene* 1991; **44**: 684–690

Cupp EW. Treatment of onchocerciasis with Ivermectin in Central America. *Parasitology Today* 1992; **8**: 212–214

Duke BOL, Zea-Flores J, Castro J *et al.* Effect of three month doses of Ivermectin on adult *Onchocerca volvulus*. *American Journal of Tropical Medicine and Hygiene* 1992; **46**: 189–192

Narita AS, Taylor HR. Blindness in the tropics. *Medical Journal of Australia* 1993; **159**: 416–420

Ogbuagu KF, Eneanya CI. A multicentre study of the effect of Mectizan (ivermectin) treatment on onchocercal skin disease: clinical findings. *American Tropical Medical Parasitology* 1998; **92**: 139–145

Pakasa NM, Nseka NM, Nyimi LM. Secondary collapsing glomerulopathy associated with Loa loa filariasis. *American Journal of Kidney Disease* 1997; **30**: 836–839

Petersen S, Ronne-Ras Mussen J, Basse P. Thrombosis of the ulnar veins – an unusual manifestation of Loa loa filariasis. *Scandinavian Journal of Infectious Diseases* 1998, **30**: 204–205

Richard-Lenoble, Kombila D, Rupp EA *et al.* Ivermectin in loiasis and concomitant *O. volvulus* and *M. perstans* infections. *American Journal of Tropical Medicine* 1988; **39**: 480–483

Schulz-Key H *et al.* Treatment of onchocerciasis with ivermectin in Central America. *Tropical Medical Parasitology* 1986; **37**: 89

Toure FS, Bain O, Nerrienet *et al.* Detection of Loa loa – specific DNA in blood from occult-infected individuals. *Experimental Parasitology* 1997; **86**: 163–170

World Health Organisation Expert Committee on Onchocerciasis. *3rd Report.* Geneva: World Health Organisation, 1987; 752: 1–167

III

General Features of Trematodes

Trematodes, also known as flukes, have conspicuous suckers. Only the digenetic trematodes infect humans. They are leaf-shaped and unsegmented. Both male and female genitalia are present in each worm, except for schistosomes. They have an oral and ventral sucker. They are oviparous. The eggs (except for schistosomes) are operculated. A body cavity is absent. The space between organs is filled with fluid and a connective tissue network. The digestive system consists of a pharynx, oesophagus leading to the bifurcated intestinal ceca or crura. The intestines may or may not be branched and may reunite to form a single caecum. The anus is absent.

The male reproductive system consists of two testes (except for schistosomes), two vasa efferentia, one vas deferens, seminal vesicle, cirrus and a prostate gland. The female genital system consists of a single ovary and its duct; two vitellaria (yolk glands) and their ducts; a vestigial vagina, seminal receptacle, uterus, ootype and Mehli's glands.

The sperms, ejaculated to the genital atrium, enter the female genital system where they self-fertilize. Cross-fertilization also occurs with sperms ejaculated into the genital pore entering the vestigial vagina (Laurer's canal) of another fluke.

The excretory system consists of flame cells and collecting tubules that drain to the bladder. The waste products are finally excreted through the excretory pore at the posterior end. The nervous system consists of two cephalic ganglia giving rise to three pairs of nerve trunks – dorsal, ventral and lateral. They are connected by numerous commissures.

The trematodes require one to two intermediate hosts to complete their life cycle. The first is a molluscan host, fresh, brackish water or land snails and the second is a fish, crab, crayfish or other snails

Ingesting infected fish, crab, crayfish, snail, ant or contaminated vegetation such as water chestnut or watercress infects the definitive host. The first-stage larva is a miracidium, which hatch out from the eggs in the water or inside the snail after ingestion.

In the snail it develops into a sporocyst, redia and a cercaria. The cercaria attacks a second intermediate host or attaches to vegetation encysting as metacercaria, which is the infective form.

Schistosomes directly invade the definitive host without having a metacercaria stage.

The trematodes of medical importance can be categorized into two main types. Those primarily parasitizing tissues and those parasitizing blood. The tissue trematodes are intestinal trematodes, e.g. *Fasciolopsis buski*, the liver flukes, e.g. *Fasciola hepatica*, *Clonorchis sinensis* and *Opisthorchis felineus*, and the lung fluke *Paragonimus westermani*. The blood trematodes parasitizing blood are the schistosomes of which four species parasitize man: *S. haematobium*, *S. japonicum*, *S. mansoni* and *S. mekongi*.

The clinical picture of trematode infection depends primarily on the size and number of worms, the organs or tissue involved and the degree to which the parasites, including the eggs invade or excyst in the tissue rather than in the intestine lumen or body cavities of the host. For example, Clonorchis or Opisthorchis occurring in small numbers in the biliary passages may not produce any tissue reaction. However, in moderate or large numbers, it may produce considerable local tissue reaction but the effect on the liver as a whole is not usually serious. Fasciola, on the other hand, because of its larger size and its location in the larger proximal biliary passages may cause profound damage. The changes produced in the host may be local, systemic or both. There can be ulceration or sloughing of tissue, abscess formation and accompanied by repair with fibrosis. Systemic manifestations are usually due to absorption of antigenic by-products of the worm. The worms cause the most damage themselves in the immediate area of tissue contact. This is particularly seen with schistosomes where damage to tissue is due to perivascular reaction to the blood-borne eggs. This response of the host tissue to the eggs is mainly responsible for the important clinical manifestations of schistosomiasis. The life cycle of schistosomes is different from the other trematodes because humans are infected by penetration of cercariae through intact skin rather than through injection of metacercariae. The cercariae in schistosomes have glands whose material is used to penetrate skin and a bifurcated tail that is lost when the cercariae penetrate the skin. Once they enter the host, the organism is termed a schistosomule. The latter migrates through the tissue and finally invades a blood vessel through where they can enter the lungs and liver. In the liver sinusoids, the worms mature into adults.

Adult *S. haematobium* is found primarily in the blood vessels of the bladder, prostate and uterine plexuses, whereas *S. mansoni* and *S. japonicum* are found in the inferior and superior mesenteric vessels. Clonorchis, Opisthorchis and Fasciola species are trematodes that parasitize the biliary ducts of humans. Clonorchis and Opisthorchis are narrow elongated worms that localize in the more distant, smaller ducts of the biliary tree, whereas, *Fasciola hepatica*, which is much larger, resides in the larger bile ducts and gallbladder. Paragonimus spp. encapsulate in the lungs but may occasionally be found in other tissues. The eggs, all of which are operculated, can be found in the faeces. Except for Paragonimus eggs, which are unembryonated, the others are embryonated when laid. The mature eggs either hatch in fresh water releasing a miracidium to infect the specific snail host or is ingested by the snail before liberating the miracidium; thus occurring in both Clonorchis and Opisthorchis species. Within the infected snail the parasites go through sporocyst, rediae stages before developing into cercariae which, when released, encyst to become metacercariae in fresh water fish in the case of Clonorchis and Opisthorchis, in crayfish or crabs in Paragonimus, or on fresh water plants in *Fasciola hepatica*. Humans become infected by ingesting the metacercariae in uncooked food.

Schistosomiasis

PARASITOLOGY

Schistosomiasis is also known as bilharziasis and was named after discoverer Theodor Maximillian Bilharz. Four species cause disease: *Schistosoma japonicum*, *S. mansoni*, *S. haematobium* and *S. mekongi*. *S. intercalatum* is of less importance compared with the other four species.

Occasionally infections of *S. intercalatum* and *S. mattheei* are reported from Africa. A closely related species to *S. japonicum* called *S. mekongi*, causing infection in humans, has recently been named. People bathing in fresh water in endemic areas are at risk (Elcuaz *et al.* 1998).

Schistosomiasis is prevalent in > 200 million people all over the world and endangers > 600 million (Bergquist 1995). Schistosomes are trematodes belonging to the phylum Platyhelminthes, family Schistosomatidae. They require an intermediate host to complete the life cycle. Apart from the differences

in the snail host and final habitat, the life cycle of different species is similar (Fig. 27.1).

Mature eggs passed in stools or urine hatch in water to become miracidium (free-swimming larva). The miracidium attacks the appropriate snail host and undergoes change to sporocyst and then to cercaria (1 day life span). After 1 month in the snail host, cercariae emerge, penetrate the skin of the final host. Cercariae detach their tails, become schistosomules and gain access to lymphatics or systemic circulation. The schistosomules then pass through right heart, pulmonary circulation, the left heart and finally enter the systemic circulation.

Sexes are separate. Female lies in the gyneacophoric canal of the male and depends on the male for transportation. Both sexes have two suckers, an oesophagus and a bifurcated intestine reuniting to form a blind caecum. Males have a primitive reproductive organ. The testes are behind the ventral sucker. The female has a

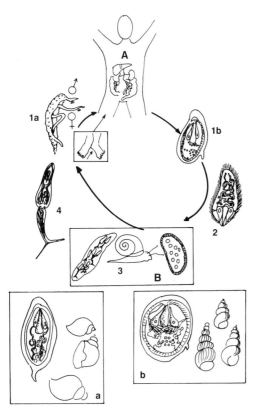

Figure 27.1 – Life cycle of schistosomiasis species. (A) Final host: man; site of the worms, the mesenteric vessels; (1a) sexually mature pair of flukes of *S. mansoni*; (b) mature egg of *S. mansoni* (lateral spine); (2) miracidium; (B) Intermediate host: aquatic snails; (3a) sporocyst of the first order (mother sporocyst); (b) sporocyst of the second order (daughter sporocyst); (2) free cercaria ('forked-tail cercaria').

single ovary, uterus and vulva leading to a genital pore near the ventral sucker. The stages in man are: a stage of invasion by the cercariae; a migration phase of the cercariae through the blood vessels to lungs and portal system; a maturation phase when the schistosomulae develop sexual maturity in the liver, intestines or bladder; and an oviposition stage when the adult schistosomes are engaged in the production of large numbers of eggs which is the cause of damage to host tissues. The adult worms do not cause any damage to the host.

Schistosoma haematobium

S. haematobium is common in the River Nile, the Middle East and many parts of India. *S. haematobium* eggs find their way into lumen of the urinary bladder. The adult worms of *S. haematobium* are found in the blood vessels of the urinary bladder, prostate and uterine plexus. Eggs

are laid in the small veins of these organs. However, eggs may be carried to the liver and other organs such as the brain, spinal cord and heart.

Schistosoma japonicum and Schistosoma mekongi

S. japonicum is confined to areas in the Far East, Japan, China, The Philippines and part of Indonesia and other small foci in Indonesia. *S. mekongi* was recently described and found along the Mekong River in South East Asia. The adult worms are found in the superior and inferior mesenteric veins. Eggs are laid in the small vessels of these organs and find their way into the intestines. Eggs of *S. japonicum* may lodge in the brain by passing through the anastomosis of the venous systems between the mesenteric and systemic veins. *S. japonicum* has a reservoir of hosts. Hence, *S. japonicum* is a true zoonosis in domesticated animals. The reservoir hosts contaminate the environment with ova.

Schistosoma mansoni

S. mansoni is widespread in the upper Sudan, East African Coast, Zambian River, South America and South Africa. The parasite matures and migrates to mesenteric or vesical veins and reach their final habitats.

PRESENTATION

The earliest manifestations are irritation at the site of entry of the cercaria. The 'cercarial itch' is due to an immune response and associated with minute haemorrhages that disappear in ~1–2 days. Cercarial itch occurs with all forms of schistosomiasis, although it is less common with *S. japonicum*.

During the period of migration, pulmonary symptoms are minimal. During the maturation period patients may develop 'Katayama' fever, which is like serum sickness, caused by immune complexes. The average time for appearance of symptoms is 27 days (Elucaz 1998) after the initial infection and is mostly seen with *S. japonicum* and to a milder extent in other forms of schistosomiasis. Katayama fever is associated with headache, rashes, lymphadenopathy, eosinophilia and dysentery, which may last for 1–2 months. It is not commonly seen in inhabitants of endemic areas.

Schistosoma haematobium

Following the stage of oviposition, the principal lesions occur in the wall of the urinary bladder. Patients present with terminal haematuria due to haemorrhage, ulceration and formation of bladder papillomata. Lesions can extend to the prostate, urethra and ureter. The symptoms are pain on micturition, with frequency and incontinence. During the fibrotic stage (Fig. 27.2) the bladder contracts and there is residual urine which is prone to infection where cystitis and pyuria can occur. Pulmonary involvement causes chronic cor pulmonale with symptoms such as cough, fatigue, haemoptysis and dyspnoea. Involvement of the brain and spinal cord can cause epilepsy and myelopathy respectively. The ultimate result of long-standing infection is chronic renal failure, renal calculi and calcification of bladder (sandy patches) (Fig. 27.3), beading of the ureters, ova and worms in uterus.

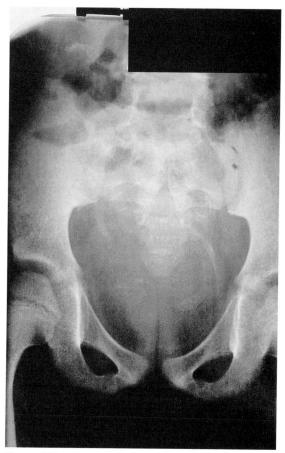

Figure 27.3 – X-ray of bladder showing calcification due to *S. hematobium*

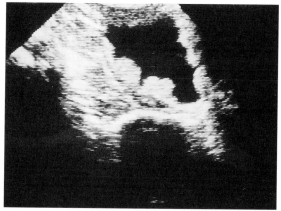

Figure 27.2 – Ultrasound of bladder showing echogenic bands of fibrosis due to schistosomiasis.

Bladder cancer

S. haematobium is associated with bladder cancers in Egypt. These cancers appear during the fourth or fifth decades. These cancers are squamous cell carcinomas with a preponderance in males. They, unlike the transitional cell carcinomas, are the most common type of bladder tumour in the Western developed world. To date, epidemiological and experimental studies confirm that there is a causal relationship between *S. haematobium* infection and bladder cancer in males (WHO 1994).

The pathogenesis of bladder cancer is related to high levels of volatile nitrosamines in schistosoma-infected Egyptian patients. It is predominantly found in *S. haematobium* infections. However, nitrosamine levels are also increased but to a lesser extent in *S. mansoni* infections. It is possible that *S. mansoni* may also play a part in multistage process of urinary schistosomiasis-associated bladder carcinogenesis (Mostapha 1994).

Bladder samples from patients with schistosomiasis-associated bladder cancer analysed for lesion O6-methyldeoxyguanosine, a promutogenic DNA agent, which was 96% versus 30–40% in the Egyptian cancer patients without schistosomiasis (Badawi 1992). Hence, alkylation damage in DNA of bladder tissue can be used as a surveillance for bladder cancer associated with schistosomiasis. This raises the possibility that antioxidants such as vitamin C and E may prevent increase in nitrosamine levels (Mostafa *et al.* 1995).

Schistosoma japonicum and *Schistosoma mekongi*

Katayama fever is more prominent with *S. japonicum* which is more severe since the female worm lays ten times more eggs than the female *S. mansoni*. Lung lesions are seen during incubation. The liver, spleen, small and large intestines are affected. Subsequently, cerebral lesions are not uncommon, presenting with Jacksonian fits. Untreated, the prognosis is bad as the disease runs a rapid course within 3–4 years, unlike *S. mansoni* where disease lasts > 30 years. *S. mekongi* is less pathogenic in comparison with *S. japonicum*. It causes hepatosplenic disease with portal hypertension. Partial immunity occurs to reinfection by *S. japonicum*.

Schistosoma mansoni

The oviposition phase affects the liver, colon and rectum. Patients present with abdominal symptoms in the form of pain and intermittent dysentery. Right lower quadrant abdominal pain is seen sometimes mimicking acute appendicitis. It is controversial whether the schistosomas cause appendicitis. Typical mucosal lesions may be demonstrated by colonoscopy. Hepatosplenomegaly is a characteristic feature and in the late stage biliary cirrhosis or 'pipe stem' fibrosis ensues with the patients developing ascites, portal hypertension and, finally, bleeding from oesophageal varices. Secondary pulmonary involvement may be seen with *S. mansoni* only after development of collateral circulation. Weakness and emaciation are more marked than in *S. haematobium*. Glomerulonephritis is a rare complication. Spinal cord involvement can occur causing myelopathy.

PATHOLOGY

Dermal schistosomiasis

Cercarial dermatitis is due to delayed hypersensitivity caused by cercarial metabolic products of the cercaria. There are granulomas and inflammatory cellular infiltrates around eggs. The Hoeppli phenomenon may be seen around the worms and eggs. This is an immune response of antigen–antibody complex deposition that is seen as radiating eosinophilic material, together with lymphocytes, histiocytes, plasma cells and giant cells in the infiltrate.

Later granulomatous inflammation is replaced by fibrosis, hyalinization and scar formation. Eggs are destroyed and calcified and gradually disappear. The living adult worm does not elicit any tissue response.

Intestinal schistosomiasis

Eggs and granulomatous inflammation are seen in the mucosa and submucosa of the intestines (Fig 27.4). Egg granulomas are seen in the subserosa and musculature. Superficial mucosal ulceration with underlying granulation tissue is seen in early stages. Adult worms can be occasionally seen in the mesenteric veins and venules of intestine and bladder. In the late stages there is thickening of the intestinal wall with induration and peritoneal and retroperitoneal fibrosis may develop.

Hepatosplenic schistosomiasis

Eggs with granuloma formation and portal fibrosis is seen in the liver (Fig. 27.5a,b) occurring more frequently in patients with HLA-A1 and B5 types. The eggs or their contents cause vasculitis and destruction of portal veins. With destruction of portal vein radicles, only bile ducts and hepatic arteries are seen in the portal tracts, a finding pathognomonic of schistosomiasis even in the absence of eggs. Lobular architecture is preserved as the pathologic changes are localized to the portal tracts – 'pipe stem fibrosis'.

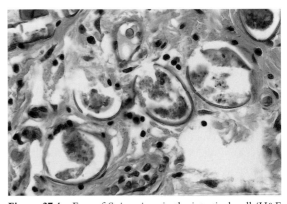

Figure 27.4 – Eggs of *S. japonicum* in the intestinal wall (H&E × 400).

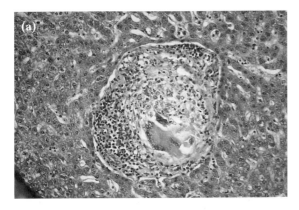

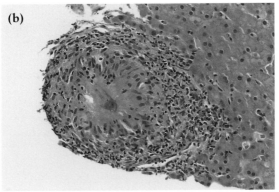

Figure 27.5 – (a) Egg granuloma of *S. japonicum* in the portal tract of liver (H&E × 200); (b) eosinophilic material with cellular infiltrate at periphery (H&E × 400).

Urogenital schistosomiasis

Eggs are most numerous in the bladder, ureters and seminal vesicles, although kidneys, urethra, prostate, spermatic cord, epididymis, testicle and penis may also be sites of egg deposition. Granulomatous inflammation and polypoid masses are found initially. These ulcerate and undergo fibrosis, followed by cicatrization, stricture and obstruction.

The urothelium may be hyperplastic with von Brunn's nests and may show mucinous columnar metaplasia, cystic degeneration or squamous metaplasia. In the late stages there is ulceration and atrophy. Calcified ova are seen throughout the atrophic epithelium giving rise to the 'sandy patches' seen at cystoscopy pathognomonic of schistosomiasis.

Schistosomal glomerulopathy

Schistosomal glomerulopathy has been described such as focal or diffuse axial, proliferative glomerulonephritis, exudative glomerulonephritis, mesangiocapillary glomerulonephritis with or without extramembranous deposits, focal and segmental sclerosis and finally amyloidosis. Response to treatment of schistosomiasis with regard to nephropathy is poor except for exudative glomerulonephritis.

Pulmonary schistosomiasis

The eggs provoke inflammatory destruction of arteriolar wall and occlude the lumen with granulomas. The inflammation causes thrombosis that heals with fibrosis, often occluding themselves.

The new vessels anastomose with the pulmonary veins, giving an angiomatoid appearance, which, in combination with endarteritis, is pathognomonic of pulmonary schistosomiasis. Granuloma may also be seen in the lung parenchyma. Fig. 27.6 shows pulmonary hypertension in chest x-ray.

Cerebral schistosomiasis

Meninges are frequently involved and the granulomatous reaction may be present as a space-occupying

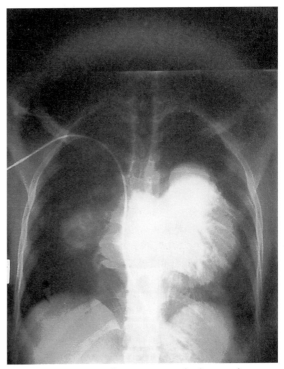

Figure 27.6 – Radiographic appearance of pulmonary hypertension with grossly dilated pulmonary artery in schistosomiasis.

lesion, Jacksonian epilepsy or cord compression – the latter when spinal medullary tissue is replaced by granulomas. Adult worms may be found in the meninges.

Renal schistosomiasis

Renal biopsy reveals mesoproliferative glomerulo-nephritis with focal mesangiocapillary change and the manifestations of cryoglobulinaemia. An auto-immune phenomenon has been attributed for the cryoglobulinaemia.

INVESTIGATIONS

1. Definitive diagnosis is made by identifying the presence of eggs in stool, urine or biopsy speci-mens. Eggs are large, non-operculated and contain the miracidium. *S. japonicum* is oval and has a small lateral knob. *S. haematobium* and *S. mansoni* are ellipsoid with haematobium having a terminal spine and mansoni lateral spine. *S. mekongi* ova are oval and minute lateral spine.

2. Schistosoma adult worms in tissue sections are characterized by a pair of worms in copula. As eggs may not be excreted it may be necessary to make the diagnosis by biopsy. Biopsy sites include rectal (high yield), bladder and liver.

3. Certain antigens associated with the gut of the adult worm, called circulating anodic antigen (CAA) and circulating cathodic antigen (CCA) may be detected by enzyme-linked immuno-sorbent assay (ELISA). This test has been a good method of diagnosing all species of schistosomia-sis (De Jong 1990, van Lieshout *et al.* 1993). The procedure is complex and needs a well-equipped laboratory.

4. Dot ELISA-type immunodiagnostic tests used in the diagnosis of several other parasitic diseases have been used for schistosomiasis. Circulating antigens and antibodies can be detected by this procedure. Detecting of antigens is preferred as it gives an index of active infection and worm burden.

5. For rapid and simple diagnosis of schistosomiasis a reagent strip assay for detection of circulating cathodic antigen in urine has been devised (van Etten *et al.* 1994). It is based on ELISA test using two anti-CAA monoclonal antibodies. It is a

good diagnostic tool for *S. mansoni* but is not a quantitative test. It can be used to assess the success of treatment.

6. White cell count for peripheral eosinophilia.

7. Cystoscopy – bladder mucosa shows calcification and papillary hyperplasia.

8. Urinary ultrasound and IV pyelogram may demonstrate obstructive uropathy.

9. Examination of ejaculates in males for *S. haemato-bium* eggs may be diagnostic when other investiga-tions are negative (Obel and Black 1994).

10. Liver function tests remain relatively normal till the end stage.

11. Liver ultrasound – changes may be minimal to thick echogenic bands of fibrous tissue extending to the lower capsule (Fig. 27.7) and marked thick-ening of gallbladder.

12. Renal biopsy if glomerulonephritis is suspected as in *S. mansoni*.

TREATMENT

- Praziquantel is the drug of choice for schistoso-miasis chemotherapy (Karanya *et al.* 1998). It is effective against all types of schistosome. Recommended dose 40 mg/kg given as a single dose or in divided doses on the same day. The drug is expensive and side-effects are uncom-mon at this dosage. However, higher doses may cause side-effects such as nausea, vomiting, vertigo, fever and ECG changes. There is usu-ally regression of the size of the spleen following treatment. Chemotherapy improves the prog-nosis even in the late stages of the disease. Persons with HIV-I infection can be treated effectively for schistosomiasis with Praziquantel (Karanya *et al.* 1998).

Hepatomegaly can be detected in 15% of pri-mary school children in some parts of Kenya with little evidence of morbidity and low preva-lence of portal hypertension and oesophageal varices. Chemotherapy given once every 3 years is sufficient to reduce the intensity of infection and hepatomegaly. School children living in areas of high prevalence and intensity of infec-tion with hepatosplenomegaly and demonstra-ble oesophageal varices, also respond to annual chemotherapy with very slow reduction of hepatosplenomegaly (Ouma 1992).

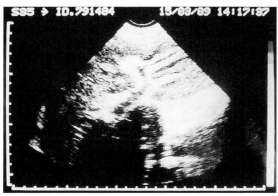

Figure 27.7 – Liver ultrasound to show echogenic bands due to marked fibrosis in liver in schistosomiasis.

PREVENTION

Provision of domestic water supply and health education is essential for the control of *S. mansoni* infection (Gryseels and Polderman 1992).

Travellers to endemic areas should be warned to take special precaution as no vaccine is available. One needs to keep away from fresh water lakes, dams, unless chlorinated and snail free. Wear high rubber boots if one needs to do any wading. If one has been exposed to infected water, it is essential to have a health check. Blood in urine or stools, fever, irritation of skin and general ill health are suggestions of infection.

Considerable reliance is now placed on community or selective chemotherapy with praziquantel. Attack of the intermediate host with molluscides is not effective for complete eradication. In China, in lake regions and marshlands, annual screening and treatment have had a significant impact on infection levels and morbidity, and community therapy has also been effective (Brindley *et al.* 1995).

Vaccines – there is no vaccine for the parasitic infection. A range of promising candidate vaccine antigens are currently undergoing independent testing and human trials will be the next step. Most schistosomiasis antigens initially identified were to *S. mansoni*. Similar developments in *S. haematobium* lag behind. However, *S. japonicum* cloned antigens have been produced (Waine *et al.* 1993). Research to candidate *S. japonicum* vaccine antigens has progressed rapidly. A number of cloned *S. japonicum* antigens are now available for testing in mice. Because of the reservoir host in *S. japonicum*, a bovine vaccine, if developed, would be the answer to control the infection. Research into

candidate *S. japonicum* vaccine antigen is in progress in China and the Philippines. Trials on rabbits have met with some success. Animal vaccination against *S. japonicum* is close to reality (Brindley *et al.* 1995).

Vaccination with radiation-attenuated *S. japonicum* cercariae in mice, rats, water buffaloes and rabbits have given a protection rate of 70–90% (Brindley *et al.* 1995).

REFERENCES

Badawi AF. PhD thesis, University of Alexandria, 1992

Bergquist NR. Controlling schistosomiasis by vaccination: a realistic option? *Parasitology Today* 1995; **11**: 191–193

Brindley PJ, Ramirez B, Wu G *et al.* Network in *Schistosoma japonicum*. *Parasitology Today* 1995; **11**: 163–165

De Jong N, Kremsner PG, Krigger FW *et al.* Detection of the schistosome circulating cathodic antigen by enzyme immunoassay using biotinylated monoclonal antibodies. *Transactions of the Royal Society of Tropical Medicine and Hygiene* 1990; **84**: 815–818

Elcuaz R, Armas M, Ramirez M. Outbreak of schistosomiasis in a group of travellers returning from Burkine Faso. *Enferm Infection of Clinical Microbiology* 1998; **16**: 367–369

Gryseels B, Polderman AM. Morbidity in *Schistosomiasis mansoni*. *Parasitology Today* 1992; **8**: 55–56

Karanya DM, Boyer AE, Strand M *et al.* Studies on schistosomiasis in Western Kenya: efficacy of praziquantel for treatment of schistosomiasis in persons co-infected with human immunodeficiency virus 1. *American Journal of Tropical Medicine and Hygiene* 1998; **59**: 307–311

Mostapha MH. Nitrate, nitrite and volatile N-nitroso compounds in the urine of *Schistosoma haematobium* and *Schistosoma mansoni* infected patients. *Carcinogenesis* 1994; **15**: 619–625

Mostafa MH, Badawi AF, O'Conner PH. Bladder cancer associated with schistosomiasis. *Parasitology Today* 1995; **11**: 87–89

Obel N, Black FT. Diagnosis of *Schistosoma haematobium* infection by examination of sperm. *Scandinavian Journal of Infectious Diseases* 1994; **26**: 117–118

Ouma JH, Mbugua GG, Butterworth AE. Morbidity in *Schistosomiasis mansoni. Parasitology Today* 1992; **8**: 55

Van Etten L, Folman CC, Eggette TA *et al.* Rapid diagnosis of schistosomiasis by antigen detection in urine with a reagent strip. *Journal of Clinical Microbiology* 1994; **32**: 2404–2406

Van Lieshout L, De Jong N, Mansour MM *et al.* Circulating cathodic antigen levels in serum and urine of schistosomiasis patients before and after chemotherapy with praziquantel. *Transactions of the Royal Society of Tropical Medicine and Hygiene* 1993; **87**: 311–312

Waine GJ, Becker M, Yang W *et al.* Cloning, molecular characterisation and functional activity of *Schistosoma japonicum* glyceraldehyde 3-phosphate dehydrogenase, a putative vaccine against *Schistosoma japonicum. Infection Immunology (United States)* 1993; **61**: 4716–4723

World Health Organisation. *Schistosomes, Liver Flukes and Helicobacter pylori.* IARC Monographs on the Evaluation of Carcinogenetic Risk to Humans, vol. 61. Geneva: World Health Organisation, 1994

28

Clonorchiasis and Opisthorchiasis

Parasitology
Presentation
   Complications
Pathology

Investigations
Treatment
Prevention
References

PARASITOLOGY

Clonorchiasis is caused by the trematode *Clonorchis sinensis* and opisthorchiasis by trematode *Opisthorchis viverrini* and *O. felineus*. Clonorchiasis is endemic in Vietnam, Japan, Korea, China and Hong Kong. *O. viverrini* is found predominantly in North East Thailand and Laos where several million people are infected. *O. felineus* infection is seen mainly in Russia and Europe. Man is infected by eating undercooked or raw fish harbouring infective metacercariae. In Thailand babies are fed raw fish mixed with other food items such as 'Koi-Pla' and may become infected as early as 3 months of age (Harinasutu 1969). The adult worm of *C. sinensis* is 10–20 × 4 mm, *O. viverrini* 6–10 × 1.2 mm, *O. felineus* 7–12 × 2 mm. They all have an oral sucker, a pharynx, which divides into two blind ceca and a coiled uterus and branched testis, ovary and seminal receptacle may be identified.

The eggs of *C. sinensis* are very small, measuring 30 × 16 × 16 μm and are operculated and with characteristic shoulders (Fig. 28.1). Opisthorchis eggs differ from *Clonorchis* eggs in their size but are very similar otherwise.

The eggs passed in faeces are ingested by an appropriate freshwater snail host specific for different species of the trematode. The egg develops through various stages: sporocyst, redia and cercaria. The mature cercaria passes out of the snail into the water. They attack the second host, which is a fresh water fish and > 100 species of fish have been identified to be secondary hosts. Crayfish has also been implicated in China as a second intermediate host. The cercariae penetrate the skin of the fish and encyst in the flesh. When man consumes raw or partially cooked fish, the encysted metacercaria ex-cyst in the duodenum and enter the common bile duct and its branches to develop into adult worms. The life cycles of both species are very similar. The life span of *Clonorchis* is 20–30 years (Fig. 28.2).

PRESENTATION

The clinical manifestations are similar in both Clonorchis and Opisthorchis infections. The features depend on the worm load, the duration of infection and complications. In mild infections patients are asymptomatic. In very heavy infections, patients may

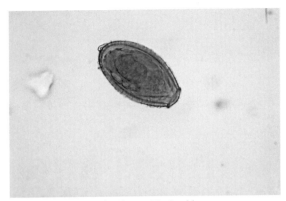

Figure 28.1 – Operculated egg with shoulder.

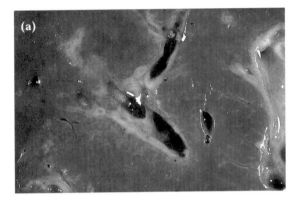

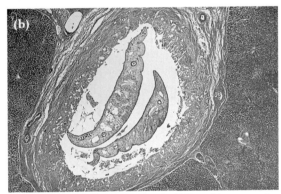

Figure 28.3 – Adult *clonorchis* worms in (a) liver; (b) cross-section of worms in bile duct (H&E × 20).

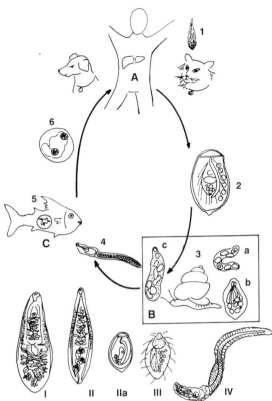

Figure 28.2 – Life cycle of *Clonorchis sinensis*. (A) (1) Final host: man and also the cat and dog (as well as household and farm animals); (2) sexually mature liver fluke; (3) egg (with miracidium) of *C. sinensis*. (B) (1) Intermediate host: snails of the genus *Bulimus*; (3a) young sporocyst; (b) mother redia; (c) daughter redia with rudiments of cercariae – cercariae that have become free. (C) (1) Intermediate host: chiefly fish with cercariae and metacercariae. (I) *C. sinensis*; (II) *O. felineus*; (a) egg of *O. felineus* with miracidium; (III) free miracidium from a snail; (IV) cercaria as it typically appears when it is swimming.

(Laik *et al.* 1968). Pulmonary hypertension is caused by micro-embolism of pulmonary vessels by necrotic tissue from the liver (Tchuikova and Pokrovski 1998).

PATHOLOGY

The fluke causes damage to the biliary tract as a result of immunological reaction, mechanical obstruction (Fig 28.3) and inflammation evoked by chemical products of the fluke. There is development of adenomatous hyperplasia of bile duct epithelium with goblet cell metaplasia. After a long period, the hyperplastic tissue is replaced by fibrous tissue, producing thickened and dilated intrahepatic ducts. The eggs are destroyed by inflammation and a granulomatous reaction occurs in

present with non-specific acute symptoms such as epigastric discomfort, fever with chills, hepatomegaly, splenomegaly and eosinophilia.

Complications

Several complications have been reported, such as sepsis, ascending cholangitis, acute pancreatitis, chronic cholecystitis, cholangiocarcinoma and polyarthritis the hepatic parenchyma, gallbladder and along the portal tracts, resulting in periductal fibrosis. The final result is biliary cirrhosis and portal hypertension. In prolonged infection, there is an increased risk of cholangiocarcinoma, but not hepatocellular carcinoma (Schwartz 1980). The carcinoma is multicentric and frequently around the parasitized bile ducts. *O. viverrini* is also a cause of cholangiocarcinoma. Early recognition of biliary hyperplasia and treatment of clonorchis sinensis is important to prevent development of cholangiocarcinoma especially in the far East (Kim *et al.* 1999).

INVESTIGATIONS

1. Demonstration of eggs in faeces, the number of which gives an index of the severity of the infection and worm burden (Elkins *et al.* 1991). A count of > 10 000 eggs/g faeces indicates heavy infection. Ova excretion is delayed for ~4–6 weeks from the time of infection. These eggs should be differentiated from *Fasciola hepatica* eggs, which are the largest operculated eggs, and *Fasciolopsis buski*, the largest intestinal fluke.
2. Duodenal aspirate is an alternative way of looking for the ova.
3. A blood count for eosinophilia is indicated.
4. Cystatin capture enzyme-linked immunosorbent assay (ELISA) for immunodiagnosis of human fascioliasis has good sensitivity and high specificity (Ikeda 1998).
5. Liver function tests, serum amylase.
6. Ultrasonography can define the extent of damage as well as the reversibility of some of the pathology after adequate treatment. Ultrasonography can define the size of the liver, gallbladder, presence of gallbladder sludge or stones, the thickness of the gallbladder wall, thickness of the portal vein radicals, suspicious malignant lesions and strictures. Ultrasonography is also useful to assess response to treatment (Mairiang *et al.* 1993). However, recent reports among egg positives shows sonography positive rate was 49.6% (Hong *et al.* 1998).
7. Although sonography, CT and direct cholangiography have been used traditionally to diagnose intrahepatic cholangiocarcinoma, magnetic resonance imaging has shown dramatic progress (Choi *et al.* 1998).

TREATMENT

- Praziquantel has revolutionized the treatment of trematode infections as a whole. The recommended dose is 40 mg/kg body weight as a single dose or in three divided doses in 1 day. This drug is rapidly absorbed from the gastrointestinal tract and is metabolized in the liver, the metabolites being excreted in the urine. Praziquantel is generally free of side-effects; however, high doses may cause nausea, vomiting, headaches, fever, seizures and ECG changes. In case of treatment failure, repeating the dose may be effective. Egg counts following the treatment after a few weeks will give a measure of the success. Repeated treatment for fresh infections may enhance immune response to parasite antigens and accelerate the pathologic changes. Surgery may be required for complications such as cholangiocarcinoma, gall stones, chronic cholecystitis.

PREVENTION

The life cycle of these flukes can be interrupted and infection prevented if all fresh water fish is adequately cooked. Night soil should be disinfected if used as fertilizers near lakes or ponds containing the secondary hosts, the snails. There should be stool examination and treatment of positive cases with Praziquantel to eliminate host reservoir and hygienic disposal of faeces to ensure interruption of transmission (Jongsuksuntigul *et al.* 1998).

REFERENCES

Choi BI, Kim TK, Han JK. MRI of clonorchiasis and cholangiocarcinoma. *Journal of Magnetic Resonance Imaging* 1998; **2**: 359–366

Elkins DB, Sithithaworn P, Haswell-Elkins MR *et al. Opisthorchis viverrini*. Relationship between egg counts, worms recovered and antibody levels within an endemic community in N.E. Thailand. *Parasitology* 1991; **102**: 283–288

Harinasutu C. Opisthorchiasis in Thailand. In *Proceedings of the 4th S.E. Asian Seminar on Parasitology and Tropical Medicine*. Bangkok: SEAMEC Centre Co-ordinating Board for Tropical Medicine and Public Health, 1969, 253–264

Hong ST, Yoon K, Lee M *et al.* Control of clonorchiasis by repeated praziquantel treatment and low diagnostic efficacy of sonography. *Korean Journal of Parasitology* 1998; **36**: 249–254

Ikeda T. Cystatin capture enzyme-linked immunosorbent assay for immunodiagnosis of human paragonimiasis and fascioliasis. *American Journal of Tropical Medicine and Hygiene* 1998; **2**: 286–290

Jongsuksuntigul P, Imsomboon T. Epidemiology of opisthorchiasis and national central program in Thailand. *Southeast Asian Journal of Tropical Medicine and Public Health* 1998; **29**: 327–332

Kim KH, Kim CD, Lee HS *et al.* Biliary papillary hyperplasis with clonorchiasis resembling cholangiocarcinoma. *American Journal of Gastroenterology* 1999; **94**: 514–517

Laik S, McFadjean AJS, Yeung R. Microembolic pulmonary hypertension in pyogenic cholangitis. *British Medical Journal* 1968; **1**: 22–24

Mairiang E, Haswell-Elkins MR, Mairiang P *et al.* Reversal of biliary tract abnormalities associated with *Opisthorchis viverrini* infection following praziquantel treatment. *Transactions of the Royal Society of Tropical Medicine and Hygiene* 1993; **87**: 194–197

Schwartz DA. Helminths in the induction of cancer. *Opisthorchis viverrini* and *Clonorchis sinensis* and cholangiocarcinoma. *Tropical Geographical Medicine* 1980; **32**: 95

Tchuikova K, Pokrovski V. Clinical and immune peculiarities of pseudo tuberculous polyarthritis against a background of chronic opisthorchiasis. *British Journal of Rheumatology* 1998; **37**: 341–342

29

Fascioliasis

Parasitology
Presentation
Pathology
Investigations

Treatment
Prevention
Illustrative Case
References

PARASITOLOGY

Fascioliasis is caused by the liver flukes *Fasciola hepatica* and less commonly *F. gigantica*. *F. hepatica,* commonly known as liver rot, can also be found in goats, cattle, horses and camels. It is primarily a zoonotic disease.

The disease is endemic in Australia (Porciv 1992, Price *et al.* 1993), China, Africa, South America and Puerto Rico. Man is infected by ingesting the metacercariae in contaminated aquatic plants such as watercress, dandelions growing in natural state and 'pakboung' (Asian water morning glory). Metacercariae are encysted cercariae, originating from the snail of the genus *Lymnaea tomentosa*, which is the intermediate host. *Lymnaea columella*, which originated from North America, has also been reported to play a part in transmission. More recently the tropical snail *L. viridis* has been found in the waterways of South East Queensland, Australia, and it appears to be a suitable intermediate host for the local strain of *F. hepatica*.

The adult worm, which is leaf shaped, measures 20–75 mm in length and 8–20 mm in width, with an anterior conical projection called the cephalic cone, which helps to distinguish it from *Fasciolopsis buski*. The spiny surface or tegument is another characteristic of this species. It has branched testes as well as an ovary and uterus. The ventral sucker is more prominent than the oral sucker (Fig 29.1). Most of the worm is occupied by a pair of branched ceca and vitellaria. The fasciola eggs hatch in water and are operculated, each egg measuring $130–140 \times 80–85 \ \mu m$ (Fig. 29.2). The free-swimming miracidia attack a suitable amphibious or aquatic snail host in which they pass through sporocyst, redia and cercaria stages. The cercariae, when they exit from the snail host, attach themselves to fresh water vegetation such as watercress and become encysted metacercariae. When man consumes uncooked water vegetation, often prepared as a green salad, infection occurs. When metacercariae excyst in the duodenum they penetrate the wall of the intestine and migrate through the abdominal cavity to the liver. The young flukes reach the intrahepatic bile ducts 7 weeks after initial infection and mature to adults in 3–4 months. Adult worms may live up to 9 years in the bile ducts, producing eggs that are carried by bile into the intestinal lumen and passed in faeces.

PRESENTATION

The incubation period is 10–16 weeks. *F. hepatica* in man has three distinct phases: hepatic, biliary and, occasionally, ectopic. There may be a latent period of 4–6

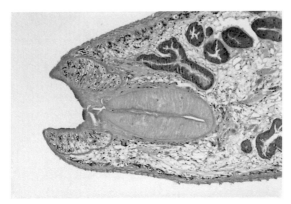

Figure 29.1 – Adult worm of Fasciola.

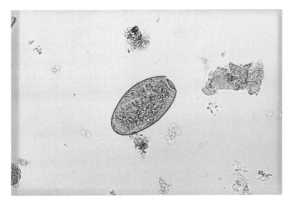

Figure 29.2 – Operculated egg of Fasciola.

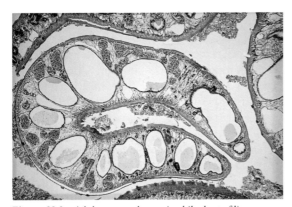

Figure 29.3 – Adult worms obstructing bile duct of liver.

weeks between the hepatic and biliary phases. However, there is no latent period if infection is recurrent.

1. Hepatic phase – during this phase, which lasts 1–3 months, the encysted metacercaria perforates the liver capsule and migrates through the liver parenchyma. Patients present with pain in the right hypochondrium, radiating to the right shoulder with fever and hepatomegaly, myalgia, arthralgia, nausea and headache. Eosinophilia is a characteristic feature. Severe subcapsular haemorrhage and frank hepatic necrosis may rarely complicate this stage. The presentation is similar to most forms of hepatitis. At this stage there are no ova in the stools.

2. Biliary phase – the final resting place of the worm is the biliary tract. During this phase the symptoms and signs are pain in the right hypochondrium, jaundice, hepatomegaly, eosinophilia and fever. The clinical picture is similar to cholestasis or ascending cholangitis. Bacterial cholangitis often plays a dominant role in the clinical course of the disease (Carpenter 1998).

3 Ectopic phase – juvenile flukes may show aberrant migration and end up in other sites such as the abdominal wall, pancreas, stomach, appendix, caecum, peritoneum, spleen, blood vessels, skeletal muscles, orbit, brain, lungs and epididymis. There is documented migration to a cervical lymph node and subcutaneous tissue (Price *et al.* 1993). Many flukes do not survive unless they reach the biliary system. The flukes in ectopic sites produce granulomatous nodules and may be calcified.

In Lebanon a condition called 'halzoun' has been described, probably being the result of an allergic nasopharyngitis to the larval flukes eaten with raw sheep or goat liver. The infected may die of suffocation.

PATHOLOGY

In the acute stages, there is tissue destruction with coagulative necrosis of liver cells and formation of abscess, patchy haemorrhages and reactive fibrosis. Microscopically, these lesions show necrosis with tissue debris, neutrophils, eosinophils, Charcot-Leyden crystals and occasional parasite eggs. Granulomata with multinucleated giant cells and histiocytes appear later on. Occasionally granulation tissue and regenerated liver cells and fibrosis can be seen in the tract caused by the parasite. Chronic infection with the parasite shows pathological changes mainly in the biliary system and gallbladder. The bile ducts are dilated and thickened and frequently contain the adult worms, occasionally completely obstructing the common bile duct (Fig 29.3). On microscopic examination, adenomatous hyperplasia of the ductal epithelium and proliferation of bile ducts is seen. Focal necrosis of liver cells with chronic inflammation, cholestasis, periportal fibrosis and hyperplasia of Kupffer cells may also be present. Multi-organ infection with *F. hepatica* is uncommon. However, severe infection can cause liver and peritoneal injuries with haemorrhagic ascites as well as pulmonary, pericardial, splenic and portal system disease (Montembault *et al.* 1997). The gallbladder may contain gallstones, fibrosis, empyema and adult worms. In cross-section the parasite resembles other flukes like Clonorchis and Opisthorchis but the presence of the cuticular spines and multiple cross-sections of the branching caecum are diagnostic features.

INVESTIGATIONS

In the biliary phase, the diagnosis may be confused with biliary obstruction due to stone, pancreatic carcinoma or cholangiocarcinoma with ascending cholangitis. However, eosinophilia in such patients should point to a parasitic infection. Several diagnostic procedures are available.

1. Examination of stool – definitive diagnosis is made by demonstration of the eggs in faeces but eggs may not always be found because the worms can be infertile or be located in ectopic sites. If eggs are scanty, biliary and duodenal drainage may be necessary for their detection. Biliary aspiration may be performed after administration of IV cholecystokinin (Gomez-Cerezo 1998).

   The Ninhydrin method of filtration is a sensitive test for ova. *F. hepatica* eggs are of the largest operculated eggs and show an indistinct operculum, which is filled with yolk cells. The eggs resemble those of *F. buski*. Multiple stool examinations are needed.

2. Serodiagnosis – this technique has improved over the years and is sufficiently specific to be a reliable routine test. It has been used in endemic areas and is especially useful in acute disease before the appearance of the eggs in stools which takes 6 to 8 weeks.

   ELISA test for fasciola is both sensitive and a quantitative test which detects antibody to excretory-secretory (ES) antigen from the adult *F. hepatica*. It is also a marker for successful treatment of *F. hepatica*. DOT-ELISA has been reported to have a 100% sensitivity and 97.8% specificity, allowing rapid diagnosis of human fascioliasis (Shahem *et al.* 1989). Cross-reactivity to schistosome has been noted. An ultra-micro-ELISA for detection of IgG

antibodies, anti-excretory-secreting antigens of *F. hepatica* has a sensitivity of 100% and specificity of 98% and cross-reactivity was shown only with *Opisthorchis felinus* (Epsino *et al.* 1997). ES 78 sandwich ELISA for eggs and parasite coproantigens and an indirect ELISA for circulating antigens and antibodies are available (Espino *et al.* 1998).

3. CT scans showing hepatic lesions suggestive of small hepatic abscesses with a subcapsular haematoma and thickening of the liver capsule may be detected by CT scan (van Beers *et al.* 1990). Parenchymal calcification may be seen as with other granulomas.

4. Sonographic investigations are very useful in the biliary stage of the disease. Irregular linear echogenic image of the fluke can be demonstrated in the biliary stage of the infection.

5. Radionuclear scanning – liver scans with ^{99m}TC or ^{198}AU may demonstrate cold areas in the acute phase.

6. Percutaneous cholangiography and endoscopic retrograde percutaneous cholangiography have demonstrated filling defects in the biliary tracts.

7. Excision biopsy of nodules – excised cutaneous nodules have been reported to reveal severe eosinophilic granulomatous lesions with foci of vasculitis and necrosis as well as the mature worm (Porciv *et al.* 1992).

TREATMENT

- Triclabendazole, which is used in veterinary medicine, has been suggested to be the agent of choice (Yilmaz 1998)
- It may be used in children and in adults. A single oral dose of 10 mg/kg given postprandial – monitor eggs in stools after 2 months. If eggs are present repeat the dose
- Complications such as ascending cholangitis should be treated with antibiotics and surgery for biliary obstruction

PREVENTION

This infection can be prevented by not consuming aquatic plants, especially watercress, by boiling drinking water in endemic areas and by thoroughly cooking sheep and goat liver. Molluscicides should be employed and sheep pastures should have proper drainage.

ILLUSTRATIVE CASE

A 39-year-old man presented with three skin nodules, the largest situated on the right chest wall, thought clinically to be sebaceous cysts. The patient worked in a slaughter house in Brisbane, Australia. The incision biopsy consisted of five greyish brown fragments, the largest 5 mm in dimension. Microscopically, one of the fragments appeared to be a larval nematode. No hooklet or scolices were observed.

A haematoxylin and eosin stained section showed a trematode 5 × 1.5 mm. The tegument contained spines of varying size and distribution. An oral sucker and a ventral sucker (acetabulum) were identifiable. The highly branched caecum extended to the posterior end of the worm. Vitellaria were present laterally and extended from the ventral sucker to the posterior end. Testes and branched ovary were not clearly discernible. No scolices or hooklets (as seen in cysticercoses) were present. The overall features were consistent with that of an adult liver fluke *F. hepatica*.

REFERENCES

Carpenter HA. Bacterial and parasitic cholangitis. *Mayo Clinic Proceedings* 1998; **73**: 473–478

Epsino AM, Padzon L, Dumemigo B *et al*. Indirect ultra-micro ELISA for detecting IgG antibodies in patients with fascioliasis. *Review Cubana Medica Tropica* 1997; **49**: 167–173

Espino AM, Diaz A, Perez *et al*. Dynamics of antigenema and coproantigens during human *Fasciola hepatica* outbreak. *Journal of Clinical Microbiology* 1998; **36**: 2723–2726

Gomez-Cerezo J, Rios-Blanco JJ, de Guevara CL *et al*. Biliary aspiration after administration of intravenous cholecystokinesis for the diagnosis of hepatobiliary fascioliasis. *Clinical Infectious Diseases* 1998; **26**: 1009–1010

Montembault S, Serfaty L, Pocrob SL *et al*. Haemorrhagic ascites disclosing massive *Fasciola hepatica* infection. *Gastroenterology Clinical Biology* 1997; **21**: 785–788

Porciv P, Walker C, Whitby M. Human ectopic fascioliasis in Australia. First case reports. *Medical Journal of Australia* 1992; **156**: 349–351

Price TA, Tuazon CV, Simon GL. Fascioliasis: case reports and review. *Clinical Infectious Diseases* 1993; **17**: 426–430

Shahem HI, Kamel KA, Fand Z *et al*. DOT enzyme linked immunosorbent assay DOT ELISA for the rapid diagnosis of human fascioliasis. *Journal of Parasitology* 1989; **75**: 549–552

Van Beers B, Pringot J, Gubel A *et al*. Hepatobiliary fascioliasis: non-invasive image finding. *Radiology* 1990; **174**: 809–810

Yilmaz H, Ones AF, Akdeniz H. The effect of triclabendazole (Fasinex) in children with fasciolosis. *Journal of Egyptian Society of Parasitology* 1998; **28**: 497–502

Paragonimiasis

PARASITOLOGY

This is a disease caused by the lung fluke Paragonimus, the major species being *P. westermani*. Five other species have recently been incriminated as human pathogens.

Man is infected by eating fresh water crabs, which are raw or undercooked. All organs of the crab can harbour the encysted metacercariae. Human infection is caused by *P. westermani* in the Far East, South East Asia, Papua New Guinea, Pacific Area, China and the Indian Subcontinent. The parasite also infects domestic and wild animals such as dogs, cats, pigs and foxes. The appropriate snail host varies according to the locality and must be available for the transmission of the disease. On both American continents, *P. mexicanus* commonly infects humans. Very rarely *P. kellicotti* can cause infection in the USA. Over 28 species of Paragonimus has been identified worldwide.

The adult worm is plump oval shaped and reddish brown in colour with a rounded anterior end and tapering posterior end, measuring 7.5–12 mm in length, 4–6 mm in breadth and 3.5–5 mm thick. The cuticle or tegument is covered with scale-like spines. There are two suckers, oral and ventral. The ventral sucker is situated slightly anterior to the middle of the worm. The most prominent structure is the pair of blind-ended intestinal caeca. The testes are lobulated and situated posteriorly. The uterus and ovaries are in the mid-portion and the vitellarian glands laterally. The excretory bladder is long and tortuous and extends from the posterior end to the pharynx.

The eggs are ovoid, yellow-brown, thick-shelled with a flattened operculum and measure 80–120 × 45–65 µm. They mature in water within 2 weeks if conditions are favourable. The free-swimming ciliated miracidium hatch out and invade appropriate fresh water snail hosts to multiply and develop and go through the stages of sporocyst, redia and cercariae. Crab and crayfish are second intermediate hosts in which the cercariae develop into encysted metacercariae. Death of infected crustaceans may release metacercaria into sources of drinking water.

Man acquires infection by ingesting raw or undercooked crustacea (Fig. 30.1; refer to life cycle). Metacercariae escape into the duodenum, penetrate the wall and migrate through the abdominal cavity, diaphragm, pleural cavity and reach the lungs. In 6–8 weeks they attain maturity in the lungs. Occasionally the parasites can arrest at any point in this migratory

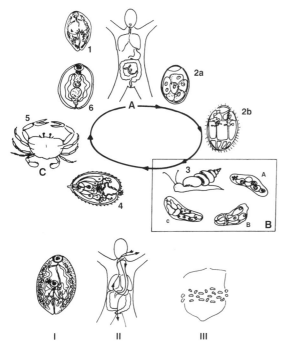

Figure 30.1 – Life cycle of paragonimus. (A) Final host: man; (1) sexually mature lung fluke; (2a) freshly laid egg (egg cell with yolk cells); (2b) a miracidium that has emerged. (B) (1) Intermediate host: aquatic snails; (3a) sporocyst; (3b) mother redia; (3c) daughter redia and free cercaria. (C) (2) Intermediate host: crabs and crayfish; (4) crab with furry chelae and metacercaria from the muscles of a crab. (I) Sexually mature lung fluke; (II) migration route of the young lung fluke in the gastrointestinal canal; (III) heart of a crab infected with metacercariae.

route and develop ectopic parasitism. In endemic areas many mammals serve as reservoir hosts and maintain the life cycle of the fluke. Eggs may be passed in the stools after rupture of the cysts or abscesses in the intestines.

PRESENTATION

The incubation period is 2–20 days.

Lung paragonimiasis

Little damage is done during the migration of the adult worm from the small intestine to the lung. In the lung, there may be mild inflammation and fibrosis that may communicate with bronchioles leading to secondary bacterial infection. Such patients may present with non-specific pulmonary symptoms such as chronic cough with bloodstained or gelatinous expectorant.

Subsequently, the patient develops shortness of breath and pleuritic chest pain. Secondary bacterial infections can result in lung abscesses, pneumonia, atelectasis, pneumothorax and pleural effusions. It may mimic pulmonary tuberculosis, and should be differentiated from other causes of lung abscesses and chronic bronchiectasis. Untreated pulmonary infection can lead to bronchiectasis. Occasionally, haemoptysis can be very severe when cysts rupture into bronchi.

X-ray of the chest may be normal in the disease or may show ill-defined pulmonary infiltrates and opacities of varying size. Later cysts, cavities, ring shadows, extensive infiltration, pleural thickening and effusions may be seen. Extensive fibrosis, bronchiectatic changes and calcification may make distinction from pulmonary tuberculosis difficult.

Extrapulmonary paragonimiasis

The migratory larvae can end up in any organ including the brain and spinal cord. The brain is a common ectopic site and cerebral paragonimiasis is common in the younger age group. Symptoms include Jacksonian-type fits, headaches and localizing signs depending on the anatomic site of involvement. Abdominal paragonimiasis can present with bloody diarrhoea, nausea and vomiting. Abscesses may also be found in the liver, spleen and abdominal cavity (Kim *et al.* 1999). Subcutaneous nodules are another manifestation of extrapulmonary paragonimiasis. These nodules measure 3–6 cm in diameter and can be found in the abdominal wall, thigh, behind the ear, head and the inguinal region. Involvement of the scrotal sac can mimic an irreducible hernia.

Differential diagnosis

Pulmonary lesions could mimic pulmonary tuberculosis, bacterial abscesses and neoplasms. Cerebral lesions should be distinguished from eosinophilic meningitis caused by Angiostrongylus, Gnathostomiasis and Cysticercosis. Tuberculus meningitis should also be considered. Skin lesions should exclude cutaneous larva migrans such as Loa loa, Onchocerciasis, Sparganosis and Gnathostomiasis. Abdominal symptoms such as diarrhoea with pain may mimic amoebiasis and malignancy. Rupture of abdominal viscera can produce an acute abdomen.

PATHOLOGY

The major pathology is seen in the lungs where the parasite is found in the pulmonary parenchyma in a subpleural location or near bronchioles. At times it can be seen within the bronchial walls causing bronchiectasis. Macroscopically, the lungs show oval mass lesions varying from 10 to 30 mm, pale yellow to reddish brown in colour. Microscopically, in the early stages, the adult worms are surrounded by an exudate of eosinophils and neutrophils. Later a fibrous cyst wall or capsule forms (Meyers and Neaffie 1976). The cyst contents consist of the worm with ova, necrotic tissue, Charcot Leyden crystals and inflammatory exudate that stains brown due to presence of haematin from haemorrhage.

When eggs enter alveoli they may become covered with eosinophilic material which can obscure the eggs, an appearance similar to corpora amylacea. Eggs can also stimulate formation of granulomas and foreign body giant cell reaction. These lesions can calcify or ossify. Pleural effusions show eosinophilia. The pathologic changes in the brain are similar to the lung lesions except that the cyst wall is thin and adult worms are rarely found (Higashi et al. 1971). There is liquefactive necrosis of brain tissue often with lysis of the worms. Granulomas with gliosis and calcification occur at a later stage.

INVESTIGATIONS

1. Ova may be found in sputum, stools, pleural fluid and cerebrospinal fluid.
2. Biopsy of subcutaneous nodules may demonstrate the adult worm.
3. Bronchial washings may demonstrate ova.
4. Counter current immuno-electrophoresis is the most satisfactory serological method of diagnosis. It can be used as a marker of the successful treatment as the test becomes negative in 6–8 months with eradication of the infection.
5. Peripheral eosinophilia associated with the infection.
6. Magnetic resonance imaging has been used as a diagnostic tool in various organs (Kim et al. 1999).

7. Genetic probes that have been developed are claimed to be as good or better than microscopic examination (Maleewong 1997).

TREATMENT

- Praziquantel – recommended dose is 25 mg/kg three times daily for 3 days, which achieves a cure rate of 95%
- Corticosteroids are recommended along with definitive treatment for cerebral paragonimiasis as there may be an exacerbation of symptoms
- Triclabendazole is an alternative drug of choice 5 mg once daily for 3 days. It is as effective as praziquantel in clearing infections and better tolerated. There was no alteration in hepatorenal functions during treatment (Calvopina et al. 1998)

PREVENTION

The reservoir hosts cannot be eliminated. Hence, in endemic areas crabs need to be thoroughly cooked before consumption, including the juices used for flavouring.

REFERENCES

Calvopina M, Guderian RH, Parades W et al. Treatment of human pulmonary paragonimiasis with triclabendazole: clinical tolerance and drug efficacy. Transactions of the Royal Society of Tropical Medicine and Hygiene 1998; **92**: 566–569

Higashi K, Aoki H, Takebayashi K et al. Cerebral paragonimiasis. Journal of Neurology 1971; **34**: 515–527

Kim MJ, Park S, Kim NK et al. Perirectal cystic paragonimiasis: endorectal coil MRI. Journal of Computer Assisted Tomography 1999; **23**: 94–95

Maleewong W. Recent advances in diagnosis of paragonimiasis. South-East Asian Journal of Tropical Medicine and Public Health 1997; **28**: 134–138

Meyers WM, Neafie RN. Paragonimiasis. In Binford CH, Connor DH (eds), Pathology of Tropical and Extraordinary Diseases. Washington, DC: Armed Forces Institute of Pathology, 1976, 517–524

IV

General Features of Cestodes

Cestodes are called tapeworms as they are ribbon-like. They are of variable length, segmented, tapelike and flattened dorsoventrally. *Hymenolepis nana* is 1–4 cm and *Diphyllobothrium latum* is 15 m long. They have a scolex or head, neck and a strobila (trunk or body). A strobila is composed of varying numbers of segments or proglottids. *Echinococcus granulosus* has three to four segments and *Diphyllobothrium latum* has 4000 segments.

Three types of proglottids are present:

1 Immature – Reproductive organs are not differentiated
2 Mature – Reproductive organs become mature
3 Gravid – Egg-filled uterus with other organs atrophied

The body wall is composed of three layers – an outer layer of resistant cuticle (integument) covered with microvilli, a subcuticular, circular and longitudinal muscle layer, and inner radially arranged tegumental cells.

Cestodes have no body cavity. The body wall and organs are filled with parenchyma, containing scattered loose calcareous corpuscles. The eggs of the order cyclophyllidea (Echinococcus and Taenia species) are double layered and contain the mature embryo with six hooklets (hexacanth embryo or oncosphere). The inner shell called embryophore has radial striations. Eggs of pseudophyllidae (Diphyllobothrium) are operculated and non-embryonated.

The reproductive system consists of double or single set of organs, genital pores located bilaterally, unilaterally or ventrally. The male reproductive system consists of testes, vasa efferentia, vas deferens, seminal vesicle and cirrus. Both cirrus and vagina open to a common genital atrium. When self-fertilization occurs, sperms go through vagina to seminal receptacle, then to spermatic duct to the ootype. Oviduct, vitelline duct, Mehli's gland also lead to ootype, where eggs are formed and fertilization takes place. Fertilized eggs are transported from the ovary to the uterus. There are no digestive organs. The cuticle may absorb semi-digested food in the intestine of host. Microvilli increase surface area of absorption. The excretory system consists of the dorsal and ventral longitudinal excretory tubules that run along the lateral margins of proglottids. Transverse excretory tubules and branches of main trunks form a network that collects waste products through terminal flame cells. The nervous system consists of cephalic and anterior ganglia with their commissures that form a rostellar ring, which is the central nervous system. All tapeworms require one or more intermediate hosts.

In the Taenia group the oncosphere develop into a cystic larva in the intermediate host. When the cyst contains only one protoscolex (miniature replica of adult) it is called a cysticercus. When multiple scolices are present it is a coenurus. When daughter cysts and brood capsules are present it is a hydatid.

Cestodes or tapeworms of medical importance can be considered in two main categories: intestinal cestodes such as *Taenia saginata* and *T. solium*; and tissue cestodes or larval forms, which cause unilocular hydatid disease (*Echinococcus granulosus*), alveolar hydatid disease (*E. multilocularis*), coenurosis (*Multiceps* species) and sparganosis (*Spirometra mansonoides* spp.).

Cestodes have complex life cycles that usually involve both intermediate and definitive hosts. In some infections like *T. solium* and *Hymenolepis nana*, man serves as both the definitive and intermediate host. The intermediate host of *T. saginata* is cattle and of *T. solium* is pig or hog. The mode of infection is via ingestion of the larval forms (cysticercus) in infected beef in *T. saginata* and infected hog in *T. solium*. The normal life span of these tapeworms is up to 25 years.

The extra-intestinal form of *T. solium* infection is far more serious than the presence of the adult worm in the intestine. Larvae or cysticercosis can be found in the brain, which, after their death, can stimulate tissue reactions with resultant epileptiform fits and abnormal behaviour, transient pareses and other neurological symptoms. (Detailed description of neurocysticercosis is described.) Surgical removal is usually recommended.

The prognosis is excellent when only adult tapeworms are present, good when the cysticerci can be surgically removed but poor when the brain is involved.

Of the larval forms invading tissue, hydatid disease is the commonest, occurring in sheep and cattle raising areas of the world including Australia. Dogs are the definitive hosts. The liver is the commonest organ involved and treatment is surgical removal of the hydatid cyst.

Alveolar hydatid is uncommon in Australia. The definitive hosts are foxes and cats.

Coenurosis is acquired by ingestion of the multiceps eggs passed in the stools of the definitive hosts, dogs and wolves, by the intermediate hosts, especially sheep, goats, cattle (herbivorous mammals). In humans most coenuri are in the central nervous system and mimic a space-occupying lesion. The cysts can rarely occur in muscle and subcutaneous tissue.

Sparganosis or infection by a sparganum (the generic term for the second stage larva or plero-cercoid) is caused by ingestion of raw, infected amphibia, reptiles, birds or mammals, or drinking water containing cyclops (the first intermediate host).

Any tissue can be involved. The most common being subcutaneous tissues and treatment is by surgical removal of the worm. Drug therapy is not satisfactory.

31

Taeniasis and Cysticercosis

PARASITOLOGY

Taeniasis is an infection caused by adult tapeworms: *Taenia saginata*, the beef tapeworm, and *T. solium*, the pork tapeworm.

Humans can act as both definitive and intermediate hosts. Cysticercosis is an infection caused by the larval stages. The larva of *T. solium* is cysticercus cellulosae, larva of *T. saginata* is cysticercus bovis. Cysticercosis cellulosae is more common than the bovine form.

T. saginata is common in parts of Africa, the Middle East, Yugoslavia and the former Soviet Union. It is also found in South East Asia, South America and Europe. *T. solium* is found in South and Central America, southern Europe, South East Asia, Central and South Africa and China. Both infections are common in communities consuming raw or partly cooked pork (*T. solium*) or beef (*T. saginata*). Human cysticercosis is widely endemic in rural areas of Latin America, Spain, Portugal, Eastern Europe, India, Spain, Africa and China. The number of neurocysticercosis cases in the USA between 1987 and 1990 has increased with an annual average of 1133 cases. Six percent of outpatients at the Neurological Institute in Mexico City had neurocysticercosis, a total of 42 000 cases in 1982 (Valesco-Scharez 1982). The secondary host stage in man occurs either by both internal or external auto-infection. External auto-infection is through ingestion of the eggs of *T. solium*; internal auto-infection occurs when segments of the adult worm from the small intestine are regurgitated to the stomach with the liberation of the oncosphere from the egg which then penetrates the intestinal mucosa, enters the blood stream or lymphatics and is carried to ectopic sites. The adult *T. saginata* measures 5–10 m and has 1000–20 000 proglottids. It is distinguished from *T. solium* by the number of uterine branches, testis and absence of an accessory lobe in the ovary. *T. saginata scolex* has four suckers and no hooklets.

Cysticerci of *T. saginata* have been reported in cattle reared on sewerage irrigated pasture (Rickard and

Adolph 1977). Up to 51% of 10–11-month-old cattle in such areas had cysticercus bovis, although the detection rate elsewhere in New South Wales is ~0.05%. Ovine cysticercosis exists in Australia in sheep and kangaroo, but man is not infected. Cysticercosis of humans due to *T. saginata* apparently does not occur.

T. solium measures 2–3 m in length and has 800–900 proglottids. The scolex is armed with a double row of 22–32 hooklets and four suckers. A mature segment measures 12 × 6 mm and contains a single set of reproductive organs.

The eggs of *T. solium* and *T. saginata* are identical and are spherical, brown and measure 31–60 μm in diameter. The inner shell is radially striated (Figure 31.1). The non-ciliated embryo has six hooklets. The adult worm lives in the small intestine of humans and gravid proglottids are expelled in chains of five or six at a time. Eggs are swallowed by the intermediate host the pig. In the small intestines of the pig, the oncosphere exits from the egg and penetrates the bowel wall to enter lymphatics and the blood stream before encysts as cysticercus in muscles and other organs. Man contracts the infection by eating inadequately cooked pork ('measly pork').

Cysticercus is white, transparent, oval or spherical and measures ~1 cm when fully developed. It contains a single invaginated protoscolex with birefringent hooklets. The cyst wall consists of an outer cuticle covered with microvilli underneath which are two layers of the smooth muscle and a row of tegumental cells within a loose parenchyma. In cysticercus bovis, the scolex is unarmed.

In the small intestine, the protoscolex evaginates and anchors to the wall to develop into an adult worm.

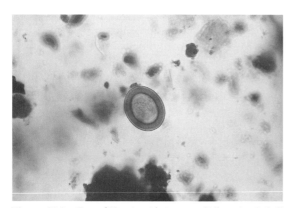

Figure 31.1 – Egg of Taenia with inner, radially striated shell and embryo with six hooklets.

Gravid proglottids and eggs begin to appear in stools 2–3 months after infection. The life cycle of *T. saginata* is similar except that intermediate host is cow or buffalo (Figure 31.2).

PRESENTATION

Taeniasis

Symptoms caused by adult worms of *T. solium* or *T. saginata* are rare or mild. Most patients are infected by a single parasite. *T. solium* survives for 25 years and *T. saginata* for 10 years.

Vague abdominal discomfort, indigestion, hunger pain, anorexia, diarrhoea and constipation can be seen. Occasionally, severe symptoms such as intestinal

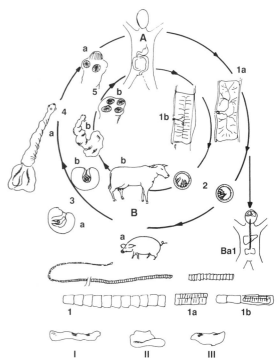

Figure 31.2 – Life cycle of *T. solium* and *T. saginata*; (a) pork (pig) tapeworm; (b) beef (cattle) tapeworm. (A) Final host: man only. Tapeworm in the small intestine; (1a) mature segment of *T. solium*; (1b) mature segment of *T. saginata*; (2) tapeworm egg (embryophore with six hooked larva). (B) Intermediate host: (a) pig; (b) cattle; (3, 4) cysticercus in different stages of evagination of the scolex; (3a) cysticercus cellulosae of *T. solium*; (3b) cysticercus bovis of *T. saginata*; (4) evaginated cysticercus stage of *T. solium* (a) and *T. saginata*; (5) scolex of the pork tapeworm (with its crown of hooklets); (b) of the beef tapeworm (without a crown of hooklets). (I–III) Phases of the movements of freshly detached tapeworm segments.

obstruction, perforation or appendicitis have been reported. Ectopic parasitism has been reported in the common bile duct, respiratory tract, uterine cavity and the nasopharynx.

Cysticercosis

The incubation period of cysticercosis ranges from a few months to 30 years. The symptoms depend on the number of cysticerci and the anatomical site of the cyst. The infection can remain asymptomatic even with heavy cyst load. Painless skin nodules may be present. The two main organs where the cysts produce symptoms are the brain, including meninges and the eye.

Cerebral

Most patients with one or two cysts remain asymptomatic unless it is localized in the motor or sensory areas, or the aqueduct. The patients can present with generalized seizures, secondarily generalized seizures or partial complex seizures (Chayasirisobhan et al. 1999) and disturbances or symptoms of raised intracranial pressure due to hydrocephalus such as headache, nausea, vomiting and visual disturbances (Figure 31.4). The meningeal form of cerebral cysticercosis can cause nerve palsies and signs of meningeal irritation and papilloedema. The patients rarely may present for the first time with a mass effect that requires urgent decompression or shunting. Acute meningitis is secondary to a rupture of a cyst. Transient ischaemic attacks (TIA) has been documented (Lee and Chang 1998).

Ocular

The cysts may affect the retina, orbit, conjunctiva, vitreous humour or the anterior chamber. Symptoms include blurring of vision, peri-orbital pain and headache secondary to glaucoma. The dead cysts cause a cellular reaction resulting in very painful iridocyclitis. Intra-ocular cysticerci may be visualized by fundoscopy. Patients with ocular cysticercosis often develop cataracts.

Skin and other organs

Skin lesions vary from 1 to 2 cm in diameter. They are painless nodules or papules and firm in consis-

tency. Differential diagnosis includes other painless soft tissue masses such as neurofibromas. Cysticercosis can invade peripheral nerves and can rarely be seen in skeletal muscle, liver and kidney. They may be asymptomatic. Cysticercosis of the breast has been reported in an Australian woman who had been on Yomesin (an antihelminthic drug), probably resulting in auto-infection (Leggett 1983). Cysticercosis of tongue and buccal mucosa has been reported (Saran et al. 1998).

PATHOLOGY

Cysticercosis

Regardless of the location, the pathologic changes are very similar. When the cyst is viable, no inflammatory reaction is seen. There is only compression of the surrounding tissue with mild fibrosis. When the cysticercus is dead or degenerated, an extensive inflammatory reaction occurs with infiltration by neutrophils, lymphocytes, plasma cells, histiocytes and rarely, eosinophils. In the late stages, a granulomatous reaction is seen with histiocytes, epithelioid cells and foreign body giant cells. The lesions finally undergo fibrosis and calcification. The cysticercus may vary in size depending on its maturity and location. They are usually 1 cm in diameter but may be larger – 3–10 cm, when space allows, e.g. in the ventricle of the brain. The parasite is characterized by a single invaginated protoscolex in a fluid-filled cystic cavity. Microscopically, protoscolex may show suckers, hooklets and a branched tract. The triple layered cyst is composed of a ciliated cuticle, musculature and tegumental cells with scattered calcareous corpuscles (Figs 31.3a and 31.3b).

Cerebral cysticercosis may be meningeal, ventricular, parenchymatous or mixed forms. A racemose variety is also described in the basal and subarachnoid space and in the ventricles. No protoscolex is present and the symptoms are probably secondary to degenerative changes. Hydrocephalus is due to arachnoiditis in the meningeal form and inflammation of the foramina of Luschka and Magendie. The cysticercus may also act as a ball valve or may completely obstruct the aqueduct of Sylvius causing a non-communicating hydrocephalus.

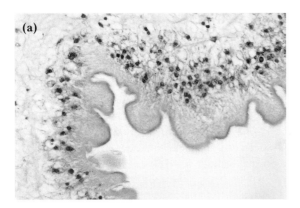

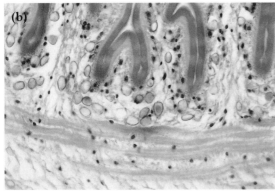

Figure 31.3 – (a) Triple layered cyst composed of a ciliated cuticle, musculature and tegumental cells; (b) scattered calcareous corpuscles.

INVESTIGATIONS

Taeniasis

1. Ova are seldom found and diagnosis is made by identifying the mobile, creamy segments of proglottids in the stool.
2. ELISA assay (using excretory/secretory antigen (TSES)) for antigen or antibody can reveal *T. solium* in stools of tapeworm carriers even when proglottidis are not found. Enzyme-linked immuno-electron transfer blot (EITB) has higher specificity than ELISA.
3. DNA probes are also useful in differentiating *T. saginata* and *T. solium*.

Cysticercosis

1. Calcified cysts may be found in nearly half the patients and X-rays may show calcified areas in soft tissue.

2. EEG is normal in active neurocysticercosis, but abnormal in 50% of patients with active and mixed forms.
3. CT imaging of the head is the most useful technique when there are mass lesions or obstructive hydrocephalus. Contrast-enhanced CT may demonstrate solid cystic, or calcified lesions. MRI is superior to CT scans in the diagnosis.
4. Lumbar puncture, in the absence of raised intracranial pressure, may demonstrate thick, yellow CSF with a raised protein level, low glucose and lymphocytosis with no microorganisms on direct smear or on culture. Rarely one may obtain parasitic tissue in a blocked lumbar puncture needle.
5. Histological diagnosis is made by identifying the three layers of the worm. However, differentiation from other species may not always be possible unless the scolices and hooklets are present. Skin nodule biopsies can establish the specific diagnosis. Fine-needle aspiration is a useful method for superficial, suspected lesions (Saran *et al.* 1998).
6. Serology – enzyme-linked immuno-electron transfer blot assay (EITB) and glycoprotein antigens assay are sensitive diagnostic tests. However, cross-reactivity can occur. The EITB assay is highly reproducible and simple to perform on CSF or serum. There is no significant difference in test performance when CSF was compared with serum (Tsang *et al.* 1989).

TREATMENT

- In taeniasis, praziquantel in low dose (10 mg/kg) is the drug of choice. Internal auto-infection can occur in *T. solium* producing cysticercosis by disintegration of segments
- Personal hygiene is essential to prevent external auto-infection via the oral route
- In neurocysticercosis, surgery is the treatment of choice in patients with raised intracranial pressure. Implantation of intraventricular shunt and/or removal of cysts are surgical procedures in management. Chemotherapy should be tried before surgery if there is no urgency. Combined conservative and surgical treatment is most often applied in extraparenchymal forms and those parenchymal forms of neurocysticercosis where symptoms persist despite antihelminthic

treatment. Dexamethasone would be beneficial in cases with raised intracranial pressure

- Albendazole is the drug of choice. It causes death of the cysts and clinical improvement in the symptoms. Recommended dose 15 mg/kg/day for 30 days. It is not recommended in pregnancy although it is relatively free of side-effects. Albendazole therapy results in significantly faster increased resolution of solitary cysticercosis and appears to reduce the risk of late seizure recurrences (Baranwal *et al.* 1998). Albendazole therapy causes adverse reactions in about one-third of patients with a persistent solitary cysticercus granuloma in the form of headache, vomiting or recurrence of seizures

- Praziquantel is the second drug of choice. Recommended dose is 50 mg/kg/day for 14 days. When combined with dexamethasone it has given 98% clinical improvement (van Dellen and McKeown 1988). However, praziquantel for neurocysticosis can cause severe headache and seizures.

- Disseminated myositis could be induced by praziquantel in disseminated muscular cysticercosis (Takayanagni and Chimelli 1998). Steroids may be beneficial

- Intra-ocular and intraventricular cysts are not affected and should be removed surgically (Robles *et al.* 1987)

- On commencement of chemotherapy there can be exacerbation of symptoms due to inflammatory responses to dying cysts. Dexamethasone is beneficial but it may affect the anticysticercidal drug level

- Patients with seizures will require anti-epileptic treatment. In patients who have epilepsy and only calcified cysts in the brain, chemotherapy is not indicated and only anti-epileptic drugs are used. Corticosteroids should be given in addition to albendazole treatment or orbital cysticercosis when cysts are in close proximity to optic nerve to prevent optic neuritis (Rajshekar 1998)

- Surgery – excision of lump and histology

PREVENTION

Pork should be properly cooked to kill all cysticerci. The same applies to *T. bovis*, although this is a much rarer infection.

ILLUSTRATIVE CASE

An India-born male, 31 years of age, was admitted for repair of right inguinal hernia. Besides the hernia, a lump on the right side of the neck was found. He had had no previous surgery. He was on Betaloc for his hypertension.

The lump noted 1 year previously was sometimes painful. It measured 1–2 cm in diameter and was in the posterior triangle of the neck. It was non-tender, mobile and solid, with a cystic component.

The excised lump consisted of two pieces of cream-coloured tissue, the larger measuring 10 mm in its greatest dimension. Microscopic sections showed an encysted protoscolex of cysticercus in skeletal muscle with suckers, hooklets, a branched tract and triple layered cyst wall. Scattered calcareous corpuscles were also seen (Figure 31.5a and 31.5b). These features were diagnostic of cysticercus cellulosae (larval stage of *T. solium*).

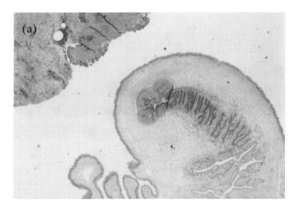

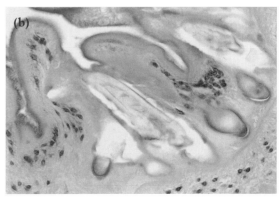

Figure 31.4 – Cysticercus cellulosae; (a) sections of encysted protoscolex of cysticercus in skeletal muscle (H&E × 40); (b) hooklets (H&E × 200).

REFERENCES

Baranwal AK, Singhi PJ, Khandelwal N *et al.* Albendazole therapy in children with focal seizures and single small enhancing computerized to onographaphlic lesions. A randomized placebo-controlled, double blind trial. *Paediatric Infectious Diseases Journal* 1998; **8**: 696–700

Chayasirisobhan S, Menoni R, Chayasirisobhan *et al.* Correlation of electroencephalography and the active and inactive forms of neurocysticercosis. *Clinical Electro Encephalography* 1999; **30**: 9–11

Lee SI, Chang GY. Recurrent brainstem transient ischemic attack due to neurocysticersosis: a treatable cause. *European Neurology* 1998; **40**: 174–175

Leggett CAC. Cysticercosis of the breast. *Australia and New Zealand Journal of Surgery* 1983; **53**: 281–283

Rajshekar V. Incidence and significance of adverse effects of albendazole therapy in patients with a persistent solitary cysticercus granuloma. *Acta Neurologica Scandinavia* 1998; **98**: 121–123

Rickard MD, Adolph AJ. The prevalence of cysticerci of *Taenia saginata* in cattle reared on sewerage irrigated pasture. *Medical Journal of Australia* 1977; **11**: 525–527

Robles C, Sedano AM, Vargas-Tentori N *et al.* Long term results of praziquantel therapy in neurocysticercosis. *Journal of Neurosurgery* 1987; **66**: 359–363

Saran RK, Rattan V, Rajwanshi A *et al.* Cysticercosis of the oral cavity: a report of five cases and a review of literature. *International Journal of Paediatric Dentistry* 1998; **8**: 273–278

Takayanagni OM, Chimelli L. Disseminated muscular cysticercosis with myositis induced by praziquantel therapy. *American Journal of Tropical Medical Hygiene* 1998; **59**: 1002–1003

Tsang VC, Brand JA, Boyer AE. An enzyme-linked immuno-electron transfer blot assay and glycoprotein antigen for diagnosing human cysticercosis (*Taenia solium*). *Journal of Infectious Diseases* 1989; **159**: 50–59

Valesco-Scharez M, Bravo-Bechelle MA, Quirasco F. In Flisser A (ed.), *Cysticercosis. Present State of Knowledge and Perspectives.* London: Academic Press, 1982, 21–43

Van Dellen JR, McKeown CP. Praziquantel in active cerebral cysticercosis. *Neurosurgery* 1988; **22**: 92–96

32

Echinococcosis (Hydatid Disease)

Parasitology
  E. granulosus
  E. multilocularis
Presentation
  E. granulosus
  E. multilocularis
Pathology
  E. granulosus
  E. multilocularis

Investigations
  E. granulosus
  E. multilocularis
Treatment
  E. granulosus
  E. multilocularis
Prevention
References

PARASITOLOGY

Hydatid disease is caused by larval tapeworm of the genus *Echinococcus*. The four species causing human infection are *E. granulosus*, *E. multilocularis*, *E. oligarthus* and *E. vogeli*. *E. granulosus* is the most common species, the second being *E. multilocularis*.

E. granulosus (cystic hydatid disease)

Cystic hydatid disease is endemic practically in most states of Australia, some more than others. The disease exists in both continents of America but is more common in South America, some parts of Africa, some Baltic countries and in New Zealand. Three distinct strains of *E. granulosus* are now identified in Australia. They are the domestic strain with sheep, dog cycle (on the Australian mainland); sylvatic strain with dingoes, wallabies and kangaroos (on the Australian mainland) and Tasmanian strain with sheep, domestic dog cycle.

E. granulosus is found mainly in rural dogs, which are fed offal of sheep. There is concern in certain parts of Australia regarding the sylvatic strain. It is not really known to what extent the increase in prevalence of the disease in the feral dog population (the sylvatic cycle) has affected the domestic cycle. Domestic dogs can become infected by feeding on macropods, and sheep can be infected from *E. granulosus* eggs deposited in the pastures of infective canids (Reichel *et al.* 1994). Hunting dogs can be infected by feasting on kangaroo and pig offal left in the bush by illegal shooters and pig hunters.

The mode of transmission of echinococcosis to man is by ingestion of the eggs passed in the faeces of dogs. Man is an intermediate host. Cattle, swine and goats can be accidentally infected with the larval form but this is unimportant in maintaining the cycle of infection. It is the dog–sheep cycle that is most important for continuation of the cycle. Dogs can be infected by ingestion of cysts in the flesh of kangaroos and wallabies. In Australia cattle play a small role in infection, as home killing of cattle is uncommon. Hydatids have been described in horses in the UK and with importation of horses, there is a possibility of introducing this additional source of infection and the establishment of a feral cycle. The *E. granulosus* adult worm measures 3–6 mm in length with a scolex, neck and a strobila with three-to-four segments representing immature, mature and gravid segments. The scolex bears four suckers, rostellum and two rows of hooklets. The eggs are indistinguishable from other *Taenia* eggs.

The ova may remain viable on the ground for > 6 months under favourable conditions, and they are resistant to freezing and disinfectants. This survival is reduced to 2–3 weeks in the hot season. The eggs may be present on dog faeces, fruits and vegetables, and is dispersed by wind, flies and beetles. Prevention of ingestion of offal by dogs and prevention if entrance to sheep pastures is a key issue in the control of hydatic disease in man.

Hexacanth embryos hatch in the duodenum of the intermediate host, pierce the intestinal wall and enter the portal circulation. Most are retained in the liver capillaries but some pass to the lungs. A few may enter the systemic circulation and be carried to virtually every organ in the intermediate host. After entering an organ, the oncosphere (hexacanth embryo) develops into a fluid-containing bladder, the hydatid cyst with thousands of protoscolices. When the intermediate host dies, infected organs may be ingested by definitive host where the protoscolices evaginate and grow into adult worms in the intestine. The life span of adult is 6 months and hydatid cyst may persist for many years (Fig. 32.1).

E. multilocularis

E. multilocularis is the cause of the alveolar form of hydatid disease. The disease is confined to the Northern hemisphere, found most commonly in northern Japan, Alaska, Europe, the former Soviet Union, Canada, the UK and the USA. Large series of patients have also been reported in Switzerland. *E. multilocularis* in foxes is on the increase in Germany although there are few reports of clinical cases in humans, probably due to low pathogenicity of the parasite strains.

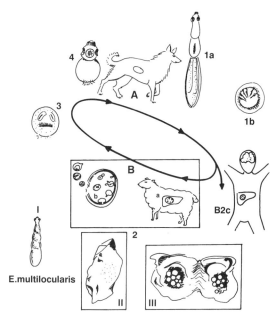

Figure 32.1 – Life cycle of Echinococcus. (A) Final host: dog (and other Canidae); (1a) *E. granulosus*; (b) embryophore, six-hooked larva ('oncosphere'); (B) intermediate host: sheep (for *E. granulosus*); (2a) liver with *Echinococcus* cyst (bladderworm stage); (b) diagram of an *Echinococcus* cyst with daughter cysts and scolices (compare with Fig. 3); (2c) man as the (secondary) intermediate host (echinococcosis); organs most often infected: liver, brain three and four isolated scolices; three invaginated, four evaginated scolex. (I) *E. multilocularis*, sexually mature worm; (II) human liver infected by the larva of *E. multilocularis*; (III) hydatid cyst of *E. granulosus* opened up; daughter cyst visible.

The definitive and intermediate hosts of *E. multilocularis* are different from that of *E. granulosus*. The definitive host of *E. multilocularis* are the foxes, canine and cats, and microtine rodents such as deer mice are the intermediate hosts. Man is accidentally infected by eggs through contaminated water, vegetables and fruit or by handling fox furs. Humans do not provide optimal conditions for development of the parasite.

E. multilocularis measures 1.2–3.7 mm. Eggs are indistinguishable from *E. granulosus* or other Taenia eggs. The life cycle is similar to *E. granulosus*.

PRESENTATION

E. granulosus

In the majority of cases of abdominal hydatid disease, the mode of presentation is by accidental discovery of an abdominal mass, detected by the patient, or doctor during clinical or special investigations. Hydatid is also common in children. The most common site in adults is the liver (60%) followed by lung (25%). Other rare sites include the brain, kidney, spleen and pancreas. In a series from the Royal Prince Alfred Hospital, Sydney, 40% of patients with lung hydatid had hydatid in the liver, while 24% with hydatid in the liver also had hydatid in the lung (Little 1976). In children, the cysts were more in lung (65%) than liver (35%), and in a few cases both organs were involved. Hydatid cysts have been found in rare sites such as the heart (Lopez-Rios *et al.* 1997).

Symptoms depend on size and location of the hydatid cyst. Hepatic lesions may not cause symptoms for years but a cerebral or bone lesion may be symptomatic in the early stages. Liver hydatids grow ~1 mm/month and can be secondarily infected by bacteria. Clinical manifestations appear when cysts reach ~10 cm in diameter and cysts become palpable at ~20 cm in diameter.

The clinical presentation of liver hydatid is abdominal pain and discomfort (Fig. 32.2). However, in a few cases the presentation is acute with biliary pain and/or jaundice. Jaundice is caused by rupture of the hydatid contents into the biliary duct system. Hydatids have also been detected following motor vehicle accidents with an acute abdomen due to compression-type seat belt injury. Secondary infection of the cyst may simulate a liver abscess. Sudden rupture of the cyst will precipitate anaphylaxis or peritonitis and dissemination of hydatid disease in the host (Lewall 1998). Hydatid disease in lung presents with cough, malaise, chest pain, and haemoptysis. In one series 20% of patients with pulmonary hydatid cysts presented with

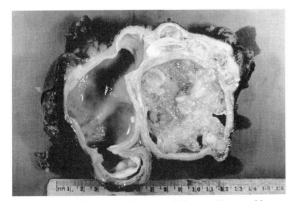

Figure 32.2 – Liver hydatid removed from a 70-year-old man presenting with abdominal pain.

urgent complications whereas this is much lower with liver hydatid disease (Little 1976).

E. multilocularis

The clinical manifestation of *E. multilocularis* mimics malignant disease in the liver. In stage 1 of the disease, which can last up to 10 years, there are no symptoms or signs. In stage 2, which can also last up to 10 years, there are clinical manifestations of hepatomegaly, jaundice and abdominal pain. In advanced cases, ascites and anaemia are common. The natural history of the disease is one of gradual progression in the liver and spread to other tissues including brain and bone. Death is secondary to liver failure. Patients may live > 16 years after diagnosis.

PATHOLOGY

E. granulosus

The wall of the hydatid cyst is composed of two layers: the outer cuticular layer is called the ectocyst (Fig. 32.3a). Characteristically, it is a laminated hyaline membrane that may be the only remaining evidence of a degenerated or dying hydatid cyst. The membrane is elastic and curls up when the cyst ruptures or is incised; and the inner layer is the germinal layer or endocyst. This membrane is the vital layer of the cyst that gives rise to brood capsules and secretes hydatid fluid.

The brood capsule is a vesicular structure protruding from the germinal layer into the cyst cavity. Inside the capsule, 5–20 protoscolices develop. They consist of an invaginated head or scolex with four suckers and a circle of hooklets.

From the brood capsule, daughter cysts are formed. These possess an outer protective layer in addition to the germinal layer. Inside a daughter cyst, brood capsules and protoscolices develop. In the cyst or daughter cyst, some of the brood capsules may detach from the germinal layer (Fig. 32.3b), others may rupture and release the protoscolices. The free brood capsules, scolices and loose hooklets may form a granular deposit at the bottom of the cyst, collectively called hydatid sand.

Cysts containing daughter cysts may hypermature and due to starvation, the cyst dies to become a mummified inert lesion. The cysts may rupture, can be clinically silent or communicate with another adjacent

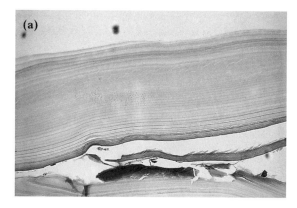

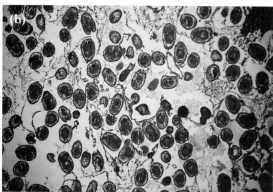

Figure 32.3 – (a) Laminated membrane; (b) detached brood capsules.

organ such as gallbladder causing obstructive symptoms. Rupture directly to abdominal or pleural cavity may cause anaphylaxis (Diebold-Berger 1997).

Host tissue reaction to the parasite varies in different organs. The surrounding parenchymal tissue gradually shows compression atrophy and the cellular reaction is gradually replaced by fibrosis, e.g. in the liver a relatively thick fibrous layer is formed around the hydatid and is known as a pericyst. The pericyst or adventitia in other organs is thinner than that in the liver and is absent in bone cysts.

Most hydatid cysts in the liver (80–85%) are located in the right lobe. The pulmonary hydatid is frequently seen in the right lung. In the central nervous system, the cysts are most frequently located in the cerebrum, especially the parietal lobe and preferentially in the white matter. Cerebellum and hypophyses are rarely involved. In the spinal cord, the lesion is usually due to direct extension from a vertebral hydatid cyst. Immune complex deposits in kidneys can cause mesangioproliferative glomerulonephritis.

E. multilocularis

Minor differences in morphology are seen between cystic and alveolar hydatid disease. In *E. multilocularis* the limiting membrane is thin and the germinal layer may bud externally proliferating in many directions to produce the characteristic multilocular or alveolar cyst. There is little fluid in the cysts with many vesicles embedded in a dense connective tissue stroma.

INVESTIGATIONS

E. granulosus

1. Histological – occasionally with a cyst rupturing into bile duct, intestine or bronchus, protoscolices, hooklets or even daughter cysts may be detected in stool, vomitus or sputum respectively. However, final diagnosis usually depends on laparotomy or direct histologic examination of the excised cysts with Giemsa staining of hooklets and scolices in cyst fluid (Lopez-Rios *et al.* 1997).

   If protoscolices are not identified, the pathologist should look for acid-fast hooklets (birefringence on polarizing microscopy), fragments of the laminated layer or calcareous corpuscles.

2. Plain X-ray of chest or abdomen – lung hydatids appear as round mass lesions, and abdominal X-rays may demonstrate a calcified ring 'eggshell sign' in the liver (Fig. 32.4) and elevation of the diaphragm. The pulmonary lesions do not calcify but the 'water lily' sign is pathognomonic of pulmonary echinococcosis when a broken membrane is seen floating on the air–fluid level.

3. Radiological scanning – liver hydatids show up as filling defects and will distinguish from other solid masses by flow studies with [99m]Technetium. The disadvantage of this imaging technique is that it is not possible to accurately localize the lesion, and proper images of left lobe lesions may de difficult to obtain.

4. Ultrasonography – liver hydatids are well demonstrated by the characteristic appearance on ultrasonography. The detection of daughter cysts is more helpful in ultrasound diagnosis. Single cysts without daughter cysts cannot be distinguished from simple liver cysts.

5. CT – useful method of localizing the lesion in the liver, especially from surgical point of view. The investigation will outline liver hydatids very well.

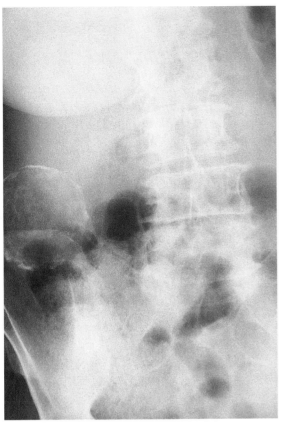

Figure 32.4 – X-ray of abdomen to show 'egg shell' sign.

It will also demonstrate involvement in the abdomen beyond the liver.

6. Pulmonary angiography – demonstrates that the pulmonary cysts are avascular.

7. Serological tests available are complement fixation test, immuno-electrophoresis (IEP). The presence of 'ARC 5' provides a specific serological test for hydatid disease, latex agglutination (LA) and indirect haemagglutination test (IHA) and ELISA. Immuno-electrophoresis is probably the best test. The complement fixation test usually becomes negative 12 months after surgery and IHA shows a 4-fold fall in 2 years. Enzyme-linked immuno-electron transfer blot (EITB) test – recommended by the US Center for Disease Control, Atlanta, GA. It detects 98% of parasitologically proven cases with two or more cysts and is 100% specific (Tsang *et al.* 1989). The sensitivity of this technique is between 60 and 80% if there is only a single Echinococcus lesion. It has been compared with other immunological assays and is presumed to be the current test for the diagnosis of cysticer-

cosis (Tsang and Wilson 1995). The cytologic material could be examined by polymerase chain reaction (Diebold-Berger 1997).

8. Comparison of protein banding pattern of *E. granulosus* (protoscolices) by isoelectric focusing on thin layer polyacramides gel has been used to identify the species, and perhaps identify the source of transmission.

E. multilocularis

1. Plain X-ray – diffuse calcification may be seen in X-rays of chest and abdomen.

2. Imaging such as radionuclide scanning, ultrasonography and CT shows diffuse infiltrative space-occupying lesions.

3. Liver function tests show elevation of liver enzymes and total bilirubin.

4. Serology is as for hydatid disease. Immuno-electrophoresis (ARC 5) will be positive.

TREATMENT

E. granulosus

Medical

- Praziquantel 15 mg/kg twice daily for 6 days has a cure rate of 70–80%. It has a greater protoscolecidal activity than benzimidazoles. Higher doses for longer periods and repeated treatment are necessary for cerebral cysts. Dexamethasone used in combination has a beneficial effect (Taylor *et al.* 1989)

- Albendazole 10–15 mg/kg for 1 month for four cycles with a 15-day rest between the cycles has resulted in partial or complete response in 80–90% of patients. Toxic effects are alopecia, neutropenia and hepatotoxicity

- Albendazole plus praziquantel is more effective than monotherapy with albendazole in the preoperative treatment of intra-abdominal hydatidosis (Cobo *et al.* 1998). With medical management monitoring the serology with immuno-electrophoresis assesses the improvement. Fever and allergic reactions to dying cysts may be seen in the first 2 weeks of treatment. The cysts usually disintegrate and become fibrosed after 2 months of treatment

Surgical

- Surgery is advocated for lung cysts, liver cysts and ocular cysts. For lung cysts surgery involves excision of the adventitia and extension of the cysts by inflating the lung affected, referred to as 'hydatid birth operation'. For liver cysts, Aaron's suction cone device has minimized complications. The suction device is placed on the surface of the cavity through which surgery is performed and hydatid material is removed and biliary communications are sutured (Kune *et al.* 1983). Ocular cysts are rarely amenable to chemotherapy. Needle aspiration of cyst fluid before surgery is recommended. Post-operative serological tests and immuno-electrophoresis should be done to monitor the success of the treatment.

E. multilocularis

Medical

- Treatment with mebendazole increases the life expectancy in patients with alveolar hydatid disease. It is also a useful adjunct to surgery (Ammann 1991). The toxic effects of mebendazole are alopecia, neutropenia and impaired liver function. The development of alopecia is an indication to withdraw the drug.

Surgical

- Surgery is the treatment of choice if performed on suitable cases. The diseased part of the liver is removed en bloc. *E. multilocularis* of the liver is almost incurable but an aggressive surgical approach can result in long lasting palliation. Liver transplant, if disease is confined to the liver, may be considered.

PREVENTION

Hydatid disease is a preventable disease. The preventive measures implemented in Tasmania, New Zealand and Western Australia has been a great success. Effective disposal of infected sheep offal is of paramount importance to break the sheep-dog-man cycle. Regular administration of antihelminthic agents such as praziquantel to rural dogs is 100% effective. Veterinary surgeons should examine rural dogs for *E granulosus*. If sheep are killed on farms there should be dog-proof fences and pits to dispose the offal. Dogs should be kept in a closed enclosure or chained at night and should not have access to vegetable gardens. Children should be prevented from playing with strange dogs particularly in rural areas.

REFERENCES

Ammann RW, Swiss Echinococcus Study Group. Improvement of liver resectional therapy by adjunct chemotherapy in alveolar hydatid disease. *Parasitology Research* 1991; **77**: 290–293

Cobo F, Yarnoz C, Sesma B *et al.* Albendazole plus praziquantel versus albendazole alone as a pre-operative treatment in infra-abdominal hydatidosis caused by *Echinococcus granulosus*. *Tropical Medical International Health* 1998; **3**: 464–466

Diebold-Berger S, Khan H, Gottstein B *et al.* Cytologic diagnosis of isolated pancreatic hydatid disease with immunologic and PCR analysis: a case report. *Acta Cytologica* 1997; **41**: 1381–1386

Kune GA, Jones T, Sali A. Hydatid disease in Australia. *Medical Journal of Australia* 1983; **2**: 385–388

Lewall DB. Hydatid disease: biology, pathology, imaging and classification. *Clinical Radiology* 1998; **53**: 863–874

Little JM. Hydatid disease at Royal Prince Alfred Hospital 1964–1974. *Medical Journal of Australia* 1976; **24**: 903–908

Lopez-Rios F, Perez-Bamos A, de Augustin PP. Primary cardiac hydatid cyst in a child cytologic diagnosis of a case. *Acta Cytologica* 1997; **41**: 1387–1390

Reichel MP, Lyford A, Gasser B. Hyperendemic focus of echinococcosis in N. E. Victoria. *Medical Journal of Australia* 1994; **160**: 449

Taylor DH, Morris DL, Reftin D *et al.* Comparison of albendazole, mebendazole and praziquantel chemotherapy of *Echinococcus multilocularis* in the Gerlie model. *Gut* 1989; **30**: 1401–1405

Tsang VCW, Brand JA, Boyer AE. An enzyme-linked immuno-electrotransfer blot assay and glycoprotein agents for diagnosing human cysticercosis (*Taenia solium*). *Journal of Infectious Diseases* 1989; **159**: 50–59

Tsang VCW, Wilson M. *Taenia solium* cysticercosis, an underrecognized but serious public health problem. *Parasitology Today* 1995; **11**: 124–126

33

Sparganosis

PARASITOLOGY

Sparganosis is caused by infection with the larval forms of spargana, a cestode worm belonging to the genus Spirometra.

Three species cause disease (*Spirometra mansonoides*, *Diphyllobothrium* spp. and *Sparganum proliferum*). Sparganosis is worldwide in distribution. *Spirometra mansoni* occurs in South East Asia, Japan and China with scattered cases in South America and is the commonest larval form in humans. Man is an accidental, second intermediate host. Humans are infected by consuming uncooked flesh of snakes, frogs and birds containing the spargana. Drinking contaminated water containing the infected Cyclops can infect man. The eggs are passed in faeces from the definitive hosts, cats and dogs. In some parts of the world frog poultices are applied on to wounds and sore eyes as a healing technique (Cross 1994) and this forms another source of infection.

The adult worms of *S. mansonoides* and *S. theileri* (East Africa) are ribbon-like ivory white and opaque. They are found in domestic and wild canines and felines. They measure 3–60 cm in length, 0.1–1.2 mm wide, 0.5–1.75 mm thick and segments number 200–300. The anterior end is broad, bearing a groove or bothrium. There is no scolex hooklets or internal organs. The body wall is composed of an outer integument 5–15 μm thick containing microvilli on the ridged surface and two layers of smooth muscle with a row of radially arranged tegumental cells. The egg is pointed, measuring 67 × 37 μm, with a conical operculum. The life cycle is outlined in Fig. 33.1.

PRESENTATION

The invaded tissue becomes oedematous and painful. The death of the sparganum produces an intense inflammatory reaction. The lesions that are superficial produce swelling, redness, induration and tenderness. The anterior abdominal wall is a frequent site. The eye can be affected with marked swelling of eyelids, pain and irritation. Spargana may be found in the subconjunctival tissue or cornea, with corneal ulceration. Visceral sparganosis, though uncommon, can be more serious than superficial sparganosis. Cerebral sparganosis can produce seizures and localizing signs and rarely cerebral haemorrhage (Jeong *et al.* 1998). Spinal cord lesions cause paraparesis (Kudesia *et al.* 1998). Aberrant spargana have been found in the lung, kidney and bone (Nakamura *et al.* 1990). Infection with the proliferative variety of spargana called *S. proliferum* can cause widespread lesions and may be fatal.

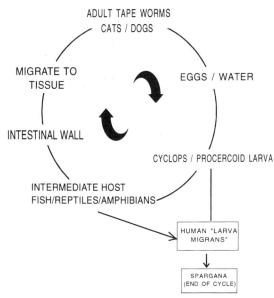

ADULT TAPE WORMS
CATS / DOGS

MIGRATE TO
TISSUE

EGGS / WATER

INTESTINAL WALL

CYCLOPS / PROCERCOID LARVA

INTERMEDIATE HOST
FISH/REPTILES/AMPHIBIANS

HUMAN "LARVA
MIGRANS"

SPARGANA
(END OF CYCLE)

Figure 33.1 – Life cycle of sparganosis.

Differential diagnosis

Sparganosis can be mistaken for cysticercosis, guinea-worm filaria including *Loa loa*, gnathostomiasis, larval flukes, and subcutaneous paragonimiasis. The distinction is made by examining the worm under a dissecting microscope or on histological sections and by serology.

PATHOLOGY

The spargana are ivory white in colour, have a smooth glistening coat and undulating movements. In the subcutaneous tissue, a tender mass or fibrous cyst can form which, on microscopy, shows an eosinophilic, granulomatous lesion where the grooved head of the worm and calcareous corpuscles can be identified. The live worms in tissue cause honeycombing and, if in lymphatic channels, lymphoedema. When they die, they elicit an acute inflammatory response. If this occurs in the orbit, it can destroy the eye. Itching pustules can develop in the subcutaneous tissue from which the sparganum can be discharged . In the brain it causes a mass lesion with spargana enclosed in acute inflammatory exudate resembling an abscess (Kudesia *et al.* 1998).

S. proliferum differs from non-proliferating sparganum in that it multiplies by contiguous budding and branching giving rise to thousands of larvae in human tissues which can be identified by multiple cross-sections of the parasite instead of the single symmetric larva.

INVESTIGATIONS

1. Confirmation is by biopsy, and identification of the worm that has a solid body with absence of suckers, hooklets and presence of a deep groove on the head.
2. Serology-ELISA test on cerebrospinal fluid and blood has high sensitivity and specificity.
3. Eosinophilia can be as high as 40%.
4. In cerebral sparganosis, for exclusion purposes, serological tests for cysticercosis, paragonimiasis, amoebiasis, schistosomiasis, hydatid disease, strongyloidiasis and HIV should be done.
5. Spect scan – there is an increased uptake of ^{99m}Tc-HMPAO in the parasite infected regions of the cerebrum (You *et al.* 1997).
6. Computerized axial tomography (CT) and magnetic resonance imaging (MRI) of the brain may show a single contrast-enhancing lesion with surrounding oedema. This can be mistaken for a glioma.

TREATMENT

- Praziquantel has been used but it is not very effective (Chai *et al.* 1998). However, it was used on a patient with a suspected lesion of the skin, who also had cerebral sparganosis lesions cleared after 2 weeks of treatment. Dose 120–150 mg/kg in divided doses over 48 h
- Surgical removal is practised widely for skin lesions and cerebral lesions. The lesion in the brain is described as a pale nodule, well circumscribed and can be excised completely (Munckof *et al.* 1994). In the rare proliferating type of sparganosis, surgical removal is very difficult

ILLUSTRATIVE CASE

A 32-year-old female complained of a migrating subcutaneous swelling in the left iliac fossa, which became painful. On exploration, a worm was removed with the surrounding tissue.

The excised specimen consisted of adipose tissue measuring 25 × 15 × 15 mm with a central elongated, thin cavity 1 mm across, encircled by fibrous tissue together with a white translucent, flat segmented worm-like structure with a bulbous thickening at one end measuring 75 mm long and up to 1 mm wide (Figure 32a–c).

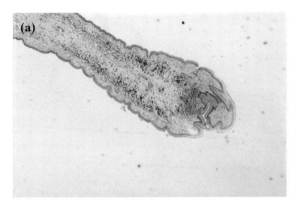

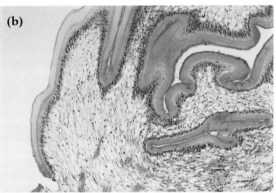

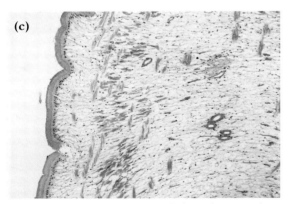

Figure 33.2 – (a) Characteristic morphology of worm with no scolex or internal organs; (b) the anterior end is broad with a groove. Note the absence of a scolex (H&E × 400); (c) body wall with ridged outer tegument beneath which are two layers of smooth muscle, stromal calcareous bodies and muscle strands (H&E 400).

Histologic sections showed a cestode worm with irregularly ridged tegument (pseudosegmentation) measuring 5–10 mm in thickness with a suggestion of a faint microvillous (brush) border. Two layers of smooth muscle and a row of cells were seen beneath the tegument. The loose stromal tissue contained smooth muscle strands and calcareous bodies. No scolices or internal organ structure were present. Within the subcutaneous tissue was a necrotic cavity surrounded by a granulomatous reaction with prominent inflammatory cell infiltrate including eosinophils and lymphocytes. The appearances were those of a sparganum (third larval stage, also called plerocercoid) of *Spirometra*, which is a tapeworm of cats and dogs.

REFERENCES

Chai JY, Yu JR, Lee SH *et al.* Ineffectiveness of praziquantel treatment for human sparganosis. A case report. *Seoul Journal of Clinical Medicine* 1988; **29**: 397–399

Cross JH. Parasitology in Vietnam. *Parasitology Today* 1994; **10**: 247–248

Jeong SC, Bae JC, Hwang SH *et al.* Cerebral sparganosis with intracerebral haemorrhage – a case report. *Neurology* 1998; **50**: 503–506

Kudesia S, Indira DB, Sarada D *et al.* Sparganosis of brain and spinal cord: unusual tapeworm infestation (report of two cases). *Clinical Neurological Neurosurgery* 1998; **100**: 148–152

Munckof WH, Grayson ML, Susil BJ *et al.* Cerebral sparganosis in an East Timorese refugee. *Medical Journal of Australia* 1994; **161**: 263

Nakamura T, Hara M, Matsuoka M *et al.* Human proliferative sparganosis. *American Journal of Clinical Pathology* 1990; **94**: 224–228

You DL, Tzen KY, Kao PF *et al.* Cerebral sparganosis: increase uptake of technetium-99m-HMPAO. *Journal of Nuclear Medicine* 1997; **38**: 939–941

34

Coenurosis

Parasitology
Presentation
  Pathology

Investigations
Treatment
References

PARASITOLOGY

Coenurosis is a rare infection caused by the larval cestode of the genus *Multiceps*, which affects the brain, spinal cord and eye. There are other species that are pathogenic to humans in some parts of the world and occasionally parasitize the subcutaneous tissues.

Most reported cases of coenurosis are from tropical Africa and South Africa. Occasional sporadic cases have been seen in the USA, UK and France and in migrants to Australia.

The adult worm measures 40–60 cm in length and has four suckers with an armed rostellum on the scolex. Each gravid proglottid measures 8–10 mm in length and 3–4 mm in width. It resembles all other taenia species and ranges from 31 to 36 mm in diameter. The larva or coenurus is white or grey, globular or sausage-shaped and has a thin-walled cyst measuring from a few to 20 mm in diameter. The unilocular cyst contains 50–100 protoscolices that develop from the germinal layer or inner lining of the cyst wall. These protoscolices project into the cyst cavity filled with jelly-like fluid. The adult worms inhabit the intestine of the carnivorous definitive host (either dog or wolf). They pass eggs, which in turn are ingested by the intermediate host which are herbivorous mammals such as sheep, goats, cattle and horses.

They swallowing eggs passed by the definitive host, mainly dogs and infect humans. The eggs hatch out in the small intestine of the intermediate host and the oncosphere penetrates the intestinal wall, enters the blood circulation, then migrates to organs such as the brain, eye and subcutaneous tissues. When the infected organs of the intermediate hosts are eaten by a dog or wolf (the definitive host), the protoscolex invaginates and grows into an adult worm, thereby completing the life cycle (Figure 34.1).

PRESENTATION

The clinical presentation depends on the site of the cyst. The sites involved are brain, eye and skin. The cerebral type of infection is seen more often in adults, and the ocular and skin lesions in children. Children are more prone to direct inoculation of the skin and eye as they play on the ground. Cerebral coenurosis is generally insidious in onset and more chronic in onset. The cysts are in the subarachnoid space. There may be signs of raised intracranial pressure due to obstruction of the cerebrospinal fluid pathway. If the cysts are in the cerebral hemisphere, the presentation is one of localizing signs such as epilepsy, pyramidal tract lesions, sensory symptoms or cranial nerve palsies. Cysts may involve the spinal cord with its attendant

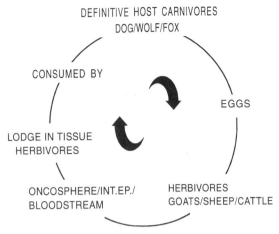

DEFINITIVE HOST CARNIVORES
DOG/WOLF/FOX

CONSUMED BY

EGGS

LODGE IN TISSUE
HERBIVORES

ONCOSPHERE/INT.EP./
BLOODSTREAM

HERBIVORES
GOATS/SHEEP/CATTLE

Figure 34.1 – Life cycle of Coenurosis.

clinical manifestations. Sciatic neuritis has also been reported.

Ocular manifestations are secondary to orbital or intra-ocular lesions such as subretinal or intravitreal. These lesions may mimic neoplastic lesions in children, such as retinoblastoma. Orbital lesions present as nodules in the extrinsic ocular muscles and eyelids or may be found in the subconjunctival system. On eye examination worms present in the anterior chamber or vitreous may be seen. Subcutaneous nodules are painless, and measure up to 5–6 cm in diameter and are commonly found in the trunk, neck, head and limbs. These lesions can be misdiagnosed for other nodular lesions such as neurofibromas, lipomas and ganglia. Coenurus has also been found in muscles (Ing *et al.* 1998).

PATHOLOGY

The adult worm provokes a basal arachnoiditis and chronic leptomeningitis. The severity depends on the viability of the parasite, with minimal cellular reaction seen to the live coenurus and a prominent inflammatory cellular infiltrate consisting of lymphocytes, plasma cells and eosinophils around the degenerated worm. A thin rim of fibrous tissue with a foreign body giant cell reaction gradually circumscribes the inflammation and dead worm. Adhesions of the leptomeninges with loculation of cerebrospinal fluid form the so-called 'racemose cyst'. When the coenurus is located in the brain, the surrounding cerebral parenchymal tissue shows significant gliosis, spongiosis

and microcalcification (Michal *et al.* 1997). A ventricular coenurus may cause ependymitis, subependymal nodular gliosis, the latter also known as ependymal glial granulation. When the eyes are involved there can be panophthalmitis, retinochoroiditis and even detachment of the retina. On microscopic examination, there is focal necrosis and granulation tissue infiltrated by leukocytes, plasma cells, histiocytes, eosinophils and neutrophils. The coenurus, when it is viable, can be readily identified by its triple layered cyst wall and calcareous corpuscles in a loose parenchyma but the most important feature is the presence of several protoscolices. However, the dead coenurus disintegrates and the only identifiable structures may be remnants of hooklets and fragmented cyst wall.

INVESTIGATIONS

1. Histologic examination – the only way of a definitive diagnosis is the identification of the coenurus or the cyst larva with its multiple protoscolices without daughter cysts or brood capsules. (A *cysticercus* contains only one protoscolex, and a hydatid has daughter cysts and brood capsules.) The site of infection is also important as the coenurus is seen mostly in the brain and eye, whereas cysticercus and hydatid can be seen in many other organs. Tape worm cysts, if found in the brain, are often 'sterile', that is without protoscolices in the cyst cavity. Therefore, when only the cyst wall and parenchyma is seen, it is difficult to distinguish between cysticercus cellulosae and Multiceps, as both are identical. In these cases a specific identification of the coenurus relies on the geographic distribution, organ involvement and the measurement of hooklets.

2. Cerebrospinal fluid examination – may show an increase of protein and immunoglobulins and a reduction of glucose.

3. Eosinophilia – rarely seen and serologic tests cross-react with other cestodes.

4. Computed tomography or magnetic resonance scan – can be used for suspected cerebral lesions. They provide localization of lesions but are not specific for diagnosis of coenurus species.

TREATMENT

Treatment is surgical. There are no reports of anti-scolicidal drugs that are effective, and praziquantel, albendazole and mebendazole have not been found to be effective. Praziquantel will kill the coenurus but the subsequent inflammatory response can cause severe complications (Ibechukwa and Onwukeme 1991).

REFERENCES

Ibechukwa BI, Onwukeme KE. Intra-ocular coenurosis: a case report. *British Journal of Ophthalmology* 1991; **75**: 430–431

Ing MB, Schantz PM, Turner JA. Human coenurosis in North America: case reports and review. *Clinical Infectious Diseases* 1998; **27**: 519–523

Michal A, Regli F, Campiche R *et al.* Cerebral coenurosis. *Journal of Neurology* 1977; **216**: 265–272

V

Arthropods

35

Myiasis

Parasitology
  Cordylobia anthropophaga
  Dermatobia hominis
  Gastrophilus spp (Botflies)
  Hypoderma bovis
  Calliphora nociva spp
  Chrysoma bezziana
  Oestrus ovis

  Sarcophaga
  Anthomyiidae
Presentation
Investigations
Treatment
  Cutaneous Myiasis
  Aural Myiasis
References

During my journey a man on one of the stations complained to me of a dull pain in his ear, and as if something moving in it … by pouring brine into the ear a large white maggot crept out, and afterwards some smaller ones. (Bennett 1984)

PARASITOLOGY

Myiasis refers to infestation of the body by larvae of fly species. The types of myiasis are recognized according to the body parts involved, namely, cutaneous and mucocutaneous, nasal, aural, ophthalmic and intestinal.

The larvae of the fly Diptera feed on the hosts of dead or living tissue. If the development takes place on a living host they are specific obligatory parasites. If the larvae grows in dead tissue (but can occasionally infest living tissue), they are semi-specific or facultative parasites. The third group is accidental deposit of eggs in excreta or decaying organic matter or in foodstuff. The majority of obligatory parasites are botflies.

The three types of fly maggots that produce myiasis are:

1. Obligatory ones where invasion of tissue is essential for their development, e.g. *Dermatobia hominis* (botfly), *Cordylobia anthropophaga*, *Gastrophilus* spp. (horseblots or Warble flies), *Hypoderma bovis* (cattle bots or warble flies).
2. Facultative ones are species of *Sarcophaga*, *Cochliomyia* (screw worm), *Calliphora* and *Wolfhartia*.
3. Accidental type where eggs or larvae are scattered accidentally, e.g. genus *Oestrus*. In humans *O. ovis* are accidental parasites.

A few documented cases of accidental external ophthalmomyiasis caused by *O. ovis* (sheep nasal bottle fly) has been occasionally reported in Australia. Man may act as an accidental host for the fly, which is widely distributed in Australia.

From an epidemiological point of view and the potential threat to agriculture, medical officers who find larvae in patients, especially in travellers, should contact the nearest Medical Entomology Unit. *D. hominis* is a serious pest of cattle in South America and has caused great losses to the cattle industry.

Cordylobia anthropophaga

Also known as the tumbu fly found in tropical Africa, *C. anthropophaga* has been imported to Australia. It is large, yellow brown in colour and measures 7–12 mm in length. They are mostly active at dawn and dusk. At other times they rest in dark places in huts. Humans can be infected. The female lays 100–300 eggs in sandy ground or on clothing contaminated with urine or faecal matter. The minute larvae that hatch out remain upright awaiting a suitable host. They are sensitive to heat and vibration. When they attach to man or dogs it takes only 1 min to penetrate the skin by means of buccal hooks. Usually the skin of thighs, buttocks, neck and head is involved. A skin nodule develops at the site of the bite. The painful skin nodule or boil eventually bursts, the larvae fall to the ground and pupate in 24 h. Finally the adults hatch out in 10–20 days.

Dermatobia hominis

D. hominis is a large bluish-grey coloured fly measuring 1.5 cm in length. The eggs are laid on foliage or on other insects such as female mosquitoes (*Psorophora* spp.), Lutzii flies and ticks. The eggs adhere to the thorax of these insects and are carried to suitable hosts such as cattle, dogs and humans. The larvae hatch out and enter the skin in 5–10 min. A small nodule develops at the penetration site. The first stage larvae is cylindrical and contain a circlet of spines. The second stage larvae is pyriform and contains stout, backwardly directed spines on the globular anterior part. The posterior portion is narrow and has the respiratory siphoun. A warble appears at the site of the bite that grows to 2–3 cm in diameter. The larvae take 6–12 weeks or more to develop in man. Finally, it drops to the ground and pupates. After 3–4 days the adult fly emerges. The long larval development time increases the opportunity for *D. hominis* to be carried from one country to another. It has been reported in travellers from Australia (Fields 1981, CDI 1994).

Gastrophilus spp. (botflies)

The larvae cause cutaneous lesions similar to the larva migrans of helminths. The larvae produce a tunnel with the infected tissues. Human cases have been reported, including ophthalmomyiasis. The *Gastrophilus* of the horse pass all or part of their life cycle in the intestines, causing no damage except for occasional gastrointestinal symptoms. The larvae leave via anus to develop further in the soil. Pupation takes place in the soil. Humans are rather unsatisfactory hosts for the larva and causes a cutaneous creeping eruption similar to cutaneous larva migrans caused by helminths.

Hypoderma bovis

Flies of the genus *Hypoderma* botflies causes dermal myiasis in humans in the USA. The lesions are similar to *Gastrophilus* spp. but less serpiginous (Salamon *et al.* 1970). They bore more deeply into subcutaneous tissue and produce an inflamed swelling resembling a furuncle.

Calliphora nociva spp. or blowfly

Calliphora nociva spp. or blowfly are found in houses and they can seek out even slightly tainted meat. The fly deposits ova in wounds of cattle or other domestic animals. It can affect sinuses of humans with bad, offensive smelling sinuses. The larvae can cause destruction of palate, pharynx and nose, forming fistulous tracts. They are also found in the ear. *C. nociva* found in Australia is an ovo viviparous native blow fly. The larvae are ~8–9 mm in length and have been reported in aural myiasis (Morris and Weinstein 1986).

Chrysoma bezziana

These flies are found in Old World tropics of Africa, Asia and the Pacific Islands, as well as Australia where the climate is suitable. They tend to lay eggs in head wounds and can cause tissue destruction. The female lays her eggs in the batch in a cutaneous ulcer, or on the gums and nasal sinuses. The larvae hatch in 8–10 h, burrow into tissues, moult in 12–18 h and burrows more deeply the second and third day, and larvae leave the wound on sixth or seventh day.

Oestrus ovis (botflies)

The larvae are found in some states of Australia; flies are obligatory parasites, invading the nasal and frontal sinuses of sheep. The female adult fly squirts her larvae to the facial area of the host. Humans working on farmland can get accidentally infected, affecting the eyes superficially, particularly the conjunctivae and the eyelids. The larvae can cause severe irritation in the eyes. They also have the potential to invade the nasal sinuses. The larvae develop over 12 months in the sheep. The larvae are 1–2 mm long and 0.5 mm broad. The female fly ejects about 50 larvae where humans are infected by aerial transmission.

Sarcophaga (flesh fly)

There are > 100 species of the fly *Sarcophaga*. The adult flesh flies feed on faeces and decaying flesh such as fish or meat. The female deposits 40–80 first-stage larvae. The larvae penetrate the tissue and produce symptoms according to the site of invasion. Humans can be infected accidentally. They have an affinity to invade bleeding tissue or wounds oozing pus (Morris and Weinstein 1986). The larvae of *S. haemorrhoidalis* may be swallowed by humans in food and may become temporary parasites in human intestines.

Anthomyiidae

Flies of the genus *Anthomyiidae* deposit eggs near the urethral meatus, and the larvae pass up the urethra causing very little damage except for urethral irritation.

PRESENTATION

Clinical presentation in humans depends on the site of the infection.

External ophthalmomyiasis

This generally commences soon after the larva enters the eyes. The patient experiences a gritty feeling in the eye with severe irritation. The larvae can invade the lacrimal canaliculi and marked lacrimation can result. No damage is seen by larval penetration. Rarely, the larva may burrow into the eyeball and may lead to optic atrophy. Intestinal myiasis rarely causes symptoms and larvae or eggs may be evacuated in the faeces. Urogenital myiasis causes dysurea, irritation in external genitalia. Lung myiasis is rare, causes ill-defined shadows on X-ray and causes cough and purulent sputum.

Cutaneous myiasis is found on the unprotected skin and the larvae produce a tunnel perpendicular to the skin (Garcia and Bruckner 1993). On examination, the skin lesions look like pimples that become sore and gradually enlarge, becoming more painful and discharging dark blood. This may be mistaken for various dermatological conditions, unless a careful travel history is taken. The larva of *D. hominis* takes ~3 months to complete its life cycle in humans. At the end of this period it migrates to the skin surface and falls to the ground. The larval life of *C. anthropophaga* is much shorter and larvae leave the host in ~10 days. Human infestation most frequently occurs in scalp, legs, forearms and face. Rarely the larvae may migrate from scalp through the anterior fontanelle and enter the cranium in infants.

INVESTIGATIONS

1. In cutaneous or mucocutaneous lesions, remove the larvae as mentioned under treatment, or from the ear.
2. Place in a Petri dish (blood agarplate). Identification depends on examination of the larval stigmal plate. The maggots removed from different sites should be referred to an entomology unit for identification.

TREATMENT

Cutaneous myiasis

If there is a suspicion of a maggot, the wound should be smeared with petroleum jelly. The maggot suffocates and is forced to leave the wound (Burgess and Cowan 1993). The wound heals once the maggot has left. Most Africans are aware of the problem and some prefer to leave the larvae to exit naturally since attempts to remove the larvae, except under proper surgical methods, can result in the rupture of larvae and sepsis.

Removal of larvae is achieved by swabbing or irrigation of the conjunctival sac. Oily cocaine drops have been applied to the eyes, thereby immobilizing the larvae. Recovery of the eye is within 24 h.

Aural myiasis

Maggots may need to be removed from the auditory canal under a general anaesthetic. The use of normal saline with direct manipulation and suction can remove viable maggots (Burgess and Cowan 1993).

REFERENCES

Anon. Interception of larvae on an exotic fly pest in skin lesions on Australian travellers. *Communications Diseases Intelligence* 1994; **18**: 229–230

Bennett G. *Wandering in New South Wales*. London: Bentley, 1834, **1**: 294

Burgess NRH, Cowan CO. *A Colour Atlas of Medical Entomology*. London: Chapman & Hall, 1993

Fields S. Myiasis in an Australian abroad. *Medical Journal of Australia* 1981; **1**: 581–582

Garcia LS, Bruckner DA. *Diagnostic Medical Parasitology*, 2nd edn. Washington, DC: Microbiology, 1993, 454

Morris B, Weinstein P. A case of aural myiasis in Australia. *Medical Journal of Australia* 1986; **145**: 634–635

Salamon PF, Catts EP, Knox WG. Human dermal myiasis caused by rabbit botfly in Connecticut. *Journal of the American Medical Association* 1970; **213**: 1035–1036

36

Scabies and Pyemote Mite Infection

Scabies
    Presentation
    Pathology
    Investigations
    Treatment

Pyemote Mite Infection
    Parasitology
    Presentation
    Investigations
    Treatment
References

SCABIES

Scabies is a skin disease caused by an acarid *Sarcoptes scabiei*, commonly known as the itch mite. 'Scabies is an ancient disease which probably afflicted the Hebrews in the Old Testament era. Aristotle, Galen and early Latin writers may have been familiar with the disease' (Myers and Conner 1976).

Scabies caused by *S. scabiei* var. *hominis* is a universal ectoparasitic disease. It may be seasonal. In Europe the incidence is highest in winter. It is transmitted from person to person by direct contact, contaminated clothing as well as by sexual contact. The mite can survive for several hours, which provides sufficient time to infect a person. It is endemic within the Aboriginal communities in Australia with a 30–65% prevalence among school children (Connors 1994). Scabies is strongly associated with overcrowding. The female mites invade beneath the stratum corneum of the skin to lay their eggs. Scabies lesions have been implicated

in facilitating spread of infections such as hepatitis B in children (Harris *et al.* 1992). The 'Norwegian itch' is a more virulent form of scabies that often causes epidemics and sheds many more organisms. Animal scabies is caused by *Sarcoptes* spp., which is closely related to the human type and is found in domestic and wild animals. It may be transferred to man by intimate contact with animals but the lesions are far less itchy and typical burrows are not present.

The female mite *S. scabiei* var. *hominis* is 330–450 × 250 μm. The male is half the size. The body is covered by hairs and spines and has transverse ridges arranged parallel on the dorsal surface. It has four pairs of short legs, two anteriorly and two posteriorly. The egg measures 100–150 μm.

In 3–5 days the hexapod larvae hatch out, moult three times and mature in 10–14 days. The female *Sarcoptes* deposits eggs and faeces as they burrow in the epidermis for up to ~2 months.

Presentation

The clinical presentation is mainly skin irritation with burrows in the skin up to 3 cm in length. It is commonly found below the neck, the interdigital web spaces in the hands, wrists, nipples, penis, scrotum and in the buttocks. The itching is maximum at night and causes excoriation of the skin sometimes with secondary infection caused by streptococci. Acute post-streptococcal skin infection can lead to acute post-streptococcal glomerulonephritis.

Pathology

The tract or burrow is seen in the stratum corneum of the epidermis (Fig. 36.1). A lymphocytic infiltrate is seen beneath the burrow. The malpighian layer in the vicinity shows oedema with vesicle formation. The mite or eggs are not usually found in the skin in ordinary scabies; however, in Norwegian scabies, plenty of mites and ova are seen virtually filling the corneal layer. In the itchy nodules and papules chronic inflammatory cells and prominent eosinophils are found around the superficial vascular plexus and sweat glands. No parasites have been identified in sections of these nodules.

Investigations

1. Definitive diagnosis is made by demonstration of the mite in skin scrapings.
2. Biopsies taken from the blind end of the burrow are most diagnostic. When the scrapings are treated with potassium hydroxide on a slide, the mite, ova or its fragments can be seen on microscopy.

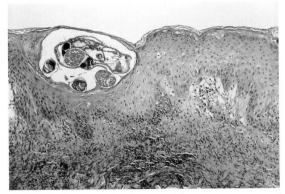

Figure 36.1 – *Sarcoptes* in a burrow of the stratum corneum of skin (H&E × 40).

Treatment

Treatment is based on complete eradication by scabicides, antibiotics to eliminate Group A Streptococcus infection, antipruritic agents and the elimination of the mite from bedding, clothing and furniture.

- Permethrin 5% for children – for children < 2 years apply to neck down; for children < 6 months, consult doctor before using permethrin (Connors 1994)
- Crotamiton 10% for children < 6 months
- Benzyl benzoate 25% for adults from neck downwards. It is an irritant to the eyes and should be applied 8–12 h before bathing after testing on a small area of skin before application
- 5% Permethrin is used if lesions are extensive, or in the case of Norwegian scabies.
- All skin lesions should be scrubbed before application of ointment
- Recently, ivermectin only has been used PO 200 μg/kg in a single dose and is 100% effective. It is particularly useful in these patients with secondary eczematization and excoriations for whom the topical treatments causes irritation (Offidani *et al*. 1999)
- All contact persons should be treated
- All linen should be washed in hot water
- Antipruritic agents and penicillin (if the patient is not allergic) are used to eliminate streptococcal infection. Failure of treatment is often due to improper application of the scabicide, and occurrences of multiple lesions in children, particularly when these occur on the palms and/or soles (Taplin *et al*. 1991)

PYEMOTE MITE INFECTION

Parasitology

Pyemote mites are ectoparasites of insects. Man is only accidentally infected. The mite does not burrow into the skin. Pyemotes are also found in certain agricultural areas such as the cotton and grain industry. Outbreaks of this ectoparasitic infestation have occurred throughout the world. The pyemote mite can parasitize on maggots of cotton seed moth and wheat. An outbreak of an itchy dermatitis was reported in the Australian Queensland Country Hospital of

Toowoomba, which was attributed to Pyemote mites from a sorghum field with a grain store in close proximity to the hospital (Letchford *et al.* 1994).

The female Pyemote mite is ~0.3 mm long; the male is 0.15 mm long. The sex can be distinguished by the pseudostigmatic organs in the female, found between the first and second pair of legs on the ventral aspect. The female gravid abdomen may have up to 300 young mites that reach full maturity. Males are born first and they assist in the birthing of the females and then fertilize them. The females thereafter move to find an insect larval host. There are several Pyemote mites that are still unnamed.

Presentation

The main clinical presentation is a very agonizing itchy dermatitis. It is found mainly in the trunk and the extremities. It may resemble scabies but there are no burrows. The rash may be papular, erythematous or vesicular. The dermatitis has been referred to as 'hay itch', 'straw itch', 'grain itch' and 'barley itch' (Alexander 1984). The differential diagnoses are insect bites, scabies and contact dermatitis. It is possible that infections of this nature are missed and treated as contact dermatitis. A clue to the diagnosis is contact dermatitis-like lesions in several people in the same environment and an awareness of this infection.

Investigations

1. It is very unusual to make a diagnosis by identifying the organism on skin scrapings or biopsy. Skin biopsies will demonstrate a chronic inflammatory reaction. Only one of 30 patients demonstrated a mite on skin scrapings (Letchford *et al.* 1994).

2. Hence, environmental specimens of hay, grain, cotton, etc. should be examined for ectoparasites and identified by an entomologist.

Treatment

There is no specific treatment available. Patients should be treated symptomatically with local antipruritic agents such as calamine lotion. It is essential to fumigate the environment by mite repellents. It is a self-limiting disease provided the source is found and necessary action taken to destroy the mite.

REFERENCES

Alexander JO'D. Pyemotes infestations. In *Arthropods in Human Skin.* Berlin: Springer, 1984, 317–324

Connors C. *Scabies Treatment.* Northern Territory Communicable Disease Collection, vol. 2. 1994

Harris M *et al.* Skin infections in Tanna, Vanuatu in 1989. *Papua New Guinea Medical Journal* 1992; **35**: 137–143

Letchford J, Shungs I, Farrell D. Pyemotes species strongly implicated in an outbreak of dermatitis in Queensland country hospital. *Pathology* 1994; **28**: 330–332

Myers WM, Conner DH. Scabies. In Binford CH, Connor DH (eds), *Pathology of Tropical and Extraordinary Diseases*, vol. II. Washington, DC: Armed Forces Institute of Pathology Fascicle, 1976, 615–617

Offidani A *et al.* Treatment of scabies with Ivermectin. *European Journal of Dermatology* 1999; **9**: 100–101

Taplin D *et al.* Community control of scabies. A model based on use of Permethrin cream. *Lancet* 1991; **337**: 1016–1018

Pediculosis

PARASITOLOGY

Pediculosis refers to infestation by lice. There are three species of lice: *Pediculosis humanus*, the body louse, *P. capitis*, the head louse, and *Phthirus pubis*, the crab louse, all belonging to the order Anoplura.

Body lice (*P. humanus*) are associated with poor hygiene and poor socio-economic conditions usually experienced by refugees. The pubic louse (*P. pubis*) is mainly sexually transmitted but can also be acquired by contaminated clothing and bed linen. Head lice (*P. capitis*) occur widely, unrelated to hygiene or socio-economic status. It is transmitted from person to person, especially among school children due to their close contact including sharing combs and hats. In some parts of the world with cold and temperate climates, *P. humanus* var. *corporis* is an efficient vector of relapsing fever, typhus and trench fever.

Lice are obligate ectoparasites. They are dorso-ventrally flattened, wingless insects, greyish or light brown in colour measuring 5 mm in length, *P. capitis* being slightly smaller than *P. humanus*. The body consists of a head and thorax with dark brown claws. The mouthparts are structured for sucking and piercing. The antennae are long and clearly seen as they are the same length as the head. The three pairs of legs each end in a tarsal claw adapted for grasping hair (Fig. 37.1).

When eggs ('nits') are laid they are firmly adherent to a single hair or, in the case of *P. humanus*, on clothing fibres. They hatch and go through several nymphal stages (after moulting) before becoming adults.

P. pubis is found in the genital and inguinal region and rarely on other body hair, but not on the scalp. It is short and stout with huge claws on the second and third pair of legs, which help it to cling to hairs (Fig. 37.2). Eggs are attached to hairs but not to clothing. They hatch in 7–8 days. The nymphs undergo three moults in ~13 days and become adults.

PRESENTATION

The common presentation is pruritus of the scalp and body. The pubic louse causes itchiness in the pubic and thigh regions and with skin excoriation. Infestation of eyelashes may be accompanied by blepharitis. The pubic louse can be seen attached to pubic hairs and occasionally to the eyelashes. The head and body lice cause severe discomfort. Itching and excoriation leading to secondary bacterial infection of the skin, are often associated with impetigo.

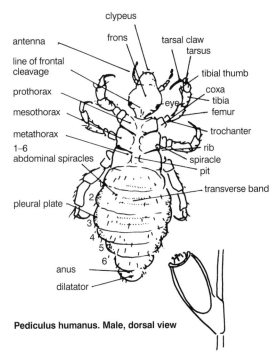

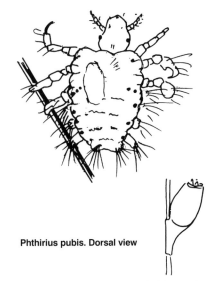

Pediculus humanus. Male, dorsal view

Figure 37.1 – Schematic diagram of *Pediculosis humanus* and egg ("nit") adherent to hair.

Phthirius pubis. Dorsal view

Figure 37.2 – Schematic diagram of *Phthirus pubis* and egg ("nit") adherent to hair.

Secondary treatment of head lice within 7 days is necessary to eradicate the lice. If left longer the remaining lice will be well enough developed to transfer to another host (Dawes *et al.* 1999).

TREATMENT

- Permethrin cream (5%) or lotion (1%) applied to the body or hair kills lice in one treatment (Taplin *et al.* 1986, Di Napoli *et al.* 1988), which should not be washed off for at least 2 h (Ares-Mazas *et al.* 1985) to ensure killing of the lice. It is not indicated if there is acute scalp inflammation or a history of pyrethrin and/or pyrethroid sensitivity (Chouela *et al.* 1997). In the UK the head lice are resistance to permethrin and are therefore of no value
- Co-trimoxazole was tried on patients infested with pediculosis in Egypt. Except for eggs (nits), prolonged use was needed to free the patient from adult and nymphoid stages (Mossy *et al.* 1996)
- Cabaryl (carylderum, Dertiac-C, Suleo-C) is almost 100% effective in the UK
- Malathion (Derbac-M, Prioderm, Quellada-M or Suleo-M) is also very effective and recommended as the first choice

There is no danger of neurotoxicity as the drugs cannot bind to neuroreceptors.

PREVENTION

Clothes should be washed in hot water (> 60°C) and then fumigated or treated with an insecticide for body lice. Prevention of reinfestation of head lice involves treatment on a community basis. Insecticidal powder should be used on clothing or articles which come into contact with the head, and subsequently washed. Individual and isolated treatments for pediculosis are useful, but massive complete and simultaneous treatments lead to a significant decrease in infestation prevalence. Careful inspection of the entire scalp with a powerful light source and lenses with big magnification is essential (Chouela *et al.* 1997).

REFERENCES

Ares-Mazas E, Casal Porto M, Sela Perez MC *et al.* The efficacy of permethrin lotion in *Pediculosis capitis. American Journal of Dermatology* 1985; **24**: 603–605

Chouela E, Abeldano A, Cirigliano M *et al.* Head louse infestations. Epidemiologic survey and treatment evaluation in Argentinean school children. *International Journal of Dermatology* 1997; **36**: 819–825

Dawes M, Hicks NR, Fleminger M *et al.* Evidence based case report: treatment for head lice. *British Medical Journal* 1999; **318**: 385–386

Di Napoli JB, Austin RD, Englender SJ *et al.* Eradication of head lice with a single treatment. *American Journal of Public Health* 1988; **78**: 978–980

Mossy TA, Ramadan NI, Mahmoud MS *et al.* On the efficacy of co-trimoxazole as an oral treatment for *Pediculosis capitis* infestation. *Journal of the Egyptian Society of Parasitology* 1996; **26**: 73–77

Taplin D, Meinking TL, Porcelain SL *et al.* Permethrin 5% dermal cream. A new treatment for scabies. *Journal of the American Academy of Dermatology* 1986; **15**: 995–1001

Tungiasis

Parasitology
Presentation
  Complications

Pathology
Treatment
References

PARASITOLOGY

Tungiasis is caused by penetration of human skin by the flea *Tunga penetrans* (syn. chigoc flea, jigger flea). It is prevalent in Central and South America, the Caribbean Islands, tropical Africa, the Seychelles, Pakistan and the West Coast of India. The prevalences of *T. penetrans* L. in inhabitants within five townships in south-western Trinidad, West Indies, were between 17 and 31%.

The mature free-living female is ~1 mm long with a flattening of the body from side to side. At the posterior end are pointing hairs and setae. It has long, large legs but no wings. After copulation the male flea dies but the female begins a pattern of jumping up to 35 cm above the ground that persists at intervals till it dies or penetrates the skin of a warm blooded animal. After penetration she becomes engorged with blood and developing eggs. The abdomen swells and becomes spherical and finally reaches ~1 cm in diameter, making the head and tail relatively tiny (Fig. 38.1). The epidermis of the skin surrounds the flea, which is oriented with its head down. The tail opens to the exterior through a hole in the epidermis. Eggs and excrement are discharged through this (Conner 1976). This opening probably enables the flea to breathe. The cuticle is thick with a prominent hypodermal cell layer and the flea has a system of branching tracheae, the blood distended intestines, reproductive tubes with ova and a minute, dwarfed head (Fig. 38.2). A thick band of striated muscle is seen extending from the cuticle near the head along the long axis to the cuticle at the external orifice. The proboscis extends into the dermis. The flea reaches maximum size in 1 week.

PRESENTATION

Although fleas attack any part of the body, the feet and legs that are most exposed are often involved, particularly ankles, instep and between the toes. The early lesion is seen as a tiny black spot, which later enlarges to a red, itchy and painful papule. When the lesions are subungual they are particularly painful.

Complications

Sepsis may be associated with *T. penetrans* infections. *Streptococcus pyogenes*, beta-haemolytic streptococcus (not group A), *Klebsiella aerogenes*, *Enterobacter agglomerans*, *Staphylococcus aureus*, *Escherichia coli* and a bacillus sp. *Clostridium tetani* was not isolated (Chadee 1998).

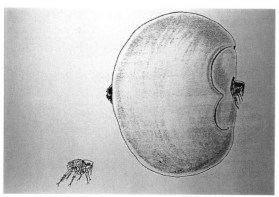

Figure 38.1 – Comparison of the size of the non-gravid with the engorged *Tunga penetrans*.

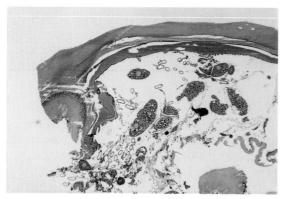

Figure 38.2 – Tungiasis. A section of skin with breached epidermis, thick cuticle of flea showing the hypodermal cells, branching tracheal and reproductive tubes.

PATHOLOGY

The epidermis is breached and the dermis is congested, containing a cellular inflammatory infiltrate of lymphocytes, plasma cells and eosinophils. The flea collapses after the eggs are extruded, with an underlying crater filled with a fibrinopurulent exudate. The base can later become re-epithelialized, with the collapsed flea and keratinous debris sloughing off.

TREATMENT

The flea should be removed intact by continuously removing or peeling back the surrounding keratin with a sharp needle. The crater is then cleaned and dressed. If the flea is ruptured, the contents elicit an intense inflammatory reaction.

REFERENCES

Chadee DD. Tungiasis among five communities in south-western Trinidad, West Indies. *Annals of Tropical Medical Parasitology* 1998; 92: 107–113

Conner DH. Tungiasis. In Binford CH, Conner DH (eds), *Pathology of Tropical and Extraordinary Diseases*, vol. II. AFIP fascicle, 1976, 610–614

VI

Bacterial Infections

Atypical Mycobacteriosis

MICROBIOLOGY

Atypical mycobacteriosis caused by several species of mycobacteria involve many organs and disseminated disease in humans. There is an increase in those who use immunosuppressive drugs and organ transplants. It is an important disease entity in the countries where mycobacteriosis is under control.

Atypical mycobacteria are present in the environment and have been isolated from fresh and coastal water, swimming pools, tap water, soil, dust and milk. They can contaminate laboratory specimens. The mode of infection in man is by aerosol or direct contamination through the skin. There is no evidence of person-to-person transmission. A limited number of familial clusters suggest a point source outbreak or human transmission. About 40 atypical mycobacteria have been identified of which ~17 are pathogenic to humans. Most of these have been cultured. They tend to be pathogenic in immunocompromised patients, patients with chronic debilitating disease such as bronchitis, healed tuberculosis, emphysema, silicosis, diabetes and malignancy.

All mycobacteria are acid-alcohol fast and stain red with the Ziehl-Neelsen stain. A characteristic feature is that the strains have considerable amount of lipids in the cell wall. These organisms multiply in cells of organs, macrophages and also extracellularly. They divide slowly and preferentially at low temperatures. A few are fast growing organisms. They also have the characteristic feature of persisting as dormant forms in chronic pathologic processes. Specific atypical mycobacteria have a predilection for specific organs such as lungs, skin, eyes, ears, lymph glands, pericardium, brain, bones, joints and kidneys. Some strains of the atypical mycobacteria are relatively new and may be isolated from sputum and gastric contents of normal people. Repeated isolation of the organism in a patient with the appropriate signs and symptoms are essential before considering them as pathogenic.

Atypical mycobacteria pathogenic to man are:

- *M. marinum*
- *M. genavense*
- *M. avium-intracellulare* (Battey bacillus)
- *M. abscessus*
- *M. ulcerans*
- *M. xenopis*
- *M. avium intracellulare* and *M. scrofulaceum* (MAIS complex)
- *M. haemophilum*
- *M. chelonae*
- *M. terrae*
- *M. fortuitum*
- *M. kansasii*
- *M. smegmatis*
- *M. vaccae*
- *M. malmoense*

(*M. avium* and *M. intracellulare* are considered together as distinction is difficult.)

Microscopic examination does not help in differentiating these different species. Culture and biochemical tests are essential. Unlike *M. tuberculosis*, which is 'niacin positive', atypical mycobacteria are 'niacin-negative'. Runyon classified the atypical mycobacteria according to reaction to light and production of pigment and the rate of growth.

M. ulcerans infects the skin and subcutaneous tissue and grows best ~32°C. It is also found in Africa, Mexico, New Guinea and Northern Indonesia and is referred to as 'Toro ulcer' and 'Bairnsdale ulcer'.

Cases of ocular keratitis have been reported in contact lens wearers, probably from water containing *M. chelonae*. *M. chelonae* grows rapidly at 25–40°C and produce aryl sulphate in 1–3 days. Septic arthritis due to *M. marinum* was reported in 40 patients who had previously been in good health but had been handling fish or were involved in aquatic activities (Harth *et al.* 1994). *M. marinum* is commonly found in seafood handlers who puncture their skin with sharp parts of fish and in those who abrade their skin in swimming pools or in aquariums. Bronchoscopy-associated *M. xenopi* infections has occurred because the hot water tank supplying the water in which the bronchoscopes were disinfected with gluteraldehyde was contaminated with organisms (Bennett *et al.* 1994). Tenosynovitis due to mycobacteria other than tuberculosis is a hazard of water sports.

M. fortuitum abscess has been documented in a patient receiving corticosteroids for sarcoidosis (Faulk 1995). The incidence of disseminated *M. kansasii* infection is higher among immunosuppressed patients and has a worse prognosis. *M. genavense* is a mycobacterium described recently and so far identified only in a person with advanced HIV disease. The reservoir of this pathogen has not been identified (Shafran *et al.* 1995). *M. genavense* infection, presenting as a space-occupying lesion of the brain, has been reported in a patient with AIDS (Berman *et al.* 1994). *M. genavense* may be responsible for > 10% of disseminated non-tuberculous mycobacterial infections in patients with AIDS (Pechere *et al.* 1995). Disseminated *M. scrofulaceum* is a rare disease and has been recorded in AIDS patients with chronic ulcerative and nodular skin lesions and pulmonary cavitation. In AIDS patients atypical mycobacteria produce significant pulmonary lesions when patient immunity is greatly reduced and also causes disseminated disease. Pericardial effusion has been reported to occur in up to 38% of patients with AIDS. *M. kansasii*, which causes mainly pulmonary and disseminated infections in immunocompromised patients, is the organism responsible for pericarditis (Moreno *et al.* 1994). Other atypical mycobacterial organisms causing disseminated disease are *M. marinum* complex (Monforte *et al.* 1995), *M. xenopi* and *M. chelonae* (Shafran *et al.* 1995).

M. marinum infection of skin has been reported in patients with lymphoma who have also had AIDS (Hanan *et al.* 1994). Mycobacterial infections other than tuberculosis is reported in patients who are immunocompromised, but do not have AIDS, such as patients having continuous abdominal peritoneal lavage (CAPD), renal, heart and liver transplant patients. It has also been reported in patients with hairy cell leukaemia.

Atypical mycobacteriosis of the skin is more common than tuberculous infections of the skin. The common atypical mycobacteria causing skin infections are *M. marinum*, *M. fortuitum*, *M. chelonae*, *M. ulcerans* and less commonly are *M. haemophilum*, *M. avium-intracellulare*, *M. kansasii* and *M. bovis* (bacillus of Calmette and Guérin).

The most common mycobacterial agent is the *M. avium-intracellulare* group and occasionally *M. kansasii* and *M. fortuitum*.

The occurrence of a human mycobacterial susceptibility gene has been postulated in a report on a familial immune defect predisposing to disseminated atypical mycobacterial infection in six children (Levin *et al.*

1995). There were two families with two brothers in each family affected. The patients affected, including their parents, had production of tumour necrosis factor-α in response to endotoxin and defective Gamma-interferon. The T-cell response to mycobacteria was reduced. Others have reported on familial disseminated atypical mycobacterial disease and there seems to be a genetic component to this. Identification of the defect could lead to better understanding of the genetics and susceptibility to mycobacterial infections (Newport and Levin 1994). Four of eight children in a Pakistani family died of immune deficiency (Levin *et al.* 1995), two children developed symptoms after BCG vaccination and one child had *M. avium* infection and all had motility of monocytes towards chemotactic stimuli diminished and monocyte derived dendritic cells (Mooij *et al.* 1993) and showed a poor ability to form cellular clusters and defective upregulation of MHC Class II molecules on these cells.

PRESENTATION

Pulmonary disease

Pulmonary disease is generally caused by *M. kansasii* and MAIS complex. *M. kansasii* is considered the most virulent of non-tuberculous mycobacteria. Unlike tuberculosis there is no contact history. The disease caused by these organisms is found in lungs already affected by obstructive airways disease, silicosis, bronchiectasis or previous tuberculous infection. The disease is generally slowly progressive with symptoms such as cough, fever, haemoptysis similar to tuberculous infection. The infection causes cavitation. Cavitary lung disease, which is diagnostic of pulmonary infection in HIV-negative patients, is documented in < 50% of HIV-positive patients. Rarely, the disease may be rapidly progressive or may be disseminated. Radiological features are similar to those seen in tuberculosis. Unusual presentations simulating a tumour obstructing segmental bronchi have been reported (Quieffin *et al.* 1994). Rarely, *M. malmoense* can cause lung infection and simulate a tumour (Yoganathan *et al.* 1994). Tuberculin reaction is generally weakly positive.

Lymph glands (scrofula)

Infection of lymph glands is common in children between the ages of 2 and 8 years. It is more common

than *M. tuberculosis* infection of the lymph glands. *M. malmoense* adenitis has been reported in a child of 5 years. The common lymph glands infected are in the neck and the nodes are mostly unilateral and may be cold or hot. The mode of infection is probably occult trauma to the dermal or oropharyngeal mucosa.

The glands may be very large, not painful or tender, and can produce a bull neck which may interfere with breathing and swallowing. If untreated, chronic draining sinuses are formed with scarring. The histopathological features of scrofula are similar to *M. tuberculosis*. Investigations are not very helpful.

Dermatological lesions

Multiple cutaneous abscesses may occur in immunocompromised patients following dissemination by blood caused by the *M. haemophilum*, *M. fortuitum* and *M. chelonae*. *M. fortuitum* and which are rapidly growing organisms found in soil and water, may infect dirty puncture wounds as well as postoperative wounds, and cause osteomyelitis of sternum, peritonitis in patients on CAPD, and infection of breast prosthesis. The skin may be involved via a sinus tract in osteomyelitis or following haematogenous dissemination of organisms such as *M. kansasii* and *M. avium-intracellulare* which predominantly affect the lung.

M. marinum infection has an incubation period of 2–8 weeks. It is called swimming pool granuloma. The skin lesions are nodular or papular and the common sites are feet, hands, elbows and ankles. Small lesions may heal or progress to involve deeper structures, such as tendons and bones or spread through lymphatics simulating sporotrichosis. The healing process may take months or years if untreated.

M. ulcerans, *M. haemophilum* and *M. marinum* have fastidious temperature requirements within the narrow range of 30–32°C, as such these organisms do not produce systemic disease at the normal body temperatures.

In *M. ulcerans* the subcutaneous lesions are mainly in the limbs. They begin as erythematous, elevated cutaneous lesions, which enlarge over several weeks. A vesicle forms and breaks down to produce an ulcer. The ulcer has a white necrotic slough and the border is scalloped or undermined. Even with large ulcers there are no systemic manifestations, the patients look well and there is no regional lymphadenopathy in half the patients. Strangely enough the ulcers are not malodorous. The adjacent skin may even appear normal despite the large ulcer. Ulcers can remain for many years and may eventually heal. The differential diagnosis of ulcers include bite by scorpions or venomous insects such as spiders that produce necrotic ulcers and tropical phagadenic ulcers, the most common ulcer in the tropics, painful malodorous and do not show acid-fast bacilli.

Ophthalmic lesions

Keratitis has been caused by non-tuberculous mycobacteria. They are an unusual cause of keratitis. It has been reported in users of hard contact lenses. Non-contact lens users who have a procedure such as blepheroplasty or radial keratotomy may also contact the infection. The organisms in a few patients are *M. smegmatis* and *M. chelonae*, a rapidly growing environmental mycobacterium.

Disseminated atypical mycobacterial infection

In one series non-tuberculous mycobacterial disease (NTM) was diagnosed in nearly 9% of 350 AIDS patients at autopsy (Monforte *et al.* 1995). Nearly all had positive blood cultures for *M. avium* complex. Sixty-five percent of those who had NTM at autopsy and the common organs involved were lymph nodes, bone marrow, spleen, followed by liver, gastrointestinal tract, lung, brain and kidney (Monforte *et al.* 1995). Bacteraemia in the initial stages is associated with non-specific symptoms such as fever, anaemia and weight loss. This is followed by specific organ involvement. Pericarditis has been reported in nearly 38% of patients with AIDS and the possibility of mycobacterial pericarditis should be considered (Moreno *et al.* 1994). *M. genavense* may produce a mass lesion in the brain resulting in convulsions (Berman *et al.* 1994). In 54 patients with HIV who developed disseminated infections caused by *M. genavense* the common symptoms were fever, weight loss, diarrhoea, anaemia and several of these patients had hepatosplenomegaly. Infection with *M. genavense* may account for > 10% of disseminated non-tuberculous mycobacterial infections in HIV-infected patients (Pechere *et al.* 1995). Common manifestations of non-tuberculous mycobacterial infections in solid organ transplant recipients include cutaneous lesions, tenosynovitis and joint infection.

PATHOLOGY

In Buruli ulcer there is extensive coagulative necrosis involving the dermis and underlying fat. Cellular filtration is sparse. There may be a septal panniculitis with a mixed inflammatory cell infiltrate at the margins. Numerous acid-fast bacilli are usually found in clumps in the necrotic tissue extracellularly. Granulomas may be seen in recurrent or longstanding lesions. Granulomatous reaction at the ulcer margins is a feature of healing. Caseation is not seen. Dystropic calcification can also be seen.

In swimming pool granuloma inflammation is usually confined to the dermis with additional subcutaneous involvement in sporotrichoid form. The features could range from an acute suppurative process to poorly formed granulomas. Caseation is absent. In a minority of cases acid-fast bacilli which are longer and fatter than *M. tuberculosis* is seen.

The histopathology of other species is not specific. Presence of poorly formed granulomas which include areas of acute suppurative foci in the dermis with extension at time to the subcutaneous tissue needs investigation for atypical mycobacteriosis. In *M. avium* and *M. intracellulare* acid-fast bacilli are in abundance.

INVESTIGATIONS
Pulmonary disease

1. Definitive diagnosis requires repeated isolation of the same species of atypical mycobacterium from sputum in those patients having signs and symptoms similar to tuberculosis. These mycobacteria may be saprophytes in the respiratory tract. The sputum should be cultured.

Lymph glands

1. Chest X-rays in scrofula are normal and Mantoux may be positive or negative.
2. Cultures are necessary to prove the diagnosis in scrofula. Ziehl-Neelsen stain may demonstrate a large number of bacilli. Cultures should be performed at 31°C and takes 6–8 weeks to grow.

3. New skin tests with non-tuberculous mycobacteria antigens and the polymerase chain reaction (PCR) method has been used in Japan for early diagnosis of non-tuberculous mycobacterial lymphadenitis.

Dermatological lesions

1. Biopsy specimens of skin lesions may demonstrate features described under pathology.

TREATMENT

Pulmonary disease

- *M. kansasii* infection can be treated with a 9-month course of rifampicin and ethambutol (Research Committee 1994). Organisms are sensitive to rifampicin and ethambutol but resistant to isoniazid and pyrazinamide. Reinfection and relapse can occur after a course of treatment.
- *M. intracellulare* is resistant to antituberculous drugs. A combination of three to six drugs is recommended. Among these the new macrolides clarithromycin or azithromycin are recommended as a component of the combination therapy. They should not be used alone (Rapp *et al.* 1994). The drugs that should be considered in the treatment are clarithromycin, ciprofloxacin, amikacin, minocycline, sulphonamides, erythromycin and traditional antituberculous agents.

Lymphadenitis

- Antituberculous treatment is not essential. For lymph gland infection, scrofula treatment of choice is total excision of the infected nodes (Venkatesh *et al.* 1994).

Dermatological lesions

- The treatment for *M. marinum* includes ethambutol plus rifampicin, minocycline, doxycycline or sulphamethoxazole-trimethoprim or amikacin. Among these, ethambutol plus rifampicin seems very promising, with a cure rate of 100% in five patients. It was more effective than minocycline (Edelstein 1994). The duration of treatment

varied from 6–8 months for ethambutol and rifampicin or at least 2 months after lesions disappear (Edelstein 1994). Most antibiotics need to be used for several months. Clarithromycin was reported to be potent against *M. marinum* (Bonnet *et al.* 1994). Other forms of treatment are surgical excision, cryotherapy, X-ray, Grenz rays and irradiation. The dose of ethambutol is 25 mg/kg/day and rifampicin 600 mg/day. Adverse reactions to these drugs should be carefully monitored. Cholestatic hepatitis has been reported in a patient who received clarithromycin therapy for *M. chelonae* pulmonary infection (Yew *et al.* 1994)

- Treatment of ulcers caused by *M. ulcerans* with antibiotics has not been beneficial. The most successful treatment is debridement, excision and skin graft

Mycobacterium chelonae

- M. chelonae is an organism resistant to most drugs. It responds to treatment with clarithromycin and ciprofloxacin. Duration of treatment could be up to 6 months. Dose of ciprofloxacin is 750 mg twice daily and clarithromycin 500 mg twice daily (Mubashir *et al.* 1994). Surgical treatment, if possible, may be necessary
- For *M. abscessus* infections, clarithromycin together with other drugs is recommended for treatment (Mushatt and Witzig 1995)
- *M. fortuitum* is a rapidly growing organism and aggressive surgical treatment with antibiotics such as azithromycin, amikacin, doxycyline, minocycline, sulphamethoxazole and sulphamethoxazole-trimethoprim is necessary. Conventional antituberculous drugs have no significant activity against rapidly growing mycobacteria, and several drugs with proven *in vitro* activity should be utilized

Ophthalmic lesions

- Successful treatment with amikacin, doxycycline, topical ciprofloxacin for *M. chelonae* keratitis has been reported (Probst *et al.* 1994). Topical application of amikacin and ofloxacin has not been used for *M. smegmatis* (Probst *et al.* 1994). Partial success with topical imipenem, ciprofloxacin and erythromycin in *M. chelonae* infection has been achieved although subsequent relapse have occurred

- Lamellar keratectomy is the treatment of choice for patients unresponsive to medical therapy (Hu 1995, Tseng and Hsaio 1995). Performing penetrating keratoplasty for intractable non-tuberculous mycobacterial keratitis early can reduce the patient's suffering (Tseng and Hsaio 1995)

Disseminated atypical mycobacterial infection

- Disseminated *M. kansasii* infection has a worse prognosis in immunosuppressed patients. Chemotherapy includes traditional antituberculous drugs such as rifampicin, ethambutol, erythromycin, minocycline, doxycycline while it is resistant to isoniazid and *p*-aminosalicylic acid. When rifampicin is used serum concentration of many drugs is reduced and plasma concentration of other medications should be monitored (Joos *et al.* 1998). In *M. avium* complex the new macrolides, azithromycin and clarithromycin are promising in this infection. It is recommended that clarithromycin is included in the combination of drugs for treatment of disseminated infections in AIDS patients (Rapp *et al.* 1994). The appropriate antibiotic for *M. genavense* is not known. However, it is stated that the treatment regimen for *M. avium* complex may be beneficial. *M. scrofulaceum* in AIDS patients is susceptible to clarithromycin, ethambutol and clofazimine. Empirical therapy with two or more drugs should be considered. *M. xenopi* is a slow growing scotochromogen which is sensitive to most of the antituberculous drugs. Isolates of *M. chelonae* are susceptible to sulphamethoxazole-trimethoprim, doxycycline, erythromycin and ciprofloxacin, and recent studies suggests that clarithromycin should be included in the initial treatment (Tebas *et al.* 1995)
- Familial disseminated atypical mycobacteria – treatment with antibiotics has been unsatisfactory. Treatment with Gamma-interferon was associated with improvement (Levin *et al.* 1995)

REFERENCES

Bennett SN, Peterson DE, Johnson DR *et al.* Bronchoscopy associated *Mycobacterium xenopi*, pseudoinfections. *American Journal of Respiratory Critical Care Medicine* 1994; **150**: 245–250

Berman SM, Kim RC, Haghighat D *et al.* *Mycobacterium genavense* infection presenting as a solitary brain mass in a patient with AIDS. Case report and review. *Clinical Infectious Diseases* 1994; **19**: 1152–1154

Bonnet E, Debat-Zoguereh D, Petil N *et al.* Clarithromycin a potent agent against infections due to *Mycobacterium marinum* [Letter]. *Clinical Infectious Diseases* 1994: **18**: 664

Conner DH, Myers WM, Krieg RE. Infection by *Mycobacterium ulcerans*. In Binford CH, Conner DH (eds), *Pathology of Tropical and Extraordinary Diseases*, vol. 1. Washington, DC: Armed Forces Institute of Pathology, 1976, 226–243

Edelstein H. *Mycobacterium marinum* skin infections. Report of 31 cases and review of literature. *Archives of Internal Medicine* 1994; **154**: 1399–1314

Faulk CT, Lesher JL Jr. Phaeohyphomycosis and *Mycobacterium fortuitum* abscess in a patient receiving corticosteroids for sarcoidosis. *Journal of the American Academy of Dermatology* 1995; **33**: 309–311

Hanan LH, Leaf A, Soeiro R *et al.* *Mycobacterium marinum* infection in a patient with the acquired immunodeficiency syndrome. *Cutis* 1994; **54**: 103–105

Harth M, Ralph ED, Faraawi R. Septic arthritis due to *Mycobacterium marinum* [Review]. *Journal of Rheumatology* 1994; **21**: 957–960

Hu FR. Extensive lamellar keratectomy for treatment of non-tuberculous mycobacterial keratitis. *American Journal of Ophthalmology* 1995; **120**: 47–54

Joos AAB, Frank UG, Kascha W. Pharmacokinetic interaction of clozapine and rifampicin in a forensic patient with an atypical mycobacterial infection. *Journal of Clinical Pharmacology* 1998: 83–85

Levin M, Newport MJ, D'Souza *et al.* Familial disseminated atypical mycobacterial infection in childhood. *Lancet* 1995, **345**: 79–83

Levin M, Newport MJ, D'Souza S *et al.* Familial disseminated atypical mycobacterial infection in childhood. A human mycobacterial susceptibility gene? *Lancet* 1995; **345**: 72–83

Monforte Ad'A, Gori A, Vago L *et al.* Atypical mycobacterial disease findings at autopsy in a cohort of 350 patients in Milan, Italy. *Journal of Infectious Diseases* 1995; **172**: No 3 901

Mooij P, Simons PJ, de Haan-Meulman M *et al.* The effect of thyroid hormones and other iodinated compounds on the transition of monocytes into veiled dendritic cells: a role of GM-CSF TNF-X and IL-6. *Journal of Endocrinology* 1993; **140**: 503–512

Moreno F, Sharkey-Mathis PK, Mokulis E *et al.* *Mycobacterium kansasii* pericarditis in patients with AIDS. *Clinical Infectious Diseases* 1994; **19**: 967–969

Mubashir AZ, Klotz SA, Goldstein E *et al.* *M. chelonae* subspecies chelonae: report of a patient with sporotrichoid presentation who was successfully treated with clarithromycin and ciprofloxacin. *Clinical Infectious Diseases* 1994; **18**: 999–1001

Mushatt DM, Witzig RS. Successful treatment with multidrug regimens containing clarithromycin [Letter]. *Clinical Infectious Diseases* 1995; **20**: 1441–1442

Newport M, Levin M. Familial disseminated atypical mycobacterial disease. *Immunology Letters* 1994; **43**: 133–138

Pechere M, Opravu M, Wald A *et al.* Clinical and epidemiologic features of infection with *Mycobacterium genavense*. Swiss HIV cohort study. *Archives of Internal Medicine* 1995; **155**: 400–404

Probst LE, Brewer LV, Hussain Z *et al.* Treatment of *Mycobacterium chelonae* keratitis with amikacin, doxycycline and topical ciprofloxacin. *Canadian Journal of Ophthalmology* 1994; **29**: 81–84

Quieffin J, Ponbeau P, Laaban JP *et al. Mycobacterium kansasii* infection presenting as an endobronchial tumour in a patient with the acquired immune deficiency syndrome. *Tubercle and Lung Disease* 1994; **75**: 313–315

Rapp RP, McCraney SA, Goodman NL *et al.* New macrolide antibodies: usefulness in infections caused by mycobacteria other than *Mycobacterium tuberculosis. Annals of Pharmacotherapy* 1994; **28**: 1255–1263

Research Committee, British Thoracic Society. *Mycobacterium kansasii* pulmonary infection: a prospective study of the results of nine months of treatment with rifampicin and ethambutol. *Thorax* 1994; **49**: 442–445

Shafran SD, Taylor GD, Talbot JA. Disseminated *Mycobacterium genavense* infection in Canadian AIDS patients. *Tubercle and Lung Disease* 1995; **76**: 168–170

Tebas P, Sultan F, Wallace RJ Jr *et al.* Rapid development of resistance to clarithromycin following monotherapy for disseminated *Mycobacterium chelonae* infection in a heart transplant patient. *Clinical Infectious Diseases* 1995; **20**: 443–444

Tseng SH, Hsaio WC. Therapeutic lamellar keratectomy in the management of non-tuberculous mycobacterial keratitis refracting to medical treatments. *Cornea* 1995; **14**: 161–166

Venkatesh V, Everson NW, Johnstone JM. Atypical mycobacterial lymphadenopathy in children. Is it underdiagnosed? *Journal Royal College of Surgeons Edinburgh* 1994; **39**: 301–303

Yew WW, Chan CH, Lee J *et al.* Cholestatic hepatitis in a patient who received clarithromycin therapy for *M. chelonae* lung infection. *Clinical Infectious Diseases* 1994; **18**: 1025–1026

Yoganathan K, Elliott MW, Moxham J *et al.* Pseudotumour of the lung caused by *Mycobacterium malmoense* infection in an HIV-positive patient. *Thorax* 1994; **49**: 179–180

Tuberculosis

MICROBIOLOGY

Tuberculosis (TB) is a chronic granulomatous disease caused by *Mycobacterium tuberculosis*, affecting principally the lungs but with the propensity to involve any organ in the body. It is a global disease that is more prevalent in tropical countries.

Tuberculosis is the leading infectious cause of death worldwide with a death rate of 3 million/year. According to the World Health Organisation, deaths could rise to 4 million in year 2004 (WHO 1994) with 98% of deaths occurring in developing countries (Zumla and Corange 1998). The estimated infected population is ~1.7 billion or one-third of the world's population.

Tuberculosis has become a more serious disease today in the context of AIDS infection and the incidence of tuberculosis will steadily rise. In the USA, the risk of active tuberculosis is six times higher in HIV-seropositive patients compared with seronegative patients. It is estimated that in the Sub-Sahara and Africa ~2.4 million people are infected with both HIV and tuberculosis (Kochi 1991). Even in developed countries where control of tuberculosis is under way, an upsurgence in the incidence is anticipated with the advent of AIDS. HIV infection renders a person infected by *M. tuberculosis* much more likely to develop overt tuberculosis. About 8–10% of all cases of tuberculosis worldwide is related to HIV infection and often 20% or more in many African countries (Raviglione and Nunn 1997).

Transmission is by droplet infection, from a smear-positive patient with pulmonary tuberculosis. The tubercle bacilli are rendered airborne through coughing and sneezing and the organism should be inhaled to reach the alveolar membrane for infection to commence. Patients with smear-positive sputum are 5–10-fold more infective compared with smear-negative patients. It is most likely the maximum infectivity occurs before the commencement of chemotherapy. Persons at risk are those with chronic debilitating diseases such as alcoholics, smokers, immunosuppressed patients and those who live in overcrowded conditions and with poor personal hygiene. Only 10% of people infected by *M. tuberculosis* develop overt tuberculosis indicating good immune response to this pathogen. There is evidence that the immune response in those who do develop tuberculosis is not weak but dysregulated.

Today, transmission of *Mycobacterium bovis* through ingestion of milk or dairy products from infected cows is very uncommon. The incidence of *M. bovis* in pulmonary tuberculosis is very low and the rate remains the same. The mode of transmission is mostly by aerosol from infected cattle.

Three types of mycobacteria are causative agents for the disease in man. *M. tuberculosis* is the organism in a large majority of cases, *M. bovis* is an uncommon cause and atypical or opportunistic mycobacteria causes pulmonary and generalized infection in immunocompromised patients. The latter is discussed in a separate chapter.

The lung is the principal site of infection. The tubercle bacillus is stained by the Ziehl-Neelsen method and the bacilli stain a brilliant red as slender rods, which are slightly curved. They may be segmented or beaded and are acid-fast, which means that the stain does not disappear on adding strong acids or alcohols. Acid fastness is a characteristic feature of all mycobacteria. The organisms can be cultured in suitable media but may take 6–8 weeks or less if infection is heavy. In immune deficiency, *M. avian intracellulare* is the causative organism in the tuberculosis meningitis. In smear-positive cases one to nine bacilli may be seen in each high-power field if the sputum contains 100 000 AFB/ml. When it is ~10 000 bacilli/ml fluorescent microscopy is necessary to detect the AFB. With sputum containing < 5000 bacilli/ml, the chance of detection is only 10%.

PRESENTATION

It is essential to understand the terminology of various clinical presentations.

1. *Primary pulmonary tuberculosis* is an initial infection of lung and draining lymph nodes in persons who were originally tuberculin-negative. It is generally seen in children in areas of high prevalence. In developed countries it may manifest in adults. HIV patients can develop primary pulmonary tuberculosis.
2. *Post-primary* or *adult type pulmonary tuberculosis* occurs in a patient who, at some stage, had an immunological response to the primary infection and developed subsequent reactivating which may either be endogenous or exogenous. It is diagnosed clinically, radiologically or bacteriologically.
3. *Active tuberculosis* is diagnosed on clinical and/or radiological criteria with a positive Mantoux or histological evidence consistent with a tuberculous granuloma. A definitive diagnosis is made on culture of mycobacterium tuberculosis.
4. *Inactive tuberculosis* is diagnosed on clinical, bacteriological and radiological grounds not to be active. They are bacteriologically negative, clinically no signs or symptoms and the X-ray shadows compared with previous X-rays show it is dormant.

Pulmonary tuberculosis

In the vast majority of patients the primary infection produces no symptoms and also passes undiagnosed. The great majority of primary infections heal. In a few cases there may be a febrile illness lasting 1–2 weeks associated with a slight dry cough. Sometimes, the child may be fretful and fail to gain weight. Hypersensitivity reactions may develop with fever, phlyctenular conjunctivitis and erythema nodosum. The latter are tender cutaneous lesions on the shins, which are bluish, red and elevated and may be associated with polyarthralgia. Erythema nodosum may also be the first manifestation of tuberculosis.

The primary infection may heal without complications and extend with erosion of the hilar glands into adjacent

bronchi with collapse consolidation of a segment or a lobe or show haematogenous spread throughout the body causing miliary tuberculosis or tuberculous meningitis. Children < 5 years of age who have not had BCG vaccinations are at a particular risk of developing tuberculous meningitis as a complication of a primary tuberculous infection. The prognosis is good in primary tuberculosis occurring in immunocompetent patients in spite of its local complications if prompt antituberculous treatment is given.

Post-primary tuberculosis is often associated with the presence of risk factors in patients > 40 years such as diabetics, smokers and those with chronic obstructive airways disease, drug and alcohol dependants, silicosis, patients with gastric surgery, HIV or immunocompromised patients and health personnel who are exposed to patients with active tuberculosis.

The clinical features are usually insidious and non-specific and include symptoms such as cough with sputum. The sputum is usually mucoid in the early stages and subsequently purulent. As the disease progresses, the patients become short of breath, have fever with night sweats, weight loss and pleuritic chest pain. Haemoptysis occurs in advanced disease and may be massive if bleeding is from a large vessel in a cavitating lesion. There may be crepitations over the apices of the lung or physical signs of consolidation. Fibrosis with shift of trachea or pleural effusion can also be seen. Rarely, a pneumothorax may be the presenting feature. It is not unusual that some have no symptoms and may be diagnosed on a routine or incidental chest X-ray.

Pleural tuberculosis and empyema

Pleural effusion is secondary to a direct extension of pulmonary tuberculosis in a host who has hypersensitivity to tuberculoprotein. It may occur in primary or post-primary tuberculosis. It is essential to consider a tuberculous aetiology as patients develop pulmonary tuberculosis within 5 years, even if the effusion resolves spontaneously. Patients present with sudden onset of chest pain and shortness of breath. A large pleural effusion, especially in a young migrant with a positive tuberculin test, should be considered to have tuberculosis until disproven.

Tuberculous empyema – empyema and bronchopleural fistula are complications of untreated tuberculosis, secondary to rupture of pulmonary lesion into the pleural space.

Laryngeal and endobronchial tuberculosis

Tuberculosis of the larynx is associated with advanced post-primary tuberculosis. The presentation is that of laryngitis with hoarseness which does not regress. The bronchial mucosa may be implanted by tubercle bacilli causing tuberculous bronchitis. Cough and minor haemoptysis occurs and the patients are highly infectious.

Lymph node

About 30% of cases of tuberculosis annually are cases of extrapulmonary tuberculosis. About 12.7% of reported cases of tuberculosis occur in the lymph nodes and they are more common in persons < 40 years. It is also more common in females with a female:male ratio of 2.5:1. The majority of patients are immigrants from countries with a very high incidence of tuberculosis such as South East Asia and South East Europe. Single or multiple nodes may be involved and cervical lymph nodes are a common site. They are generally not tender, varying in size from 1 to 4 cm in diameter (Fig. 40.1). Occasionally it may break through the skin, discharging caseous material with sinus formation. In the Australian-born population it is reported that the organism responsible for lymph node infection is an atypical mycobacteria whereas in the migrant population, the organism is predominantly *M. tuberculosis*. Transient unilateral enlargement of glands is seen in primary tuberculosis.

Massive mediastinal lymph node enlargement may be seen in Asian migrants even without pulmonary shadows. Hence, a strongly positive tuberculin reaction in an Asian migrant with hilar lymphadenopathy should suggest tuberculosis and a mediastinal biopsy should be performed for confirmation.

Pericarditis

Tuberculous pericarditis may be secondary to spread from a mediastinal lymph node or from tuberculous pleurisy. The effusion is an exudate. Patients present with pericardial pain. A pericardial rub may be present.

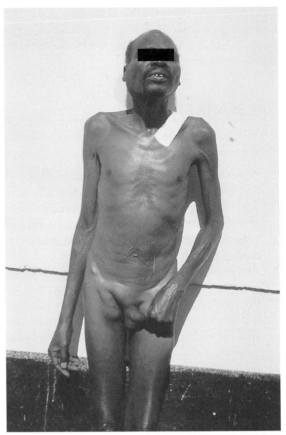

Figure 40.1 – Illustrates disseminated tuberculous lymphadenitis in a 50 year old African man.

Few patients develop pericardial tamponade which is life threatening. Constrictive pericarditis is a late presentation. Fig 40.2 shows tuberculous pericardial effusion.

Urinary tract

In the very early stages there are no symptoms. The common presenting symptoms are dysuria, frequent microscopic haematuria, loin pain or backache. Frank haematuria may occur. In the very late stages there may be cold abscesses in the loin and chronic renal failure.

Female genital tract

In females secondary amenorrhoea may be a presenting feature of tuberculous endometritis and salpingitis. It is not always associated with renal tuberculosis. Other features are pelvic pain, dyspareunia and vaginal discharge.

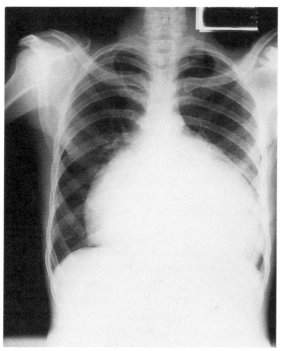

Figure 40.2 – X-ray appearance of pericardial effusion in tuberculosis.

Male genital tract

In males genital tract involvement is secondary to renal tuberculosis. Bacilli reach the prostate, epididymis and seminal vesicles. There may be nodularity or beading of the epididymis with pain, swelling and irregularity of testicular surface. Sinus formation may occur later.

Central nervous system

Involvement may be in the form of tuberculosis meningitis, tuberculoma or both. Tuberculous meningitis is secondary to acute miliary spread or rupture of a primary focus in the brain. It tends to occur before immunity to tuberculin has been established in infancy or childhood, or with a loss of immunity in old age (Fernando and Fernando 1993). The common sites for tuberculoma are cerebellum, basal ganglia and frontoparietal regions (Howells 1969).

The initial clinical presentation is a prodromal stage of headache, irritability, behavioural changes and lethargy. Signs of meningeal irritation, vomiting, stiff neck and seizures follow this. Cranial nerve lesions are seen in about one-quarter of the patients. Other localizing signs are hemiparesis, paraplegia and aphasia. Raised intracranial pressure and papilloedema may be seen. If untreated, patients become comatose and may develop decerebrate rigidity. Choroid tubercles may be seen on fundoscopic examination. With history of contact in infants and children and a positive tuberculin test with cerebral symptoms, tuberculous meningitis should be considered. In the differential diagnosis consider acute bacterial, acute viral meningitis and in immunocompromised patients, consider cryptococcal meningitis. A five category scoring system at presentation usually predicts the outcome. In patients presenting as Grade 3 or less the prognosis is extremely good. Of 15 patients presenting in Grade 1–3, 14 recovered fully (Watson et al. 1993). Overall, the mortality rate for central nervous system tuberculosis is ~15–30% or more.

Gastrointestinal tract and peritonitis

Three forms of disease affecting the gastrointestinal tract are described – ulcerative tuberculosis, hyperplastic tuberculosis and tuberculous peritonitis.

Both human and bovine tuberculous bacilli may cause intestinal tuberculosis. It is very uncommon today to see bovine tuberculosis in developed countries. Infection with the human strain may occur in patients with a normal chest X-ray. However, > 50% of patients with abdominal tuberculosis have pulmonary tuberculosis.

The onset is insidious with lower abdominal pain, low grade fever, weight loss and diarrhoea. In advanced disease, the symptoms would be secondary to haemorrhage or perforation. On examination, there is often a mass in the right iliac fossa, anal ulceration, fistulas or an anorectal abscess. The differential diagnosis is carcinoma of colon, Crohn's disease, amoeboma and schistosomiasis.

Peritonitis – tuberculous peritonitis may occur in the absence of tuberculous enteritis. Infection can be from a pulmonary focus or reactivation of latent tuberculous foci. In tropical countries, tuberculous peritonitis is a major cause of ascites.

The presentation is one of insidious onset of ascites, abdominal distension, low-grade pyrexia, anorexia, loss of weight and abdominal pain, which is usually not severe. On examination, there is evidence of fluid in the peritoneal cavity, hepatosplenomegaly and oedema of lower limbs. A dry form of tuberculous peritonitis may present with palpable masses due to matted omentum and lymph nodes. Peritoneal calcification may occur

(Fig. 40.3). Prognosis is good with complete resolution of the disease and resorption of the fluid.

Bone

The common sites are the spine and the hip. The disease is rare in Australia, however, it is by no means rare in the migrants from developing countries. Pott's TB of the spine usually involves the mid-thoracic spine. The presentation is generally one of pain in the spine or hip, angulated kyphosis or neurological deficit. Rarely, a cold abscess may be present in the groin. Onset of paraplegia is an emergency and requires urgent neurosurgical consultation to determine whether decompression is essential. Tuberculosis of joints is confined mainly to weight bearing joints such as hip and knee.

Cutaneous

Primary

Cutaneous tuberculosis is rare. The cutaneous lesions are due to tubercle infection of the skin, hypersensitivity or involvement of skin due to extension from adjacent organs. The cutaneous lesions of TB are primary tuberculous complex, lupus vulgaris, lupus verrucosus, scrofuloderma, tuberculosis cutis orificialis and tuberculosis paronychia.

Tuberculous complex consists of a tuberculous chancre on the face, eyes, hands or knees. The lymph glands draining from the chancre are enlarged. The chancre persists as a patch that is indurated with a little blood-stained discharge. The primary chancre slowly heals and the draining lymph glands break down, forming a scar. Mantoux reaction changes from negative to positive. Biopsy shows granulomatous inflammation with tubercle bacilli.

Lupus vulgaris comprises flat nodules. Ulceration may occur. Fig 40.4 shows a lesion in the forearm. It is commonly found in the butterfly area of the face and can destroy the nasal cartilage. It arises from exogenous, contiguous or haematological spread of the bacilli from another tuberculous form such as a tuberculous gland. Lesions show tubercles in the upper dermis with bacilli together with a proliferation of T-cells and Langerhans cells. Lupus vulgaris can be psoriasiform in appearance. Contracture from scarring below the eye causes an ectropion. Parrot-bill or simian deformities may arise due to destruction of the alae and septum of the nose.

Lupus verrucosus is secondary to inoculation of the skin of an adult with tubercle bacilli. It occurs in the hands, buttocks and has a warty surface. Differentiation from viral warts and lichen planus verrucosus is necessary. The former do not show dusky discoloration, while lichen planus is very itchy and occurs on the shins.

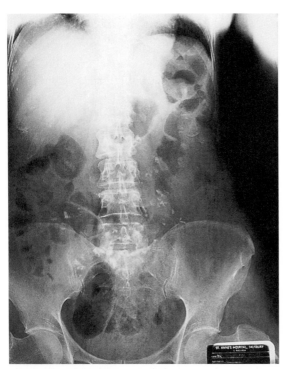

Figure 40.3 – Shows peritoneal calcification in tuberculous peritonitis in abdominal x-ray.

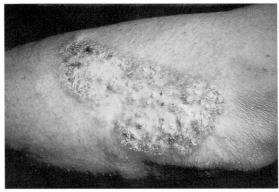

Figure 40.4 – Lupus vulgaris in an African male.

Scrofuloderma is tuberculosis of the skin secondary to tuberculosis of underlying lymph nodes, bones or joints. The commonest site is the neck, secondary to tuberculous lymphadenitis. The mass of matted infected lymph nodes breaks down and a sinus is exposed. There is caseation with numerous tubercle bacilli. The condition heals with irregular scarring.

Tuberculosis paronychia are very painful infections of the nail beds. They ulcerate and heal by scarring.

Tuberculosis cutis orificialis represents spread from adjacent organs. This may be from tuberculosis of anus spreading to the scrotum, spreading to the skin around the anal orifice, from tuberculosis of epididymis and testis, from pulmonary or laryngeal tuberculosis spreading to the nose, palate, tongue, floor of the mouth or lips. The ulcers are painful and shallow with undermined edges.

Tuberculides

Tuberculides are symmetrical cutaneous hypersensitivity responses to internal tuberculosis which respond to antituberculous drugs. These are erythema nodosum, erythema induratum, lichen scrofulosorum and papule necrotic tuberculides.

Erythema nodosum is a non-specific hypersensitivity reaction to many infections and drugs. They are found over the skin in the legs and are indurated and tender.

Erythema induratum – these are dusky and painful, occurring in the lower half of the legs in young women producing 'billiard table-like legs'. The lesions

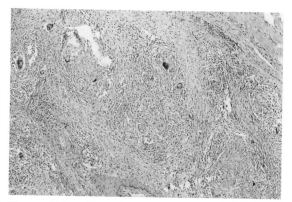

Figure 40.5 – Typical tubercle with epithelioid cells, Langhans giant cells, fibrosis, lymphocytic infiltration and cental caseation (H & E × 40).

may break down, forming undermined and ragged ulcers. Differential diagnosis includes sarcoidosis, where ulceration is unusual.

Lichen scrofulosorum – the lesions are lichenoid papules, usually in children with tuberculous lymph nodes, bones or joints. They are often grouped together. Mantoux reaction is strongly positive.

Papulonecrotic tuberculides – these can be discrete, inflamed papules which undergo central necrosis, ulcerate and scar. The lesions occur in the trunk and limbs. Some of these lesions are truly tuberculous and others tuberculide.

Ophthalmic

Tuberculosis may affect any part of the eye. The diagnosis is difficult. Phlyctenular keratitis, chorioretinitis, uveitis are the common manifestations. Phlyctenular lesions are considered to be hypersensitivity reactions. In tuberculous meningitis ophthalmic examination for choroid tubercles are diagnostic.

Adrenal

This is rare and is not the commonest cause of Addison's disease. Spread is haematogenous from a pulmonary lesion. The cortex is mostly affected. There is a fair amount of damage by the time diagnosis is made and chemotherapy at this stage may not restore complete function.

Miliary

This is a very severe form of tuberculosis. It is common in infancy and childhood before sensitivity to tuberculin has been established. It is a disseminated form of tuberculosis that spreads by blood stream and lymphatics from any active tuberculous focus in the lung. Classically, it arises from the primary infection and spreads through the blood stream.

The presentation is usually sudden in onset with fever, breathlessness, cyanosis, altered levels of consciousness and signs of meningeal irritation. The clinical appearance is similar to that of a septic patient. The liver and spleen may be enlarged. Patients become rapidly anaemic.

Subacute or cryptic miliary

This is a very difficult condition to diagnose and diagnosis is often made only at autopsy. The presentation is that of pyrexia of uncertain origin without any focal signs. The elderly and immunosuppressed are prone to this type of infection. They are very ill, cachectic and may have lymphadenopathy or serous membrane involvement. Treatment is given on suspicion of the diagnosis after the institution of the necessary investigation, as for miliary tuberculosis.

Disseminated non-reactive

Disseminated non-reactive tuberculosis is a very rare form of tuberculosis due to massive, widespread dissemination of organisms without granuloma formation with pancytopenia developing within a few days. The prognosis is poor and response to chemotherapy is unsatisfactory in this form of tuberculosis.

HIV patients

In patients with HIV/AIDS, the T-cell-mediated protective effect diminishes, thereby developing opportunistic infections. The hypersensitive tissue response is also poor and normal pathological processes such as caseation and fibrosis may not take place effectively. Such patients have a large number of acid-fast bacilli in the infected tissues. Where prevalence of tuberculosis is high, the chances of HIV patients contracting tuberculosis is high and the reverse is equally true, i.e. there is a high positivity of HIV-infection among tuberculous patients.

Post-primary and adult forms of tuberculosis in HIV patients – in the early stages of HIV infection, the clinical presentation may be similar to non-HIV infected patients. Pulmonary infection is the common presentation.

The clinical picture will be more complicated in the late stages of HIV infection. There is a greater incidence of extrapulmonary tuberculosis in HIV infected patients. Furthermore, other opportunistic infection and malignancy complicate the clinical picture. Lymph node involvement of the mediastinum is common.

Radiological diagnosis is not typical as there are no hypersensitivity reactions in the lung and a few cavities and diffuse linear shadows may be present.

PATHOLOGY

Pulmonary

In primary tuberculosis (TB), when an individual acquires infection for the first time, a single lesion known as the Ghons focus forms. It is usually situated subjacent to the pleura in the lower part of the upper lobes and upper part of the lower lobes. It is an area of grey-white inflammatory consolidation of ~1–1.5 cm diameter. Initially it is granulomatous and then becomes soft with central caseous necrosis by the 14th day. Tubercle bacilli are seen at this stage both lying free in the lesion or within macrophages. The bacilli can spread via lymphatics to regional lymph nodes causing similar lesions; the combination of pulmonary and nodal lesions known as the Ghon complex.

In the great majority of cases, the pulmonary lesion undergoes shrinkage with fibrosis, calcification and sometimes ossification. There is finally a fibrous scar with puckering of pleural surface. The bacilli may be dormant for years in these lesions. Progression of primary TB is rare and more likely to affect children. The primary lung lesion can enlarge rapidly and erode into the bronchial tree giving rise to satellite lesions. There is enlargement of tracheobronchial lymph nodes and air flow can be hampered. There can also be miliary spread with death from tuberculous meningitis.

Secondary tuberculosis occurs in a previously sensitized individual as a result of reactivation of the primary lesion often following lowered immunity. The lesions commence in the apical or posterior segments of one or both upper lobes and is a caseous consolidation measuring 1–3 cm. They can also occur in other parts of the lung.

Microscopically, the typical reaction is a tubercle or granuloma formation with epithelioid cells, Langerhans giant cells, fibrosis, lymphocytic infiltration and central caseation (Fig. 40.5).

In immunosuppressed patients, necrotic foci containing plentiful bacilli with little or no cellular reaction is seen. Large cavitating lesions may erode into bronchi.

The apical lesions can arrest with fibrocalcification, progress and spread to other areas, involve the pleura with pleural fibrosis, adhesions, effusions or empyema, erode into bronchi with organisms being coughed up and further disseminated to the trachea, larynx etc., be swallowed leading to intestinal TB, or the organisms can enter lymphatics and blood with spread to distant organs – miliary tuberculosis. A definite diagnosis should be made only when typical mycobacterium are seen in characteristic lesions; or when they are isolated by culture.

Lymph nodes

Tuberculosis lymphadenitis presents the whole spectrum of the histopathology from small tubercle, caseous necrosis, fibrosis and calcification. Involvement of lymph nodes is usually secondary as in hilar and peribronchial due to drainage from bronchogenic pulmonary tuberculosis.

Pericardium

Tuberculous pericardial lesions can be trivial and transient to serious and progressive, arising from adjacent organs (mediastinal lung or bone) most commonly retrograde lymphatic spread from tracheo-bronchial lymph nodes. Metastatic dissemination also occurs. It is characterized by a fibrous exudate, the epicardium covered by thick blood stained shaggy fibrin arranged in ridges. Pericardium can become leathery as the disease progresses with resultant fibrosis. Tubercles can be seen in both the parietal and visceral pericardium with yellowish white layer due to coalescence of caseous necrosis. Effusion occurring soon after fibrin formation can be from a few millilitres to several litres. The fluid contains blood, fibrin and caseous debris. The adherence of the pericardial layers can result in localized pockets of fluid. Microscopically typical granulomata can be seen. Later stage calcification can occur with resultant constrictive percarditis.

Urinary tract

Tuberculous pyelonephritis occurs by haematogenous spread from lung and other foci, caseous foci form in renal cortex with extension to medulla and papillae with ulceration in the lesion progresses causing hydronephrosis and spread to the lower urinary tract. The opposite kidney can also be involved. In miliary tuberculosis kidney is involved as other organs but renal impairment is not significant.

Female genital tract

The commonest cause of granulomatous salpingitis is due to *M. tuberculosis* where the fallopian tube is dilated and wall is thickened with the lumen filled with pus. On microscopic examination typical caseating granulomas are seen with adhesion of plical and epithelial hyperplasia mimicking adenocarcinoma. Tuberculous endometritis can occur after tubal infection and shows small sparse granulomas without caseation.

Placental tuberculosis occurs rarely as a complication of miliary spread in the mother.

Male genital tract

Tuberculosis of the testis is usually with involvement of the epididymis. Discrete tubercles in the testis are seen in miliary tuberculosis. Epididymal tuberculosis is usually unilateral and associated with pulmonary and genito urinary tuberculosis. Earliest lesions are seen as discrete or confluent yellowish, necrotic areas in the globus minor consisting of characteristic tubercles or inflammatory reaction of polymorphs, plasma cells, monocytes, epithelial cells including multinucleated giant cells and many acid-fast bacilli. Early lesions may regress and calcify or progress to involve the entire epididymus. When the tunica vaginalis is invaded serosanguinous or purulent exudate develops.

Central nervous system

Tuberculous leptomeningitis, especially in children, is mostly part of a generalized miliary tuberculosis; and in adults in association with pulmonary tuberculosis. In early stages, a scant diffuse and grey white exudate (sometimes with faint green tinge) is seen. Later 1–3 mm discrete grey nodules are found along the leptomeningeal blood vessels. In chronic disease the exudate is more prominent at the base of the brain. Microscopically, lymphocytes, large mononuclear cells and small caseous necrotic foci are seen with serum and fibrin in exudate in addition. Giant cells are less frequent. Acid fast bacilli are numerous or scanty. The leptomeningeal vessels exudates have lymphocytes in their walls and may show reactive endothelial hyperplasia. Sometimes thrombosis resulting in infarcts may occur in the brain and spinal cord.

Tuberculous encephalitis shows either multiple small granulomas up to 1 cm or 5 to 6 cm solid foci with 'growth rings' formed by layers of granulation tissue. The larger lesions are common in cerebellum.

Gastrointestinal tract and peritoneum

Tuberculous gastroenteritis follows advanced open pulmonary disease with widespread lesions in disseminated disease.

In isolated lesions ileocaecal or anal region is involved commonly and rarely oesophagus, stomach or intestine. The granulomas must be distinguished from sarcoid, syphilis, fungal and parasitic infections.

Tuberculous peritonitis is a manifestation of disseminated disease, association with intestinal involvement or in females secondary to genital disease. It can produce wide spread dense adhesion.

Bone

Most common site of extrapulmonary tuberculosis is bone with 1% of patients with pulmonary tuberculosis developing skeletal involvement. The major sites are spine and hips, knees, ankles, small bones of hands and feet are also involved. The basic lesion is a combination of osteomyelitis and arthritis, the latter arising haematogenously or by extension from epiphysial bone. Bone destruction and repair seen in pyogenic osteomyelitis is not seen in tuberculous osteomyelitis. Histologically classic tubercle granuloma is seen.

Cutaneous

In early lesions of primary tuberculosis a mixed dermal infiltrate of neutrophils, lymphocytes and plasma cells followed by necrosis and ulceration. Caseating granulomas form weeks later. Bacilli can be demonstrated easily in early lesions but is sparse after granulomas form.

In lupus vulgaris, the granulomas are in the upper and mid-dermis and have a tendency to confluence. Sometimes a granuloma resembles a sarcoid. In verrucosa lesions, hyper keratosis and pseudo epitheliomatous hyperplasia of the epidermis with caseating granulomas in the mid-dermis where acid-fast bacilli can be demonstrated.

In scrofuloderma epidermis is atrophic or ulcerated with underlying abscess formation including caseous necrosis extending to involve the subcutis. Smears from the areas are more rewarding in demonstrating bacilli than in tissue sections.

In orificial tuberculosis ulceration with underlying caseous granolomas are seen.

In tuberculids features of erythema induratum, lichen scrofulosorum and papulonecrotic tuberculids are seen. Erythema induratum shows a lobular panniculitis with tuberculoid granulomas in the lower dermis. In Lichen scrofulosorum non-caseating tuberculoid granulomas in the upper dermis has a perifollicular and eccrine localization. Bacilli are not usually demonstrated. In papulonecrotic tuberculid ulceration and necrosis with occasional granulomas are seen. Fibrinoid necrosis of vessels including thrombosis can be seen. Bacilli are difficult to see in routine stains for acid-fast bacilli.

Adrenals

Bilateral destructive adrenocortical tuberculosis is the classic cause of Addison's disease. Both glands enlarge and are replaced by caseous granulomas.

Miliary

The lung is studded with firm white tubercles 1 mm in diameter or caseating tubercles several millimetres in diameter. Tubercles in the upper lobe are the largest with even distribution throughout. The tubercles are more numerous and closely distributed in heavy infection and grow smaller when infection is resisted. They are mainly in alveolar septa which enlarge and caseate where later fibrous capsules are formed if patients survive. Similar lesions are found in liver, spleen, kidneys, meninges, bone marrow, lymph nodes and thyroid gland, only muscle tissue being spared.

INVESTIGATIONS

Pulmonary tuberculosis

1. The presence of any of the symptoms or signs mentioned above should merit a radiological examination.

The radiological features are those of an ill-defined opacity or opacities in the upper lobes. The opacities may be bilateral and small or large bronchopneumonic shadows. There may be consolidation of a lobe and cavitation with fibrosis. The heart and lungs are displaced to the side of the fibrotic lesion. Pleural effusion is revealed by the meniscus sign (Fig. 40.6).

2. Tuberculin test – If a child has not had BCG vaccination and shows a positive tuberculin test, the child must be assumed to have active disease.

3. If there is any abnormality of the lungs on radiology, sputum should be taken for microscopic examination and culture of tubercle bacilli on at least three occasions. Sputum should be stained by the Ziehl-Neelsen method or auramine-phenol fluorescence. Microscopy has two advantages, one where it can detect open cases and the other where diagnosis can be made. In patients who have been commenced on antibiotics, the smear may be positive but culture may be negative. 1992 statistics for Australia revealed that microscopy produced a positive result in 24.2% and culture in 54.5% of cases. Hence, ~30% of cases are smear-negative but culture-positive. The positive bacteriology can be improved if specimens from fasting, gastric washings, bronchial lavage or lung biopsy. Therefore ~40–50% of cases are diagnosed purely on radiological, clinical and tuberculin testing.

4. Sputum, gastric washings, bronchoalveolar lavage fluid and laryngeal swabs may be used for culture. PCR or DNA probes can be used to identify the acid-fast bacilli in the specimen and in culture (Galietti et al. 1992, Lebrium et al. 1992).

Identification of mycobacterial tuberculosis traditionally takes 4–6 weeks. It takes another 2–4 weeks for assessment of drug susceptibility. With the introduction of the commercial BACTEC system in the USA, the period is reduced to ~4 weeks, inclusive of drug susceptibility testing (Galietti 1992). New technologies which include high performance liquid chromatography for mycotic acid and nucleic acid probes together with the BACTEC system have reduced the period to 2 weeks, inclusive of drug susceptibility testing. However, these techniques are costly and not readily affordable (Jacobs 1994).

Polymerase chain reaction – this is a highly sensitive method of direct detection of mycobacterium or their nucleic acid components. It has a specificity

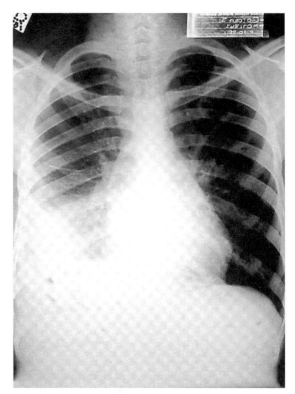

Figure 40.6 - Pleural effusion is revealed by the meniscus sign in the lung x-ray.

of 95–100% and sensitivity of 84–91% with a diagnosis available within 48 h (Jacobs 1994). It cannot distinguish drug-resistant forms from drug-susceptible organisms. However, it is useful for comparing the genetic material of a drug-resistant strain to that of a drug-susceptible strain. Identification of the Kat G and Inh A genes associated with isoniazid resistance by PCR is a significant advancement.

5. Viable mycobacteria infected with specific reported phages expressing the firefly luciferase gene produce photons (Jacobs 1994). Culture of drug-susceptible strains of *M. tuberculosis* incubated with a susceptible drug will fail to produce light after infection with the luciferous reporter phages, as the organism is now metabolically inactive. On the other hand, cultures of drug-resistant organism incubated with resistant drug after infection with reporter phage, will produce light as the organism is still metabolically active.

Pleural effusion and empyema

1. X-ray of chest
2. Tuberculin skin test

3. Aspiration – shows an exudate with lymphocytes and rarely contains tubercle bacilli on smear or culture. Cultures should be performed
4. Pleural biopsy – pleural granulomas are in ~80% of patients

Laryngeal and endobronchial tuberculosis

1. Bacteriological examination of sputum
2. The patients respond well to antituberculous chemotherapy

Lymph node

1. Aspiration, smear and culture
2. Biopsy, smear, culture and histology
3. Tuberculin skin test
4. Chest X-ray

Pericarditis

1. Tuberculous pericarditis by pericardial aspiration
2. Investigation for other sites of tuberculous infection
3. Pericardial biopsy
4. Tuberculin test

Urinary tract

1. Urine examination – sterile pyuria or haematuria is a common feature of urinary tract tuberculosis. Culture urine for tubercle bacilli
2. An IV pyelogram, will allow assessment of renal involvement, ureteric obstruction and hydronephrosis all of which may require special treatment
3. Cystoscopy allows visualization of the bladder
4. Renal function tests
5. Chest X-ray
6. Tuberculin skin test
7. Renal ultrasound examination

Female genital tract

1. Diagnosis is made by curettage, smear, culture and histologic examination
2. Other investigations include X-ray of chest and tuberculin skin test

Male genital tract

1. Examination of urine and culture
2. Tuberculin skin test
3. Chest X-ray

4. Ultrasound of testis and radiological assessment of the urinary system

Central nervous system

1. X-ray of chest as most cases are secondary to pulmonary tuberculosis.
2. Lumbar puncture and cerebrospinal fluid examination will show a low glucose, high protein, a high polymorph count initially followed by high lymphocyte count. The cell count is between 50 and 500/ml. The CSF may demonstrate a 'spider's web' clot on standing. All these features are not diagnostic of tuberculosis as viral, cryptococcal and partially treated meningitis may simulate tuberculous meningitis. Acid-fast bacilli are demonstrated in the CSF in ~19% of meningitis cases (Illingworth 1956). Rates of 85–90% have been achieved by centrifuging 10–20 ml CSF and examining the resultant thick film for 30–90 min (Illingworth 1956, Stewart 1953). CSF culture takes time for the bacilli to grow. PCR shows higher sensitivity and specificity (Kaneko et al. 1990).
3. CT scanning – this imaging technique can demonstrate tuberculous meningitis and tuberculomas. Contrast may be used. Tuberculous meningitis displays exudates in suprasellar and ambient cisterns and in the Sylvian fissure. Tuberculomas may be seen in 10% of patients with meningitis, and 30% of patients have cerebral infarction due to tuberculous arteritis, mainly in the basal ganglia (Bargava *et al.* 1982). Communicating hydrocephalus and its enhanced basal exudates can be demonstrated by CT scanning.

Gastrointestinal tract

1. Sigmoidoscopy or colonoscopy and biopsy and investigation for pulmonary tuberculosis
2. A positive tuberculin skin test
3. Stool culture for tubercle bacilli
4. Diagnosis may be made at laparotomy for obstructive symptoms. At laparotomy, in addition to obstructing masses and peritoneal lesions, lymph node biopsies should also be taken.

Peritonitis

1. There is often evidence of tuberculosis in lungs
2. Analysis of ascitic fluid shows a protein concentration of > 2.6 g/100 ml with large numbers of

lymphocytes. Tubercle bacilli are rare but centrifuged fluid should be cultured

3. Peritoneal biopsy by laparoscopic examination may be done
4. Tuberculin test which is positive
5. ESR which will be high

Bone

1. Radiological osteolytic changes are seen
2. Biopsy of bone or joint tissue should be done for histologic examination and for tubercle bacilli
3. Tuberculin test is positive
4. ESR may be elevated
5. Investigations should be performed for other sites of infection such as the lungs and computerized tomogram of the spine and myelogram will help eliminate spinal cord compression

Cutaneous

1. Diagnosis is made by bacteriological examination
2. Skin biopsy of the exudate
3. Tuberculin skin test.

Tuberculides

1. Diagnosis is established by identifying primary forms of tuberculosis
2. Positive tuberculin skin test
3. Skin biopsy

Adrenal

1. Cortisol and synacthen test
2. Abdominal CT
3. Tuberculin test
4. X-ray chest
5. Abdominal CT

Miliary

1. X-ray of chest – patients are often acutely ill even before the classical miliary nodules appear on X-ray, the latter may take up to 4–6 weeks to be detected (Fig. 40.7). Miliary nodules are very fine nodules the size of sago granules throughout the entire lung fields. Sputum examination may be negative for bacilli, however, cultures should be carried out

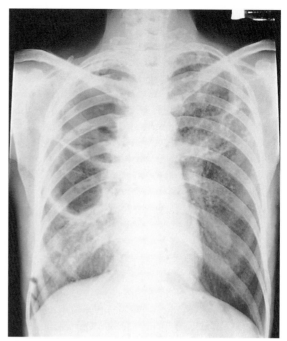

Figure 40.7 – Chest X-ray showing miliary tuberculosis.

2. Transbronchial, liver and bone marrow biopsy are other methods of diagnosis
3. The tuberculin skin test is often negative due to anergy
4. Lumbar puncture and investigations as for tuberculous meningitis should be performed

HIV patients

1. Diagnosis is based on clinical suspicion and investigations to establish the diagnosis should be instituted. These include repeated examination of sputum of smears and sputum for culture
2. X-ray of the chest may be sometimes difficult to evaluate due to multiple pathologies
3. Tuberculin testing with a 5 mm induration to 10 IU purified protein derivative (PPD) may be considered significant. However, false-negatives may occur
4. If there are cerebral symptoms, computerized tomography and lumbar puncture should be done
5. Lymph node biopsies for smear and culture are often positive in the late stages

Tuberculin test

Tuberculin is a mixture of antigenic tuberculoproteins, PPD. It is obtained from disintegrated tubercle bacilli. The principle of the test is to detect a delayed hypersensitivity reaction in a person who has been infected or those previously BCG vaccinated. The dose is a standard dose of 10 IU human PPD tuberculin. Human PPD is used in Australia. Besides the dose, one needs to take into consideration the immune response of the patient. If the host has depressed immune response (anergy) such as in immunocompromised patients, AIDS, poor nutrition, the elderly, alcoholics, any severe recent infection, sarcoidosis or malignancy, the test may well be negative. This should be borne in mind when interpreting the results.

A false-negative tuberculin test also occurs in ~15% of new active pulmonary disease and becomes positive only after the disease stabilizes. It may be negative in ~50% of patients with miliary tuberculosis. The terms positive and negative are relative. Tuberculin hypersensitivity may result from contact with non-pathogenic or atypical mycobacteria and this non-specific reaction makes interpretation somewhat difficult. A tuberculin reaction of > 5 mm induration is indicative of mycobacterial tuberculosis infection of the typical type. However, in Western Australia, Queensland and some other parts of Australia, due to a high prevalence of atypical mycobacteria, indurations of 5–9 mm are generally considered cross-reactions and an induration of 10 mm is more significant for typical mycobacterial infection (Patel and Streeton 1990). However, children who are contacts of adults with active tuberculosis should be considered infected when showing a response of 5–9 mm. A seroconversion from negative to positive Mantoux and had a history of exposure is significant of recent tuberculosis infection. People who have had BCG vaccination and show reactions of 15 mm or more may be regarded as positive and should be considered infected with tuberculosis.

If the reaction to 10 IU PPD is negative in a person suspected of having active tuberculosis, the test may be repeated using 100 IU.

TREATMENT

Grading of tuberculosis

Tuberculosis may be graded from the point of view of treatment:

1. Grade 0 – the person has not been exposed to tuberculosis and the tuberculin test is negative. Needs protection by immunization if there is a possibility of becoming infected.

2. Grade I – the person has been exposed to tuberculosis but does not have clinical tuberculosis. The tuberculin reaction may be negative if exposure is for < 3 months. Children < 1 year of age will require primary prophylaxis.

3. Grade II – the person has had an infection as indicated by a positive tuberculin test but has no clinical or radiological infection. The individual needs surveillance, periodic assessment and may require prophylactic chemotherapy if the tuberculin conversion is recent and if there are risk factors such as immunosuppression.

4. Grade III – the person has active tuberculosis based on clinical, radiological or bacteriological evidence. This is a notifiable disease in Australia and requires urgent treatment.

5. Grade IV – the person has inactive tuberculosis that may or may not have been treated. S/he may show varying reactivation. In those treated actively with modern combination of drugs, relapses are relatively uncommon. There may be reactivation among those who are untreated or if there is immunosuppression.

6. Grade V – the person is suspected of having tuberculosis and investigations have been commenced. Those individuals will subsequently be regraded.

Anti-tuberculous drugs and treatment regimen

The first line of drugs used in antituberculous treatment is isoniazid, rifampicin, pyrazinamide, ethambutol and streptomycin.

The second line of antituberculous drugs is used in proven drug resistance or where there are adverse reactions to first line drugs. Second line drugs are:

1. Ethionamide
2. Para-aminosalicylic acid
3. Prothionamide
4. Thiacetazone
5. Capreomycin
6. Kanamycin
7. Cycloserine

There is still insufficient clinical data to the fluoroquinolones in first line treatment of tuberculosis, but may find a role in multidrug resistance infection or in patients with adverse reactions to other drugs (Gillespie and Kennedy 1998). Tubercle bacilli are found in the extracellular space and small numbers of organisms are found in macrophages. The bacilli in the extracellular space actively multiply and have different metabolic rates. The aim of chemotherapy using a combination of drugs is to attack the tubercle bacilli with their different metabolic rates and eliminate mutant bacilli that may be resistant to any one drug.

Isoniazid and rifampicin are the two most active and bactericidal agents against the extracellular tubercle bacilli. Pyrazinamide acts on the relatively inactive bacilli with macrophages. Pyrazinamide is not active against *M. bovis*.

Chemotherapy should commence as early as possible. Commencement of treatment is not a problem when there is bacteriological and histological confirmation of diagnosis. However, when smears are negative and cultures are pending, a decision to treat has to be made by the attending physician in consultation with the radiologist, microbiologist or pathologist and an experienced colleague. A definitive positive tuberculin test is also helpful. The strategy for treatment of tuberculosis is based on multidrug approach to decrease resistant mutant strains and, second, the concept of two-phase therapy with initial three-to-four drugs to decrease the microbial concentration and two drugs thereafter (Ortona and Antinori 1998).

- Short-term, 6- or 9-month regimen
- Longer duration regimens – this is offered only if isoniazid and rifampicin cannot be offered together at the commencement of the treatment due to resistance or severe side-effects. These regimens are offered for up to 12–18 months.
- Intermittent supervised chemotherapy or directly observed therapy (DOT). Drug combination is administered under full supervision in single doses two to three times a week. Their efficacy is as good as daily treatment. No drug should be used as a single reagent and should not be used intermittently because of development of resistance.

The Committee of Treatment of Tuberculosis of the International Union against Tuberculosis and Lung Disease (IUATLD) has recommended the following regimen for Australia and New Zealand.

Six-month regimen

In this regimen in the first 2 months ethambutol, isoniazid, rifampicin and pyrizinamide are used and followed by isoniazid and rifampicin the next 4 months. The 6-month regimen has the maximum bactericidal effect.

Nine-month regimen

In the first 2 months ethambutol, isoniazid and rifampicin, and the next 7 months isoniazid and rifampicin. Ethambutol is a bacteriostatic agent against all the groups of bacilli. In Australia, streptomycin is rarely used and is replaced by ethambutol. If short-term therapy cannot be applied for some reason, isoniazid or rifampicin cannot be used in the initial treatment, in which case treatment must be continued for a long-term using alternative drugs.

If sensitivity is confirmed for all four drugs in 6-month regimen, at any time, usually in the first 8 weeks, then ethambutol need not be continued. Pyrazinamide should be continued for 2 months to qualify for short-term therapy. If isoniazid resistance is confirmed then the quadruple ethambutol, isoniazid, rifampicin and pyrazinamide needs to be continued beyond the initial 2 months, with close monitoring for side-effects. The success rate of the 6-month regimen is 95–98%, with few relapses.

When should the 9-month regimen be used? The British Tuberculosis and Thoracic Association in 1976 introduced the first short-term regimen. Ethambutol is added to the regimen to cover the possibility of isoniazid resistance. It is also a regimen that is useful if pyrazinamide cannot be used due to hepatitis or severe gout. It can also be used for treatment of tuberculosis caused by *M. bovis* that is resistant to pyrazinamide. For dosage refer to Table 40.1.

Longer duration regimen – If isoniazid or rifampicin cannot be used throughout the treatment, then other drug combinations should be used for 12–18 months with close monitoring of the success of the treatment. Drug administration should be under the supervision of a chest physician. The options available are:

1. First 2 months, two to three bactericidal drugs
2. Remaining period, at least one bactericidal drug with other antituberculous drugs

For second line drugs, see Table 40.2.

Intermittent supervised chemotherapy

This regimen is useful mainly in developing countries where there is poor compliance or inadequate home supervision. The intermittent therapy is effective for both pulmonary and extrapulmonary tuberculosis.

Table 40.1 – Anti-tuberculous drug regimen. Daily 6-month regimen

Drug	Duration (months)	Daily dosage Adults total dosage and children mg/kg weight Children (mg/kg)	Adults (total dose)
Isoniazid (H)	6	5	300 mg
Rifampicin (R)	6	10	< 50 kg 450 mg
			> 50 kg 600 mg
Pyrazinamide (Z)	2	35	< 50 kg 1.5 g
			> 50 kg 2.0 g
*Ethambutol (E)	2	25	15–25 mg/kg then
			15 mg/kg if continued
**Streptomycin	2	15–20	< 50 kg 750 mg
			> 50 kg 1 g

Recommendation of International Union Against Tuberculosis and Lung Diseases 1988; 63: 60–64 with courtesy.

*Not recommended for children.

**Not used in Australia.

Table 40.2 – Second-line drugs (anti-tuberculous)

Drugs	Daily dose (mg/kg) Children	Daily dose (total) Adults
Thiacetazone	4	150 mg
Sodium Para-Aminosalicylic acid	300	10–15 g
Ethionamide and Prothionamide	15–20	< 50 kg 750 mg
		> 50 kg 1 g
Kanamycin	10–15	500 mg–1 g
Capreomycin	15	1 g
Cycloserine	15	< 50 kg 750 mg
		> 50 kg 1 g

Courtesy of Recommendation of International Union Against Tuberculosis and Lung Dis 1988; 3: 60–64.

The following regimens are recommended for Australia (Patel and Streeton 1990).

1. First 2 months combination of ethambutol, isoniazid, rifampicin and pyrazinamide and 4 months of isoniazid and rifampicin. The drugs are given only three times a week for 6 months.
2. If there is initial isoniazid, ethambutol, rifampicin and pyrazinamide (i.e. 6 months course), the drugs are given three times a week.
3. Two months of ethambutol, isoniazid, rifampicin and pyrazinamide daily followed by 4 months of isoniazid and rifampicin given three times a week or 4 months of isoniazid and rifampicin two times

a week, ethambutol could be deleted if the organisms are fully drug-sensitive

For dosage of drugs used intermittently, see Table 40.3.

Side-effects of anti-tuberculous drug

Isoniazid – included in all short-course regimens, even if the organism is resistant *in vitro*. Minor side-effects that disappear in a few weeks are gastrointestinal such as anorexia, nausea and constipation. Major side-effects are hepatotoxicity, found more in the elderly and alcoholics. Alcohol is prohibited during its use. Rarely fatal hepatitis may occur.

Table 40.3 – Anti-tuberculous drugs, dosage of drugs used intermittently

Drug	Adults/***children (mg/kg)	Adult dose (mg/kg)
Isoniazid	15 three times a week	15 mg three times a week
Rifampicin	15 three times a week	600–900 mg (total)
**Streptomycin	15–20 three times a week	< 50 kg 750 mg 75 kg 1.0 g
Pyrazinamide	50 three times a week 75 twice a week	< 50 kg 2.0 g > 50 kg 2.5 g < 50 kg 3.0 g > 50 kg 3.5 g
*Ethambutol	30 three times a week 45 twice a week	– –

*Generally not recommended for children.

**Not used in Australia.

Courtesy of Recommendations of International Union Against Tuberculosis and Lung Diseases 1988; 63: 60–64.

***Do not exceed adult total dose.

Refer to Intermittent regimen of anti-tuberculous drugs in text (p221).

Peripheral neuropathy is commoner in alcoholics and diabetics. Pyridoxine in moderate doses of 10–20 mg/day but not in excess should be used with isoniazid treatment. Hypersensitivity drug reaction is generally seen in the first 8 weeks, including Stevens-Johnson's syndrome. Drugs such as Tegretol (carbamazepine), Dilantin (phenytoin) may reach high levels if used with isoniazid, due to drug interaction.

Rifampicin – a harmless side-effect is an orange discoloration of body fluids and excreta. It can cause permanent discoloration of contact lenses and lens implants. Mild side-effects are nausea and vomiting. A major side-effect is hepatotoxicity. The liver toxicity of isoniazid and rifampicin are cumulative. Assessment of liver function before and during treatment is essential. Transient elevation of enzymes is not a contraindication. A 3-fold or more rise is a contraindication. Rifampicin may show drug interactions, enhancing the clearance of warfarin, sulphonylurea and oestrogenic oral contraceptives. It can rarely affect renal function.

Pyrazinamide – a mild side-effect is arthralgia. Major side-effects include hepatitis. The risk is not increased when used in combination with isoniazid and rifampicin. Gout is a complication when the drug is used for > 6 months. Hyperuricemia is seen invariably in most patients and occasionally gouty arthritis (Koumbaniou *et al*. 1998).

Ethambutol – mild side-effects are dyspepsia, anorexia and abdominal pain. A major side-effect is neuritis, in one or both eyes. This is dose related. Vision becomes blurred and there is loss of green and red colour perception. Visual acuity diminishes. There is no abnormality seen on fundoscopy. Ophthalmic examination before and during treatment in the first 4 months is recommended. It should be avoided in children and patients with renal disease.

Streptomycin – toxicity is related to the dosage. The principal toxic effect is on the vestibular component of the 8th nerve and to a lesser extent on the cochlear component. If the patient develops ataxia or vertigo, the drug should be discontinued. This drug is not used in Australia. The drug may produce nephrotoxicity. Renal function should be assessed before treatment. Hypersensitivity reactions such as fever, rashes and haematological disorders may be seen. The drug is not recommended for patients > 60 years, and all other drugs causing toxicity or nephrotoxicity should be avoided. Patients with renal problems can still use rifampicin, isoniazid and pyrazinamide if they do not have pre-existing liver disease. The problem is more complicated with liver disease as three of the four first line drugs produce hepatotoxicity (isoniazid, rifampicin and pyrazinamide). The recommendation for such patients is to use one of these drugs at a low dose, combined with ethambutol and streptomycin and to monitor liver function.

Second line antituberculous drugs

Cycloserine – the major toxic effects include epilepsy and severe mental depression, including suicidal tendencies. This drug is rarely used.

Capreomycin – side-effects are similar to streptomycin. Both drugs are given IM. It is rarely used in the treatment of tuberculosis.

Ethionamide and prothionamide – minor side-effects are gastrointestinal upset, vomiting and diarrhoea. The drugs produce a metallic taste in the mouth. Major side-effects are hepatitis and hypoglycaemia in diabetics which are stabilized.

Non-tuberculous drugs

Other non-tuberculous drugs used in tuberculosis that have no action on the tubercle bacillus are pyridoxine and corticosteroids.

Pyridoxine – already mentioned under isoniazid.

Corticosteroids – should be used only in combination with antituberculous drugs for severe pulmonary infiltration, tuberculous meningitis, control of hypersensitivity reactions to drugs and to minimize inflammatory reaction in serous membranes. The recommended dose is 60 mg prednisolone/day, gradually tapered to 5 mg/week. Corticosteroids should not be used in patients who may have inactive tuberculosis without adequate antituberculous drugs coverage. It is wise to exclude tuberculosis, especially in patients in developing countries and those subject to transplants, before commencement or long-term corticosteroids, immunosuppressive drugs. The majority of antituberculous drugs produce toxicity in the liver and kidney.

Tuberculous lymphadenitis

The final outcome of treatment with antituberculous drugs is good. However, during treatment there may be complications such as abscess formation with discharging sinuses. This may be secondary to a hypersensitivity reaction to released tubercular protein from the macrophages. Surgery is indicated only for diagnosis or for drainage of abscess.

Pleural effusion

- As for pulmonary tuberculosis
- Corticosteroids may be used to reduce long-term sequelae of infection of the pleura
- The effusion, if large, should be fully drained

Empyema

- Surgical drainage and chemotherapy

Pericarditis

- Drainage if there is impending tamponade
- Full chemotherapy
- Steroids to minimize fibrosis

Urinary tract

- Antituberculous drugs – prednisolone at a dose of 20 mg/day initially minimizes further obstruction of the urinary tract and the progress is monitored with urography
- In the majority of cases the obstruction will be relieved
- Nephrectomy is rarely indicated except for a non-functioning kidney

Central nervous system

Chemotherapy should be commenced on clinical suspicion without waiting for confirmation. The treatment regimen is similar to that for pulmonary tuberculosis. The drugs isoniazid and pyrazinamide enter the CSF readily, with ethambutol and rifampicin to a lesser extent, but adequately (Watson et al. 1993). Streptomycin enters the CSF poorly. In children, because of the serious nature of the disease, ethambutol may be used. Although corticosteroids is generally contraindicated it is an absolute indication in treatment of tuberculous meningitis. It prevents death and cuts down residual crippling disability. Hydrocephalus may require neurosurgical intervention. The optimum duration of chemotherapy is 12–18 months.

Tuberculomas – surgical intervention is necessary for insertion of shunts for hydrocephalus, for resection of tuberculomas if causing intracranial hypertension or for specific neurological deficits. With antituberculous drugs paradoxical expansion and worsening of symptoms can manifest in tuberculoma as in tuberculous lymphadenitis. However, it is a phenomenon not seen in the whites (Watson et al. 1993).

Gastrointestinal tract

- Medical – full course of antituberculous chemotherapy for 12 months
- Surgical – resection if there are obstructive symptoms

Peritonitis

- Full course of antituberculous chemotherapy for 1 year with corticosteroids
- Prognosis is good with complete resolution of the disease and resorption of the fluid

Bone

- Medical – full course of antituberculous chemotherapy for at least 1 year
- Surgical – if there is neurological compromise which can be reversed by decompression

Cutaneous

- Treatment – as for pulmonary tuberculosis

Tuberculides

- If the hypersensitivity is due to tubercle bacilli, treatment is as for pulmonary tuberculosis

Adrenal tuberculosis

- Chemotherapy is indicated

Ophthalmic

- Ocular tuberculosis responds well to anti-tuberculous chemotherapy

Miliary and cryptic

- Antituberculous drug 9–12 months

HIV patients

A longer course of chemoprophylaxis is preferred along the usual lines of 6 months or 9 months. Drug toxicity will definitely be a problem. In Australia, the 'four drug' regimen has been used routinely for all patients. The American Thoracic Society (ATS/CDC) Tuberculosis Statement Committee now also recommends the 'four drug' regimen for such patients (Centers for Disease Control and Prevention 1993).

In areas of the USA where there is a high incidence of multiple drug resistance tuberculosis, the policy of prescribing 'five drug-' and in some areas even 'six drug-regimens' for patients with HIV infection or AIDS has been implemented. Monitoring should be performed combining close surveillance of clinical course with microbiology.

BCG vaccination should never be given to HIV-infected patients. Before vaccination of an individual care must be taken to determine risk factors for HIV. For the rest of the community, the vaccination policy remains the same. HIV testing of all tuberculosis patients is not advocated in Australia. However, it may have to be evaluated in the future. In all patients presenting with pulmonary or extrapulmonary tuberculosis, a very careful clinical evaluation to exclude stigmata of HIV infection should be prepared.

Hypersensitivity to antituberculous drugs

Hypersensitivity reactions are rash, with pruritus, fever, malaise, vomiting, myalgia, hepatosplenomegaly and rarely jaundice. It is possible to desensitize such patients. All medications should be suspended till symptoms subside. The drug responsible is identified by giving a challenge dose of each individual drug, and gradually increasing the dose. The commencing challenge dose is about one-sixth of the full daily dose. Desensitization may be required if there is no other suitable chemotherapeutic replacement in the hospital as in patient. However, desensitization is not recommended if reactions are severe such as mucocutaneous, renal or haematological reactions. The desensitization dose is about one-tenth of the challenge dose which produces a reaction (Patel and Streeton 1990). A much smaller starting dose may be required depending on the degree of hypersensitivity. The dose should be gradually increased monitoring side-effects. If reaction starts at a certain dose, then it needs to be again commenced at a lower dose. The full dose generally can be achieved in ~7 days. Antihistamines and steroids should be available during the procedure.

Drug resistance

Multidrug resistant tuberculosis is caused by a strain of *M. tuberculosis* that is resistant to two or more drugs. One definition requires resistance to both isoniazid and rifampicin. Primary drug resistance is resistance in bacterial isolates from patients who have not previously had antituberculous drugs. Hence, such patients have contracted the infection from someone who had acquired drug resistance. Rarely it may be due to mutation. It should be impressed on patients that drug resistance is predominantly due to poor compliance, inadequate dosage and the number of drugs used. It also occurs in patients with cavitatory pulmonary tuberculosis and HIV infected/AIDS patients. In 1988, 12.7% of isolates from patients in Australia were resistant to at least one drug (Dawson et al. 1991). In 1992, laboratory surveillance of *M. tuberculosis* isolates in Australia revealed 12% of the isolates were resistant to one or more drugs. Of these, 78% were resistant to one drug and 22% were resistant to two or more drugs. Isoniazid was the most common drug occurring in 7.4% of cases showing drug resistance (Dawson et al. 1991, Curran et al. 1994). The present level of drug resistance has risen compared with Commonwealth Health Department statistics of 3.8% among new cases (Howells 1969). The resistance of rifampicin was 1.2%.

It is now realized that transmission of multiresistant antituberculous drugs to primary cases can occur especially from HIV infected/AIDS patients with tuberculosis. Large-scale epidemics of multidrug resistant positive cases have been described among HIV-negative individuals.

Two important management principles are to use at least two drugs to which the organism is susceptible and to never add a single drug to a fair drug regimen (Bradford and Daley 1998).

The two major indicators of drug resistance in Australia are:

1. Previous use of antituberculous drugs and the country of origin of the migrants, such as Asia, South America and Africa. The drugs of resistance are most commonly streptomycin and isoniazid. In the 6-month regimen, isoniazid should be continued, even if there is a likelihood of resistance, as the success rate of treatment still is ~95%. If bacteriological negativity is not achieved within 3 months, an additional drug should be used and treatment continued > 6 months. In such situations the clinician should consult the relevant experts regarding the antituberculosis treatment.

2. Multiple drug resistance to three or more drugs in the first line drugs, the clinician has very little choice left. In such cases if there is no resistance to rifampicin, it should be used with another drug. Resistance rates to rifampicin at present is ~1.2% compared with isoniazid which is 7.4% (Curran et al. 1994).

It is postulated that the resistance mechanisms for isoniazid are encoded on genes. It has been identified that in *M. tuberculosis*, the gene Kat G encodes catalase peroxidase activity, causing resistance in the mutant bacillus (Zhang et al. 1992). Fatty acid synthesis for the mycobacterial wall, which is inhibited by isoniazid, is encoded by another gene Inh A and upregulation of this gene may impart resistance to isoniazid.

The two possible mechanisms postulated for resistance to rifampicin are mutation of RNA polymerase, the target of rifampicin activity and alteration in cell wall permeability which inhibits drug uptake (Honore and Cole 1993).

Chemotherapy in extrapulmonary tuberculosis

Chemotherapy of extrapulmonary tuberculosis is similar to that for pulmonary tuberculosis. The period of treatment may be extended, for the 6- or 9-month regimens. The prolongation is generally through continuing Isoniazid and Rifampicin treatment.

Approximate duration of treatment for various types of tuberculosis are:

1. Tuberculous lymph nodes – 9–12 months
2. Urogenital – 9–12 months
3. Pleural effusion – 6- or 9-month regimen
4. Skeletal tuberculosis – 9–12 months
5. Miliary tuberculosis – 9–12 months
6. Tuberculous meningitis – 12–18 months
7. Intestinal tuberculosis – 9–12 months
8. Peritoneal, pericardial – 9-month regimen
9. Genital tract – 9 months

Tuberculous treatment in pregnancy

All antituberculous drugs are toxic to the foetus and the issue of delaying treatment until after first trimester, or after delivery needs to be considered. In sputum-positive pregnant women treatment cannot be delayed, irrespective of stage in pregnancy. With other patients, the decision has to be made on an individual basis. Streptomycin should not be considered in pregnancy. There is no contraindication for the mother to nurse the newborn if she is bacteriologically negative and the infant has been given BCG. If the mother is bacteriologically positive, antituberculous drugs should render her bacteriologically negative and the infant need not be isolated if offered chemoprophylaxis with isoniazid. Once mother is bacteriologically negative the infant should be Mantoux tested, given BCG accordingly and the isoniazid can be stopped. Isoniazid-resistant BCG if available, can be used together with prophylactic isoniazid, when the mother is bacteriologically negative and isoniazid can be stopped.

CHEMOPROPHYLAXIS

Chemoprophylaxis may be required in some infected individuals with a positive tuberculin reaction but no clinical, radiological or bacterial evidence of tuberculosis. These persons are:

- Recent tuberculin converters especially children and teenagers
- Children who have been exposed to an open case of tuberculosis

- Contacts who react very strongly to tuberculin testing
- Neonates with bacteriologically positive mothers (refer to Tuberculosis in pregnancy)
- Persons who are tuberculin-positive and on steroids or immunosuppressive drugs, insulin-dependent diabetics, patients with silicosis and following gastrectomy, but with no other evidence of tuberculosis. The alternative is that of long-term surveillance
- Tuberculin-positive transplant patients
- Tuberculin-positive HIV-seropositive patients in the presymptomatic stage

ROLE OF SURGERY IN MYCOBACTERIAL DISEASE

With the contemporary multidrug regimen, the necessity for surgical management is very minimal. In pulmonary disease, the indications are bronchial stricture with bronchiectasis, tuberculous empyema and lungs which are extensively destroyed resulting in severe persistent haemoptysis. In extrapulmonary tuberculosis, surgery may be required for intestinal tuberculosis with obstruction, confirmed Pott's disease of the spine with cord compression. Urogenital tract tuberculosis may require surgery to relieve ureteric stenosis, or for removal of a non-functioning tuberculous kidney. A tuberculoma of the brain producing localizing signs may require surgical removal.

Surgery should, as far as possible, be performed only after adequate chemotherapy.

IMMUNIZATION

BCG vaccination – vaccination with bacillus Calmette Guerin, an attenuated strain of *M. bovis* was recommended by the Medical Research Council in the UK. There are different reports with regards to its efficiency. It is reported to be ~60% effective (McIntosh *et al.* 1993) but others have reported efficacy of 85–100% against tuberculous meningitis (Wunsch *et al.* 1990, Sirinivan *et al.* 1991). Routine vaccination has been phased out in Australia and New Zealand and is no longer advocated in schools. The WHO recommended neonatal BCG vaccinations as a routine, and this has also been recommended by the National Health and Medical Research Council in Australia for Aboriginal babies, and babies from high risk ethnic groups and older individuals in high risk groups (National Health and Medical Research Council Immunisation Procedure 1991). However, in developing countries those who are tuberculin-negative unless immuno-compromized should be vaccinated. One is tuberculin-negative if tuberculin response is 0–4 mm and Heaf Grades 0 and 1 (Department of Health, UK 1996).

High risk tuberculin-negative persons for whom BCG vaccination is recommended (besides the neonates mentioned above) are all hospital and ambulance staff who have patient contact, close contacts of persons with active tuberculosis, ethnic groups having a high incidence of tuberculosis and people travelling overseas for long periods to places where there is a high incidence of tuberculosis.

ILLUSTRATIVE CASES

The fatal outcome of two foreign-born patients with extrapulmonary tuberculosis, one with tuberculous meningitis and the other presenting with gastrointestinal involvement are described. Both cases were bacteriologically negative at the time of presentation and there was considerable delay in diagnosis and institution of therapy. These two cases illustrate the need for rapid commencement of therapy on the basis of clinical suspicion.

Case 1

An 84-year-old female from Punjab, India, was admitted to a local hospital in October 1989 with a history of a fall. She had arrived in Australia in 1988 and did not speak English. On admission she was febrile (38°C) with a blood pressure of 220/100 mmHg. She was drowsy but obeyed commands. There was no neck stiffness, photophobia or focal neurological deficit. Blood examination including erythrocyte sedimentation rate (ESR) was normal.

There was no abnormality on chest X-ray. Blood cultures were sterile. Urine and sputum examinations revealed no pathogens. She was commenced on ampicillin and gentamicin. Her level of consciousness started to decline. Two days after admission, neck stiffness was noted. She suffered a grand mal seizure for which Valium and Dilantin were commenced. At this stage a lumbar puncture was performed. Five millilitres of colourless cerebrospinal fluid (CSF) were obtained, it showed 2.4 g/litre protein and 1.4 mmol/litre glucose.

Pressure was 13 cm. There were 60×10^6/litre red blood cells and 20×10^6/litre white blood cells with 18 mononuclears and two polymorphs. Acid-fast bacilli were not seen and there was no growth on culture. Cerebral CT scans was not done.

The next day her level of consciousness improved. There were spontaneous movements and she obeyed commands. Mantoux test performed at this stage was positive. A repeat lumbar puncture showed 680 red blood cells and 270 white blood cells with 99% mononuclears and 1% polymorphs. No organisms including acid-fast bacilli were found. The following day she was difficult to rouse and was responding to painful stimuli only. There was no focal neurological deficit. Although there was no bacteriological confirmation, a clinical diagnosis of tuberculous meningitis was made and she was commenced on rifampicin, isoniazid, ethambutol and pyrazinamide. Ampicillin was continued. She was transferred to a major teaching hospital.

Her level of consciousness fluctuated with rapid deterioration and there was persisting hyponatraemia and hypokalaemia. She was intermittently febrile and there were increased upper limb tone reflexes and she showed Cheyne-Stokes respiration.

Cerebral CT scan done at this stage showed cortical atrophy. There was prominent bifrontal slowing in the EEG. At this stage, antituberculous therapy was stopped and she was discharged home where she died 2 weeks later. Consent for post-mortem was refused.

Case 2

A 66-year-old Hungarian male presented to the Emergency Department of another local hospital in January 1990 with colicky abdominal pain lasting from a few hours to 3 days. He had arrived in Australia in 1956 and was an ammunitions factory worker in Hungary. He was known to have had 'abnormal' chest X-rays since 1956, for which no treatment was given.

CT scan of the abdomen showed a thickened segment of small intestine. Chest X-ray showed further patchy opacities in the left upper lobe. Sputum and urine were negative for acid-fast bacilli. A laparotomy was recommended.

From January to April there was increasing ill health, night sweats, weight loss, anorexia and a productive cough. He was admitted to hospital and found to be cachectic and febrile. On examination, he had ascites with a 20 cm liver and splenomegaly. Haemoglobin was 10.19/dl and the white cell count was 15.8×10^3 with 77% polymorphs and ESR was 30 mm in 1 h. He had abnormal liver function tests and numerous acid-fast bacilli were present on blood and urine cultures. He was commenced on isoniazid, rifampicin, pyrazinamide, ethambutol and pyridoxine. Over the next few days the patient became confused, disorientated and dehydrated. On lumbar puncture, the cerebrospinal fluid had normal pressure. There were two red cells and one polymorph. Mononuclear cells were absent. The glucose was 2.4 mm/litre and the protein content was normal. An ascitic tap revealed 1500 red cells, 140 polymorphs, 100 mononuclears, 4.9 mm/litre of glucose and 90 g/dl proteins.

He was transferred to the Intensive Care Unit for enteral feeding. On the 9 April his condition deteriorated. More opacities were seen on the left side on chest X-ray. The fever had decreased. Liver functions worsened and he was found to have jaundice, ascites and encephalopathy. He was treated with gentamicin. Sputum was positive for acid-fast bacilli. Three days later, chest X-ray revealed gas under the diaphragm. A laparotomy was performed and he had multiple perforations of the terminal ileum. At surgery, 60 cm terminal ileum and 18 cm colon were removed. Liver and lymph node biopsies were taken.

Microscopic examination of sputum, urine, ascitic fluid demonstrated the presence of acid-fast bacilli. The bone marrow, liver biopsy and sections of the ileum showed caseating granulomata with the presence of acid-fast bacilli. The patient developed postoperative ileus and was started on IV isoniazid, rifampicin including IM injection of 1 g capreomicin. He developed renal failure and was transferred to another hospital for haemodialysis.

There was transient improvement of his liver function but he developed aspiration pneumonia and later pneumothorax and died soon after. Autopsy was not performed.

COMMENTS

Dawson et al. (1991) suggested that the incidence of bacteriologically positive tuberculosis in Australia is continuing at three-to-four cases/100 000 population and 40% of notifications in Australia related to patients whose bacteriological status was either negative or unknown like the present two cases.

In 1986, a survey in the USA revealed that 17.5% (3942) of all cases of tuberculosis were extra-pulmonary (American Review Respiratory Diseases 1990). Of these, 4.6% was tuberculous meningitis and 3.3% of cases had intestinal involvement. Of extra-pulmonary tuberculosis, 71.2% occurred in racial or ethnic minorities or foreign-born patients, as was the case in our two patients (Indian and Hungarian). Racial and ethnic minorities now represent a larger proportion of all cases of tuberculosis. In 1933, the incidence in non-whites was 24% and 49% in 1986. Extrapulmonary tuberculosis is more likely to be present in blacks, Asians and American Indians. There is an increased occurrence of extrapulmonary tuberculosis in HIV-infected patients. Before the advent of chemotherapy, abdominal tuberculosis was diagnosed in 70% of patients due to swallowing of infectious secretions. The distribution in 81 patients was peritoneal 41 (50.6%), ileocaecal 17 (20.9%), anorectal 16 (19.7%), lymph node 8 (9.8%) and other 1 (1.2%).

Ileocaecal tuberculosis usually presents with pain, diarrhoea and a mass lesion similar to case 2. The presence of typical caseating granulomata containing acid-fast tubercle bacilli in tissue biopsy material, together with culture studies confirmed the diagnosis.

CSF examination is necessary to diagnose tuberculous meningitis. The diagnostic yield is better if the CSF is clotted. Three or four separate collections of 10 ml of each of CSF are centrifuged and stained with Ziehl-Neelsen. The stain is positive in 10–100% of cases and the specimen must be cultured. In tuberculous meningitis, the CSF changes in response to treatment and occur over several weeks. There is an increase in glucose with a decrease in white cells and proteins.

A more practical new method of diagnosis is the use of PCR/DNA probes of clinical material to identify acid-fast bacilli in culture.

Treatment regimens do not differ for pulmonary and extrapulmonary tuberculosis. However, for tuberculosis meningitis drugs used must have adequate penetration into the inflamed CSF. Isoniazid, rifampicin, pyrazinamide and ethambutol are used in high doses together with cycloserine. As to whether these levels are adequate after 3 months of treatment is debatable. Diagnostic features in the CSF result from rupture of a tuberculous granuloma also alongside ventricles into the subarachnoid space resulting in a 'tuberculin' reaction in CSF and the characteristic CSF findings (polymorphs predominating).

Atypical CSF findings also occur in the early stages of treatment (predominance of polymorphs, rise in protein, and a positive AFB stain). Culture and smears remain positive for days after treatment. Streptomycin given IM formed part of the initial successful regimens for tuberculous meningitis, and may be used for patients who are not tolerating oral treatment. Current recommendations are for intrathecal administration of streptomycin 50 mg/day for 1 week, 50 mg every second day for a further week and followed by IM streptomycin for 3 months. The daily dose of streptomycin should not exceed 1 g for adults (15–20 mg/kg) and not to exceed 0.75 g for those weighing < 50 kg or > 50 years. Daily use for a month should be replaced by intermittent treatment thrice weekly. There is no place for streptomycin if high dose ethambutol is given. Another treatment for tuberculous meningitis is intrathecal PPD, streptokinase hyaluronidase and steroids.

Prognosis depends on age, presence of miliary TB and the clinical staging. If the patient is rational with no focal signs and no hydrocephalus, good recovery is expected. If the patient shows confusion with focal signs and hydrocephalus and stuporose major focal signs, the mortality rate is > 50%.

REFERENCES

Bargava S, Gupta AK, Tandon MS. Tuberculous meningitis, a CT study. *British Journal of Radiology* 1982; **55**: 189–196

Bradford WZ, Daley CE. Multiple drug-resistant tuberculosis. *Infectious Diseases Clinics of North America* 1998; **12**: 157–172

British Thoracic and Tuberculosis Association. Short course chemotherapy for pulmonary tuberculosis. *Lancet* 1976; **ii**: 1102–1104

Centers for Disease Control and Prevention. Initial therapy for tuberculosis in the era of multidrug resistance recommendations of the Advisory Council for Elimination of Tuberculosis. *Morbidity and Mortality Weekly Report* 1993; **42**: 1–8

Curran M, Dawson D, Cheah D. Laboratory surveillance of *Mycobacterium tuberculosis* isolates in Australia 1992. *Communicable Disease Intelligence (Australia)* 1994; 18

Dawson D, Anargyros P, Blalock Z *et al*. Tuberculosis in Australia. An analysis of cases identified in Reference laboratory in 1986–88. *Pathology* 1991; **23**: 130–134

Department of Health. *Immunisation against Infectious Diseases*, 1996 edn. London: HMSO, 1996, 219–241

Fernando S, Fernando SSE. Extrapulmonary tuberculosis – two case reports with fatal outcome. *Pathology* 1993; **25**: 214–215

Galietti F, Chirillo MG, Gulotta C *et al*. Identification of *Mycobacterium tuberculosis* and *Mycobacterium avium intracellulare* directly from primary BACTEC cultures by using acridinium-ester-labelled DNA probes. *Journal of Clinical Microbiology* 1992; **30**: 2427–2431

Gillespie SH, Kennedy N. Fluoroquinolones: a new treatment for tuberculosis? *International Journal of Tuberculosis and Lung Disease* 1998; **2**: 265–267

Honore N, Cole ST. Molecular basis of rifampicin resistance in *Mycobacterium leprae*. *Antimicrobial Agents Chemotherapy* 1993; **37**: 418

Howells G. Primary drug resistance in Australia. *Tuberculosis* 1969; **50**: 334–339

Illingworth RS. Miliary and meningeal tuberculosis. Difficulties in diagnosis. *Lancet* 1956; **2**: 646–649

Jacobs RF. Multiple drug resistant tuberculosis. State of the art clinical article. *Clinical Infectious Diseases* 1994; **19**: 1–10

Kaneko K, Onodera O, Myarake R *et al*. Rapid diagnosis of tuberculous meningitis by polymerase chain reaction (PCR). *Neurology* 1990; **40**: 1617–1618

Kochi A. The global tuberculosis situation and the new control strategy of the World Health Organisation [Editorial]. *Tubercle* 1991; **72**: 1–6

Koumbaniou C, Nicopoulos C, Vassilion M *et al*. Is pyrazinamide really the third drug of choice in the treatment of tuberculosis? *International Journal of Tuberculosis and Lung Disease* 1998; **2**: 675–678

Lebrium L, Espinase F, Poreda JD *et al*. Evaluation of non-radioactive DNA probes for identification of mycobacteria. *Journal of Clinical Microbiology* 1992; **30**: 2476–2478

McIntosh ED, Isaacs D, Oates RK *et al*. Extrapulmonary TB in children. *Medical Journal of Australia* 1993; **159**: 735–740

National Health and Medical Research Council. *Immunisation Procedure*, 4th edn. Canberra: Australia Government Publication, 1991, 110–115

Ortona L, Antinori A. Principles of therapy for tuberculosis. *Rays* 1998; **23**: 181–192

Patel A, Streeton J. Tuberculosis in Australia and New Zealand into the 1990s. *Canberra National Health and Medical Council/Australian Government Publication* 1990; **1**: 4

Raviglione M, Nunn PP. Epidemiology of tuberculosis. In Zumla A, Johnson M, Miller RF *et al*. (eds), *AIDS and Respiratory Medicine*. London: Chapman & Hall, 1997, 117–143

Sirinivan S, Chotpitauasounondh T, Suwanjuntha S *et al*. Protective efficacy of neonatal bacillus Calmette-Guerin vaccination against tuberculosis. *Paediatric Infectious Diseases* 1991; **10**: 359–365

Stewart SM. The bacteriologic diagnosis of tuberculosis meningitis. *Journal of Clinical Pathology* 1953; **6**: 241–242

Watson JDG, Shnier RD, Seale JP. Central nervous system tuberculosis in Australia. A report of 22 cases. *Medical Journal of Australia* 1993; **159**: 408–413

World Health Organisation. *TB – A Global Emergency*. Geneva: WHO, 1994

Wunsch FV, deCastilho EA, Rodrigues LC *et al*. Effectiveness of BCG vaccination against tuberculous meningitis. A case control study in Sao Paulo, Brazil. *World Health Organisation* 1990; **68**: 69–74

Zhang Y, Heym B, Allen B *et al*. The catalase-peroxidase gene and isoniazid resistance of mycobacterial tuberculosis. *Nature* 1992; **358**: 591–593

Zumla A, Corange J. Establishing a united front against the injustice of tuberculosis. *International Journal of Tuberculosis Lung Disease* 1998; **3**: 1–4

Leprosy

MICROBIOLOGY

Microbiologists at University College London Medical School extracted an amplified ancient DNA of Mycobacterium leprae *from bone dating around AD600 from a grave in the grounds of the monastery of St John the Baptist on the River Jordan. They regard their results as important to the study of medicine and establishing paleobacteriology as a new scientific approach. (Rafi* et al. *1994)*

The registered number of cases have fallen from 5.4 million worldwide in 1985 to < 1 million in 1998. This is most likely an underestimate. Six hundred and eighty-five thousand new cases were registered in 1997 (WHO 1998). The incidence therefore has changed little. The greatest concentration is in South East Asia, especially India, with a prevalence rate of 20.5/10 000, other countries being Indonesia, Myamar, Brazil, Nigeria, in some Pacific islands, tropical Africa, Central and South America, Southern Europe, Middle East and North Africa and in the Northern Territory of Australia (Valverde *et al.* 1998). With a prevalence rate

of 0.1 cases/1000 persons as a lower limit in 93 countries, an estimate of total population of 2.46 billion people are at risk (Britton and Hargrave 1993). Leprosy occurs at all ages, ranging from infancy to very old age. It has a bimodal pattern with age peaks in childhood (10–14 years) and in the fourth and seventh decades. The incidence in males is nearly double that of females, but this can vary. It is prevalent among the low socio-economic groups where there is malnutrition and poor immune status. Leprosy is transmitted from man to man. An identical *M. leprae* has been discovered in the Armadillo but transmission through this source has not been proved. It has also been found in chimpanzee, sooty mangabey monkeys and cynomolgus macaque (Britton and Hargrave 1993). The majority of people do not develop leprosy after exposure and those who develop leprosy after an incubation period of several years may only have a single lesion (intermediate leprosy) which often heals. It is often difficult to identify the source of the infection because of the long incubation period. There is sufficient evidence that in lepromatous leprosy (multibacillary type) the portal of entry is the respiratory route via aerosol spread as patients are teaming with bacilli in their nasal mucosa. Entry through other routes such as abraised skin is a possibility (Abraham *et al.* 1998). The *M. leprae* multiplies very slowly with a generation time of 12.5 days. It is an obligate intracellular bacterium. It grows best at 27–30°C, hence its predilection for cooler parts of body. There is an impaired cell-mediated immune response to *M. leprae* specially the multibacillary type. The source of impaired immune response may be due to genetic defect and has been linked to NRAmP1 'gene' (Abel *et al.* 1998).

Indeterminate lesion (IL), is the early lesion of leprosy and may heal or progress to one of the five other types – tuberculoid leprosy (TL) where the resistance to infection is high, borderline tuberculoid leprosy (BTL), borderline leprosy (BL), borderline lepromatous leprosy (BLL) and lepromatous leprosy (LL) (WHO Classification 1998) when the resistance to infection is very low. In borderline leprosy one finds features of both forms of leprosy, tuberculoid and lepromatous in same patient.

In the classification of leprosy the following criteria are taken into consideration. The number of skin lesions present the greater the immune resistance. Asymmetry of distribution of skin margin and degree of infiltration vary with the type. Lepromatous leprosy (multibacillary) affects other parts of the body such as nose, mucosa of the upper respiratory tract, the eyes, bones, tendons, muscles, male genitalia and lymph nodes. Another method of classification is by means of the Bacterial Index based on the density of bacteria in a slit skin smear (Ridley and Jopling 1966). This is graded as 0+ when acid-fast bacilli up to 100 are seen per field to grade 6+ when > 1000 acid-fast bacilli are seen per field. The higher the number of bacilli indicates poor immune response and vice versa. Paucibacillary leprosy itself is defined by five or fewer skin lesions with no bacilli on skin lesions. Multibacillary cases have six or more lesions and may be skin-smear positive.

PRESENTATION

The cardinal signs of leprosy are discoloration of skin, anaesthetic patches of skin and thickened peripheral nerves (Figs 41.1a, b and c). In light coloured skin the lesions appear different from those in darker skin.

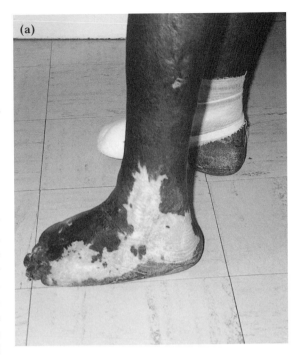

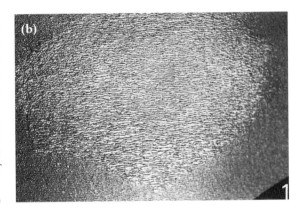

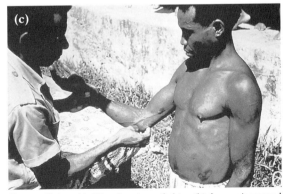

Figure 41.1 – (a) Discoloration of skin; (b) hypo-pigmented patch; (c) enlarged peripheral ulnar nerve.

Hypo-pigmentation in the former is so subtle that it can be overlooked. The clinical features are different in the clinical types mentioned.

Indeterminate leprosy

This presents as a hypo-pigmented dry macule, a few centimetres in diameter, which may be erythematous in the white skin. There may be hypo-aesthesia. It is the first sign of leprosy in a large proportion of cases and diagnosis is difficult. The lesions can be mistaken for tinea or psoriasis. In most instances true indeterminate lesions will heal spontaneously, depending on the immunity. In others, it progresses to tuberculoid or lepromatous lesions. If there is definite anaesthesia, it should be treated for presumptive leprosy or observed closely. Photographs of the lesions allow objective assessment of progress.

Tuberculoid leprosy

Tuberculoid leprosy affects the skin and peripheral nerves. Macular or papular skin lesions which are single or few, with sharp borders, are seen. The edge of the lesions may be elevated, indicating healing in the centre. They are hypo-pigmented and have a copper patch appearance in Australian aborigines. These lesions may be found in any part of the body. The lesions are anaesthetic, anhidrotic with scanty hair. Few nerves are involved and there can be some deformity of hands and feet associated with damaged peripheral nerves. The nerves commonly involved are the lateral popliteal, posterior tibial, the greater auricular, median, radial and ulnar. The combination of a thickened nerve with peripheral nerve lesions differentiates leprosy from other neurological conditions.

Lepromatous leprosy

Lepromatous leprosy has a very extensive clinical presentation, involving the skin, initially peripheral sensory nerves, eyes, cartilage of nose, liver, testis, kidney, bone mainly that of the nasal and zygomatic process, and joints of the fingers. The bacilli are found in millions in the skin and blood stream and patient has no established immunity. It is a very serious systemic disease and if untreated would be fatal.

The earliest skin lesions are macules, then the skin in the face and earlobes becomes indurated, producing the 'leonine facies' (Fig. 41.2a and b). In Australian Aborigines, the skin colour is the same. In lighter coloured races, the lesions are reddish or hypo-pigmented. There is a loss of eyelashes on the lateral aspect, described as 'madarosis'.

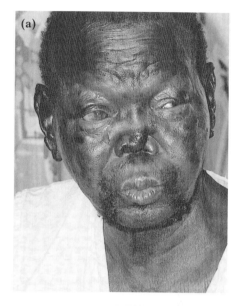

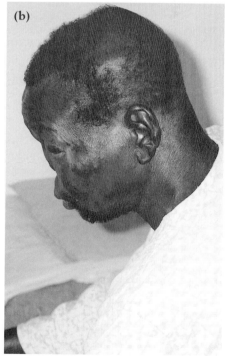

Figure 41.2 – (a) Typical leonine facies; (b) thickened earlobes.

The earliest neuronal lesion is a peripheral sensory neuropathy of the extremities that gradually progresses upwards. There is loss of sweating in the distribution of the nerves. It is impossible to find clinical signs of damage to peripheral nerves. As the disease progresses, the peripheral nerves become thickened, then hard and the patients develop muscle weakness and sensory loss. Peripheral nerves are affected symmetrically.

The mucous membrane of the upper respiratory tract is involved with epistaxis and blocked nose. Thickened nodules are found in the tongue and the palate. The bridge of the nose is eroded producing flattening of the face. The palate may be perforated. There may be hoarseness and stridor due to involvement of the larynx. Erosion of zygomatic process causes flattening of cheeks and contributes to the characteristic facial deformity.

Corneal anaesthesia results from bacillary infiltration of corneal and trigeminal nerves. Iritis and secondary glaucoma may be pointers and should be detected early to prevent blindness.

There may be swelling and shortening of joints. The digits taper towards the tips. The hands and feet are subjected to traumatic injury if there is neural involvement.

Erythema nodosum leprosum

Erythema nodosum leprosum (ENL) or (type II reaction) is an immune complex reaction occurring in affecting lepromatous and borderline lepromatous leprosy. Patients present with small tender subcutaneous nodules that persist for a few days then subside. It is associated with fever, iridocyclitis, glomerulonephritis and orchitis. Precipitating antibodies (Roche *et al.* 1990) are found in the serum and as are large amounts of mycobacterial antigens. ENL, if not controlled, can cause amyloidosis. Tumour necrosis factor and cytokines are elevated and causes systemic manifestations (Barnes *et al.* 1992).

Owing to very high bacillaemia, internal organs are bombarded by large numbers of bacilli. Bacilli found in the endothelial cells may produce an acute allergic vasculitis ('luciophenomenon').

Mid-borderline leprosy

Mid-borderline leprosy (BB) – this classification is based on immunopathological features (Ridley and Hibson 1967) widely used for research and clinical work. It was formerly known as dimorphous leprosy, which lies between tuberculoid (TT) and lepromatous (LL) leprosy. The diagnosis depends on a combination of all the clinical features and bacterial counts. The clinical picture is involvement of skin with many skin lesions not as much as in lepromatous leprosy and also a single peripheral nerve involvement. The skin lesions are symmetrical. It is an unstable category. Patients with mid-borderline leprosy whose immunity improves may become more tuberculoid but not necessarily due to treatment. In others who are untreated or inadequately treated or has relapsed may downgrade in immunity and become more lepromatous, often following a type I reaction. Hence, histology and bacterial counts are useful in assessing progress.

Borderline tuberculoid

The difference from tuberculoid lesions is that the definition of the margin of borderline tuberculoid lesions is not absolutely clear. The lesions are larger with greater numbers of lesions (even up to 25). Satellite lesions are also seen. The lesions may be less anaesthetic. The damage to peripheral nerve trunk is more extensive and they are asymmetrical, thickened and tender.

The nerves may be damaged further with an antileprotic treatment and need monitoring of the dose. Type I reactions which are cell-mediated immune reaction with oedema can occur in skin or nerves with such rapidity. Every time a type I reaction occurs, there is further damage to the nerves, manifested by pain and tenderness along the nerve and functional impairment.

Reversal reactions or type I reactions

Reversal reactions (or type I reactions) are uncommon in tuberculoid and lepromatous type. During this phase cell-mediated immune reactions to mycobacterial antigens take place in the skin and nerves, associated with oedema and hyperaemia. As a result, adjacent tissues are damaged. *M. leprae* are found in Schwann cells and this immunological hypersensitivity is responsible for loss of nerve function. It is a delayed type hypersensitivity reaction. Generally there is a balance between antigen available for immune reactions and host response.

Borderline tuberculoid leprosy is specifically prone to reversal reactions. Although the acid-fast bacilli are few, the reaction is directed against the bacterial antigens.

Borderline lepromatous leprosy

The main difference from lepromatous leprosy is that the papules and nodules are well defined. They are variable in size. Signs of nerve damage begin sooner. The peripheral nerves become thicker, sooner than in lepromatous leprosy. They are less tender than in borderline tuberculoid, as spontaneous reactions are less common.

Anaesthesia of hands, feet and cornea appear late. 'Madarosis' is infrequent. The type II reaction immune complex reactions are less but they may develop erythema nodosum leprosum and iritis.

Neural leprosy

In neural leprosy there are no skin lesions. In this very uncommon type, the clinical manifestations are those of neuritis of generally a single nerve with loss of function. Diagnosis is difficult but a nerve tender to palpation is suspicious. These cases may turn out to be borderline tuberculoid or tuberculoid leprosy.

Neurological complications of leprosy causes severe physical disability. Motor paralysis causes claw hand, foot drop and claw toes. Sensory loss causes blindness as a result of complications of anaesthesia and immunological reactions. Ulceration of feet and hands are common features in advanced disease. Autonomic disturbances can cause anhidrosis in sensitive skin.

PATHOLOGY

The pathology is influenced by the immune response, and varies from no granulomas with a superficial perivascular, peri-adrenal and perineural infiltrate in indeterminate leprosy to foamy macrophages demonstrating abundant leprae bacilli in lepromatous leprosy.

Borderline leprosy shows a wide range of appearances depending on whether it is borderline tuberculoid leprosy (BT), true borderline (BB) or borderline lepromatous leprosy (BL). The skin lesions show granulomata containing both foamy macrophages and epithelioid cells. Acid-fast bacilli are found with ease within macrophages.

In tuberculoid leprosy low numbers of *M. leprae* are seen with epithelioid granulomas, some with central necrosis around dermal nerves, giving an 'elongated' appearance.

In lepromatous leprosy the typical macular or infiltrative nodular lesions show extensive cellular infiltrate with flattened epidermis and underlying Grenz zone. The skin appendages are destroyed with foamy macrophages filled with bacilli called 'lepra cells of Virchow'. The Fite-Ferraco stain identify the numerous red staining lepra bacilli measuring 0.5×5 μm. There are a few lymphocytes of CD_4 and CD_8 phenotypes (Britton and Hargrave 1993). The nerves unlike in tuberculoid leprosy are well preserved.

Two other forms of leprosy which is reactional leprosy (type 1) and erythema nodosum leprosum (type 2) is also seen. This is described under immunological reactions in leprosy.

'Luciophenomenon' is an acute allergic vasculitis due to large number of bacilli in the endothelium of blood vessels.

INVESTIGATIONS

1. Skin smears and/or biopsy – skin and nasal smears will demonstrate large numbers of bacilli. Skin smears are obtained from small slits made in the skin. The edges of these are scraped and the tissue fluid obtained in smeared on slide and stained for the acid-fast bacilli. Biopsies should be taken from entirely within a lesion.
2. Lepromin skin test is a suspension of killed *M. leprae* prepared from heavily infected human or armadillo tissue. It is negative in lepromatous leprosy. Its usefulness is limited. A positive response in normal person is associated with immunity.
3. PCR amplification of the 531-bp fragment of *M. leprae* gene in fresh biopsies and slit skin smears has been studied in Thailand. It has been shown to have a clear advantage over both microscopic examination of slit skin smears and serological methods. It can also be used to evaluate the progress while the patient is on chemotherapy. Bacterial clearance with chemotherapy of cases that were PCR positive, gradually became negative (Wichitwechkaran 1995). Higher positive results were obtained in multibacillary lesions, and more in biopsy specimens than in slit skin smears. It has

also been useful in the very early stage of leprosy (indeterminate type). However, it is an expensive technique but a useful additional diagnostic item to conventional methods used routinely.

4. There is no useful serologic test for diagnosis of leprosy. Phenolic glycolipid 1 (PGL-1) antigen is immunologically specific to *M. leprae* and has a characteristic structure. Detection of antibody to this antigen has been tried with good results for lepromatous leprosy, but poor result for tuberculoid leprosy. A study in Thailand PCR was more useful than the serology test.

TREATMENT

The treatment of leprosy today with the multidrug regimen is very rewarding. Early diagnosis and treatment is essential for complete cure. Completely damaged nerves cannot recover completely with treatment. However, all newly diagnosed cases require treatment irrespective of the stage of the disease. Treatment today is based on multidrug therapy as recommended by the WHO in 1982. Treatment is determined on whether the lesions are paucibacillary or multibacillary and should the drug be self-administered or supervised. Therapy also is directed also at reversal reactions and erythema nodosum leprosum. Six effective, antileprosy drugs, rifampicin, dapsone, and clofazimine (the three widely used), minocycline, ofloxacin and clarithromycin. Rifampicin is mostly bactericidal (99.9%).

Paucibacillary leprosy

- Rifampicin (10–15 mg/kg) up to 600 mg/month supervised; dapsone (1–2 mg/kg) up to 100 mg/day, self administered. This treatment is continued for 6 months

Multibacillary leprosy

Lepromatous, mid-borderline and borderline lepromatous leprosy. The skin smears are positive for acid-fast bacilli.

- Rifampicin (10–15 mg/kg) up to 600 mg/month supervised; clofazimine 300 mg/month supervised; dapsone (1–2 mg/kg) up to 100 mg/day self administered; clofazimine (0.5–1 mg/kg) up to 50 mg/day self administered. Duration of treatment is 2 years. The WHO now recommends

only 12 months of treatment for multibacillary disease. However, it may be sufficient for most cases. Concern has been expressed that it may not suffice for patients with higher bacterial indices (Jacobson and Krahenbuhl 1999). During treatment, one should be on the lookout for adverse drug reactions

Rifampicin is a bactericidal drug. It produces a harmless orange colour to body fluids such as urine, tears and sweat, and contact lenses. Adverse effects are rashes, thrombocytopenia, impairment of liver function and rarely nephritis. It induces microsomal enzymes in the liver and drug level of other medications need monitoring of the drug levels of other medications. Rifampicin 600 mg once monthly rarely causes significant side-effects. Pregnant patients have safely taken dapsone and clofazimine but experience with rifampicin is limited (Wabers 1998).

1. Dapsone – adverse reactions are haemolysis, particularly if there is glucose 6-phosphate dehydrogenase deficiency, gastrointestinal intolerance and methemoglobinaemia. Patients may develop erythema nodosum leprosum. Exfoliative dermatitis is a well-known complication and can be fatal. Large doses of corticosteroids are life saving, with antibiotics for secondary infection. Dapsone has been used for many decades as the only drug for treatment of leprosy and *M. leprae* have resistance to a certain extent and should not be used alone (Britton and Hargrave 1993)

2. Clofazimine – the characteristic side-effect is on the skin, producing a skin discoloration ranging from red-brown to black, posing a cosmetic problem on the white skin. It clears when drug is discontinued. Gastrointestinal intolerance can occur

The WHO regimen has been very successful with an average lapse rate of 1% for multibacillary cases and slightly > 1% for paucibacillary cases. However, relapse rate may be higher with high bacterial indices (Bertoli *et al.* 1997).

1. Reversal reactions – a close watch for reversal reactions during drug treatment is imperative. Patients should be warned to report symptoms of acute neuritis if they develop. If patients develop acute neuritis large doses of prednisolone should be used 40–60 mg/day for 3 months and preferably 6 months.

In Zimbabwe, prednisolone is used at 30–40 mg for 1 week and tapered down over 6–12 months. Clofazimine may also be useful. Reactions may occur in 25% or more of all borderline and lepromatous patients at some time during disease

2. Erythema nodosum leprosum – short courses of prednisolone 60–100 mg for 1–2 days, taper in 8–10 days. Thalidomide is the most effective drug that rapidly controls the symptoms, if it can be used without contraindications, such as in pregnancy. In recurrent ENL Clofazimine is used as an anti-inflammatory drug. Dose 100 mg three times a day for 2 months then 100 mg/day for 6 months. Clofazimine accumulates in macrophages. A short course of prednisolone may be sufficient for ENL without neuritis. Clofazimine is not useful for acute reactions, may be of value for chronic cases. Thalidomide 300–400 mg/day will control the reactions in 48 h. The dose is tapered to 100 mg/day and every few months an attempt be made to wear off the drug altogether

- Leprosy control – in Australia leprosy has been very well controlled in the Aboriginal population. However, doctors should be vigilant of patients among the indigenous migrants who present with skin and nerve lesions. They often present to an emergency department or to the general practitioner for a completely different ailment
- In endemic areas, BCG vaccination has been used with a protective effect from 80 to 20%. BCG vaccination has a greater preventive measure in leprosy than tuberculosis. A single dose appears to be 50% protective and two doses increase protection (Bertoli *et al.* 1997). Initial studies indicates that addition of dead *M. leprae* to BCG increased the protective benefits by 18% (Convit *et al.* 1992)
- Reconstruction surgery and physiotherapy – amputation is a last resort. Reconstructive surgery is undertaken to regain function which will not be discussed further (Brand 1970). Physiotherapy should be used to improve function

ILLUSTRATIVE CASE

A 12-year-old boy from Vietnam was seen in the Department of Emergency Medicine, Liverpool Hospital, Liverpool, New South Wales, Australia. He presented with skin rash. He had arrived in Australia 2 years earlier following a short stay in Singapore. The rash had been noted 4 months before presentation. The boy had been quite well apart from this. There was no family history of leprosy and he was attending the local school.

There were numerous lesions on the legs, upper arms and trunk, mainly in the back. The skin lesions on the legs were maculopapular, slightly erythematous and mildly hypoanaesthetic. The lesions on the trunk were annular, with a raised erythematous margin, and hypopigmented hypoanaesthetic centre. The lesions in the upper arm were similar to the ones in the trunk. The lesions were not itchy.

The ulnar nerve and the greater auricular nerves on both sides were thickened. There was no sensory loss in the distribution of these nerves. The nasal mucosa was not thickened. There was no 'leonine' appearance of the face. Testicular sensation was normal. Skin biopsies were done in the Emergency Department, one from the chest wall and one from a leg.

The biopsies were reported as showing borderline lepromatous leprosy. This was classified as borderline leprosy because of the severe involvement of the nerves. The cellular infiltrate were those of lepromatous leprosy (Fig. 41.3).

Skin smears demonstrated numerous acid-fast bacilli (*M. leprae*) within foam cells on Fite stain. Routine chest X-ray, full blood count and ESR were normal.

The boy was commenced on rifampicin 350 mg/day. Two weeks later he was started on dapsone and clofazimine. The liver function tests were slightly elevated transiently while on rifampicin. He had a mild eosinophilia after commencement of dapsone. Both

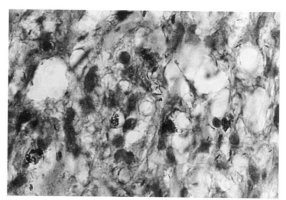

Figure 41.3 – Leprosy bacilli in macrophages (Fite stain × 100).

these changes resolved on discharge from hospital after 2 months of inpatient treatment.

The medications on discharge were:

1. Rifampicin 350 mg mane for a further 3 weeks, then cease
2. Clofazimine 100 mg twice a week
3. Dapsone 25 mg mane (6 days a week)
4. Hansolar 1.5 ml deep IMI 3 monthly

The boy was advised to attend school after a month of outpatient treatment.

Skin smears were done before discharge from hospital. Smears from the back of the chest showed no acid-fast bacilli. Right ear lobe smears showed scanty acid-fast bacilli 85% granular. The dorsum of left middle finger showed scanty acid-fast bacilli 95% granular. The dorsum of right middle finger showed very scanty acid-fast bacilli 99% granular. The skin lesions on the back were found to fade slightly at time of discharge.

On follow-up, his skin lesions showed gradual but satisfactory resolution within 3 months.

REFERENCES

Abel L, Sanchez FO, Obert J et al. Susceptibility to leprosy is linked to the human NRAMPI gene. *Journal of Infectious Diseases* 1998; **177**: 133–145

Abraham S, Mozhi NM, Joseph GA et al. Epidemiological significance of first skin lesions in leprosy. *International Journal of Leprosy* 1998; **66**: 131–139

Barnes PF, Chatterjee D, Brennan PJ et al. Tumour necrosis factor production in patients with leprosy. *Infectious Immunology* 1992; **60**: 1441–1446

Bertoli J, Pangi C, Frenchs R et al. A case study of the effectiveness of the BCG vaccine for preventing leprosy in Yangon Myanmar. *Infectious Journal of Epidemiology* 1997; **26**: 888–896

Brand PW. Tendon transfers for median and ulnar nerve paralysis. *Orthopaedic Clinic North America* 1970; **1**: 447–459

Britton WJ, Hargrave JC. Leprosy in the tropics and Australia. *Medical Journal of Australia* 1993; **159**: 326–330

Convit J, Sampson C, Zóga M et al. Immunoprophylactic trial with combined with leprosy. *Infectious Immunology* 1992; **60**: 1441–1446

Jacobson RR, Krahenbuhl KL. Leprosy. *Lancet* 1999; **253**: 655–660

Rafi A, Spigelman M, Stanford E et al. Mycobacterium leprae DNA from ancient bone detected by polymerase chain reaction. *Lancet* 1994; **343**: 1360–1361

Ridley D, Jopling W. Classification of leprosy according to immunity. A five group system. *International Journal of Leprosy* 1966; **34**: 255–273

Ridley DS, Hibson GRF. A logarithmic index of bacilli in biopsies. *International Journal of Leprosy* 1967; **35**: 184–186

Roche PW, Britton WJ, Fallbus SS et al. Operational value of serological measurements in multibacillary leprosy patients. Clinical and bacteriological correlates of antibody responses. *International Journal of Leprosy and Other Mycobacterial Diseases* 1990; **58**: 486–490

Valverde CR, Canfield D, Tavara I et al. Spontaneous leprosy in a wild-caught cyanomolgus macaque. *International Journal of Leprosy* 1998; **66**: 140–148

Wabers MFR. Is it safe to shorten multidrug therapy for lepromatous (LL and BL) leprosy to 12 months? *Leprosy Review* 1998; 110–111

Wichitwechkaran J, Karnjan S, Shuntawuttizettee S et al. Detection of *Mycobacterium leprae* infection by PCR. *Journal of Clinical Microbiology* 1995; **33**: 45–49

World Health Organisation Study Group. *Chemotherapy of Leprosy*. Technical Report No. 847. Geneva: World Health Organisation, 1994

World Health Organisation Expert Committee on Leprosy. *Seventh Report*. Technical Report No. 874. Geneva: World Health Organisation, 1998

World Health Organisation. *Chemotherapy of Leprosy for Control Programmes*. Technical Report Survey. Geneva: World Health Organisation, 1982, 675

World Health Organisation. Progress towards leprosy elimination. *Weekly Epidemiological Review* 1998; **73**: 153–160

42

Typhoid and Paratyphoid Fevers

Microbiology
Presentation
Pathology
Investigations

Treatment
Treatment of Major Complications
Paratyphoid A, B and C
Prevention
References

MICROBIOLOGY

Typhoid is an acute febrile illness caused by *Salmonella typhi*, a Gram-negative aerobic bacillus. Man is the only host infected.

Transmission is from man to man by the faecal-oral route through bacteria-contaminated water or food such as uncooked vegetables. Another source of transmission is through food handlers who are chronic carriers.

The notorious Mary Mallon had been a carrier of typhoid fever bacillus in 1907. Eight years later she was captured and had infected 50 people with three deaths while working as a New York City cook under several assumed names (Fanning 1997).

Typhoid is a global disease with > 75% occurring in Africa and South East Asia, Middle East and Latin America. In Australia, it is an exotic disease in > 90% of the reported cases, some being travellers to the Indian Subcontinent, South East Asia and Philippines. *S. typhi* infection has been reported in HIV-positive patients. In Peru, in 1991, six cases of typhoid were reported in HIV-positive patients (Gotuzzo 1991).

Increasing the pH of gastric contents such as in hypochlorhydria and eradicating normal bacterial flora sets the correct environment for typhoid bacillus to obtain a foothold in the Peyer's patches of the small intestine.

Virulence surface antigen (V1 antigen) may inhibit killing of the organism by phagocytosis. During the incubation the organism localizes in the reticulo-endothelial system and gallbladder. Septicaemia occurs subsequently when organisms enter the blood stream from reticulo-endothelial cells.

PRESENTATION

The incubation period is from 7 to 14 days. Severe headache before the onset of fever is a prominent symptom. Constipation is also a characteristic symptom. Other symptoms are lassitude, cough, anorexia, abdominal discomfort and occasionally vomiting. Diarrhoea may occur at times more common in children (Yap and Puthucheary 1998). The stepladder pattern of the temperature, with a rise in temperature in the evening and a drop in temperature in the morning, is not a true guide for diagnosing typhoid fever.

Apart from the rash (Rose spots) there are very few physical signs that suggest typhoid fever in the initial stages. The spleen may be palpable in ~30% of cases, and hepatomegaly occurs in ~30% of cases. Bradycardia is often described as a hallmark of typhoid fever is found in only half the patients. The rash occurs about the seventh day, commencing over the abdomen and then the thorax. They disappear after 2 or 3 days. Some patients may have rhonchi and crepitations in the chest. If untreated patients become more toxic, they may be dehydrated with a furred tongue, mental confusion and delirium. The patients may then lapse into coma by the fourth week. Complications set in within the third or fourth week. There is a 'doughy' feeling of the abdomen in third or fourth week.

Intestinal complications occur in ~6% of adults and less frequently in children. Complications are gastrointestinal haemorrhage and perforation. Haemorrhage occurs usually in the third week with sudden deterioration, tachycardia, tachypnoea, sweating, fall in blood pressure and anaemia. Acute perforation may occur around the end of the third or fourth week and is accompanied by abrupt onset of abdominal pain, distension, vomiting and collapse. It may sometimes be difficult to distinguish from paralytic ileus. Non-intestinal major pulmonary complications are uncommon. A mild cough with sticky sputum is the earliest symptom. This has been reported up to 85% of patients. Bronchopneumonia secondary to superimposed bacterial infection has been reported in 11% (Tong *et al.* 1972). This figure will probably be less with early diagnosis and treatment. Pure *S. typhi* lobar pneumonia is very rare. Only a few isolated reports are documented where the organism was actually cultured from sputum or from pleural fluid (Tong *et al.* 1972). Meningitis is rare and occurs in < 10% of patients and mainly in neonates. If neck stiffness is present, it is essential to perform a lumbar puncture to exclude typhoid and other forms of meningitis. Often the CSF is clear. Renal complication is uncommon and occurs mainly in children. Acute nephritis results from antigen-antibody immune complexes and very rarely may result in renal failure requiring dialysis. Renal function tests should therefore be done. The patient will be anaemic if there is an intestinal bleed. Thrombocytopenia occurs without accompanying bleeding disorders. Purpura may rarely be a feature. Infective endocarditis with *S. typhi* is very rare but cases of myocarditis have been reported.

Localized abscess formation in the pancreas has occasionally been reported following acute pancreatitis (Gard and Parashar 1992).

Peripheral neuritis, osteomyelitis, typhoid hepatitis, abortion or miscarriage in pregnancy especially in the first trimester, acute cholecystitis and alopecia have been recorded. Persistent infection in the gallbladder leads to chronic cholecystitis.

The most important late complication from the public health point of view is the carrier state due to persistence of infection in the gallbladder. Urinary carriage is very rare except where there has been a pre-existing chronic urinary infection such as from *Schistosoma haematobium*. Hence, it is important to culture the stools on separate occasions until there are six negative consecutive cultures, before patient is pronounced carrier-free.

PATHOLOGY

The infective oral dose of *S. typhi* is between 10^5 and 10^8 organisms in human volunteers. After multiplying in the intestinal lumen, organisms penetrate the mucosa and enter macrophages and disseminate in the lymphatics of the gut and mesentery in the first 2 weeks. There is hyperplasia of the reticuloendothelial and lymphoid tissue in the body. Submucosal lymphoid nodules, especially the Peyer's patches of the terminal ileum enlarge and become sharply demarcated and elevated up to 80 mm in diameter. There is enlargement of mesenteric lymph nodes, liver and spleen. If untreated, there is ulceration overlying the lymphoid tissue resulting in oval ulcers which are only mimicked by Yersinia infection. Tuberculosis gives rise to circumferential or transverse ulcers. The ulcers can heal and lymphatics can regenerate without scarring. Rarely, they perforate and cause death.

There is accumulation of macrophages to form nodular clusters. The macrophages are filled with red cells (erythrophagocytosis) and nuclear debris. Lymphocytes and plasma cells are also seen, but neutrophils, except in the region of ulceration are scanty. The peripheral blood shows a neutropenia.

The spleen is enlarged and soft with obliteration of white pulp and a pale red pulp. Microscopically, there is sinus histiocytosis and proliferation of reticulo-endothelial cells. Rarely, splenic rupture occurs. The liver contains small foci of hepatocyte necrosis and replacement with macrophages produces a 'typhoid nodule'. These nodules are also seen in lymph nodules and bone marrow.

INVESTIGATIONS

1. White cell count – leukopenia is commonly seen.
2. Cultures/identification of *S. typhi* or *paratyphi* is the Gold Standard. Several new laboratory tests are available with a view to a quick diagnosis. A single positive blood culture for the organism with the appropriate clinical picture is diagnostic for typhoid fever. In the early stage of the disease blood and bone marrow cultures are positive in the majority of patients, but negative cultures do not exclude typhoid. *S. typhi* may be cultured from stools or urine. However, at the beginning of the illness, only a small percentage will produce positive results. In the third or fourth week, patients who have not had antibiotics will have more positive cultures. Stool and urine cultures are absolutely essential after successful treatment to exclude a carrier state. Cultures of mononuclear cell-platelet layer of blood combined with separate cultures of bone marrow aspirate and rectal swab will yield a positive rate of detection of ~100% (Rubin *et al.* 1990).
3. The most commonly used serological method, the Widal test, is particularly unreliable with single titres, especially in endemic areas. It is useful if there is a fourfold rise in titres to the 'O' somatic antigen. However, it takes time during the illness to show such a rise that occurs at earliest in the second week and is therefore not useful for early diagnosis. High 'VI' capsular antibody levels is suggestive of a carrier state (Labrooy 1993). Studies done in children in an endemic area in Malaysia concluded that the Widal test in children is a sensitive and specific fever screen for typhoid with a 99.2% negative predictive value. However, the cut off points for 'O' and 'H' titres should be reduced to 1:40 or over and not 1:80 or 1:160 (Choo *et al.* 1993). Rates of positive blood cultures are less in children compared with adults (Chow *et al.* 1989).
4. Specific monoclonal antibody to group D Salmonella antigen 9 can be used in an indirect enzyme-linked immunosorbent assay (ELISA) for detecting antigens in urine. It has been described to have a sensitivity of 95% when serial urines were examined (Chaicumpa *et al.* 1992).

A dot enzyme immunoassay (EIA) that detects serum antibodies to antigen has been used in several microbial diseases and has been applied to typhoid fever (Oprandy *et al.* 1988). It is comparable with the Widal test for serodiagnosis with speed of diagnosis and simplicity (Choo *et al.* 1994).

A polymerase chain reaction (PCR)-based test was developed for rapid detection of *S. typhi* in blood specimens as a more rapid diagnostic method of typhoid fever, particularly in culture-negative cases, in Seoul, Korea (Song *et al.* 1993).

5. Phage typing – VI phage typing is useful when tracing the source of the infection for typhoid and paratyphoid infections.

TREATMENT

Several regimens of antibiotic therapy are available, some better and more expensive than others, but may not be available in developing countries. The drug resistance is high except for ciprofloxacin and ceftriaxone and fluoroquinolines.

Chloramphenicol was the first antibiotic that was used successfully. However, plasmid medicated resistant strains of *S. typhi* have been isolated against chloramphenicol. It is not the best drug today, the cure rate being ~45% (Rabbani *et al.* 1998). Amoxycillin and sulphamethoxazole-trimethoprim – the latter two being alternative forms of therapy that has been rarely used over the past 5 years. Quinolones were promising agents for the treatment of typhoid fever, but animal toxicity data on bone growth has been reported, although its relevance to children is not known. It is not used in children. It can be given PO and is also active against paratyphi infections. It also reaches a concentration of two to three times in bile compared with the drugs mentioned above, it is useful to eliminate the organism in the gallbladder. The side-effects are minimal and transient (Hafiz *et al.* 1998).

Ciprofloxacin is very effective and often first line of treatment in both adults and children. The temperature is normal in 4 days.

Ceftriaxone, a third generation of cephalosporin is safe in children and it also attains a high level in bile (Moosa and Rutlidge 1989). The disadvantage is that it has to be given IM or IV. This expensive drug is the drug of choice in developed countries. Blood dyscrasias such as agranulocytosis have been reported with the use of chloramphenicol.

- Ciprofloxacin – 24 mg/kg/day in two divided doses for 10 days. IV dose is 15 mg/kg/day (Thomsen and Paerregaard 1998)
- Ceftriaxone – 2 g/day in two divided doses for 7–14 days for adults and 75 mg/kg for child maximum 2 g for 7–14 days
- Lomefloxacin – adult dose 200 mg twice a day for 14 days (Hafiz *et al.* 1998)

The use of corticosteroids in severe cases is debatable, although there are some favourable reports.

Treatment of major complications

- Gastrointestinal haemorrhage – resuscitative methods such as Intensive Care monitoring, IVI access fluid infusion and blood transfusion
- Perforation – in cases of intestinal perforation adequate resuscitation with IV fluids, use of a nasogastric tube and laparotomy for closure of perforation seem to reduce the mortality rate (Gibney 1989)
- Carrier state – use of ciprofloxacin has improved elimination of the carrier state to > 75% (Ferrecio *et al.* 1988). Amoxycillin is much less effective than ciprofloxacin in this respect. Surgery has to be considered
- Relapses – occur in 5–20% of patients, especially where the duration of treatment has been short. They occur after ~2 weeks of cessation of treatment. Diagnosis of relapses depends on isolating the organism. The treatment is the same, provided the drug is sensitive to the organism.

PARATYPHOID A, B AND C

Paratyphoid A, B and C may cause a disease resembling typhoid. Of these, paratyphoid B is the commonest. The epidemiology and pathology is similar to typhoid fever. Paratyphoid runs a relatively milder course than typhoid and complications are less frequent. However, it may be fatal if diagnosis is missed. Relapses are less frequent. Treatment is the same as for typhoid fever.

PREVENTION

Properly controlled sewerage disposal and purified water supply, proper care of typhoid patients, detection of carrier state, proper advise to travellers, vaccination of travellers to a certain extent and surveillance of migrants from endemic areas are measures that should be taken to minimize the incidence of typhoid.

Travellers should be warned to drink safe water and consume properly cooked food in endemic areas. Two types of active vaccinations are available. The long-standing killed typhoid vaccines have to be given parentally and the oral live vaccine strain enteric coated Ty 21 (a) taken PO. The dose is one capsule 1 h before food on days 1, 3 and 5 (day 1 = 28 days before journey). The efficiency has varied from 50 to 100%. The vaccine (parenteral) is given according to age, two doses at 4–6 week intervals subcutaneous.

REFERENCES

Chaicumpa W, Rvangkunaporn Y, Burr D *et al.* Diagnosis of typhoid fever by detection of *Salmonella typhi* antigen in urine. *Journal of Clinical Microbiology* 1992; **30**: 2513–2515

Choo KE, Oppenheimer SJ, Ismail AB *et al.* Rapid serodiagnosis of typhoid fever by Dot enzyme immunoassay in an endemic area. *Clinical Infectious Diseases* 1994; **19**: 172–176

Choo KE, Razif AR, Oppenheimer SJ *et al.* Usefulness of the Widal test in diagnosing childhood typhoid fever in endemic areas. *Journal of Paediatric Child Health* 1993; 2936–2939

Chow CB, Wang PS, Leung NK. Typhoid fever in Hong Kong children. *Australian Paediatric Journal* 1989; **25**: 329–349

Fanning WL. Typhim V vaccine. *Journal of Travel Medicine* 1997; **4**: 32–37

Ferrecio C, Morris JG, Benavente L *et al.* Efficacy of ciprofloxacin in the treatment of chronic typhoid carriers. *Journal of Infectious Diseases* 1988; **157**: 1221–1225

Gard P, Parashar S. Pancreatic abscesses due to *Salmonella typhi*. *Postgraduate Medical Journal* 1992; **68**: 294–295

Gibney EJ. Typhoid perforation. *British Journal of Surgery* 1989; **76**: 887–889

Gotuzzo E, Trisancho O, Sanchez J *et al.* Association between acquired immunodeficiency syndrome and infection with *Salmonella typhi* or *Salmonella paratyphi* in endemic typhoid areas. *Annals of Internal Medicine* 1991; **151**: 381–382

Hafiz S, Habib F, Ahmad N. Typhoid fevers: treatment with lomefloxacin. *Journal of the Pakistani Medical Association* 1998; **48**: 168–170

Labrooy JT. Typhoid in 1993. *Medical Journal of Australia* 1993; **159**: 598–601

Moosa A, Rutlidge CJ. Once daily ceftriaxone vs chloramphenicol for treatment of typhoid fever in children. *Paediatric Infectious Diseases Journal* 1989; **8**: 696–699

Oprandy JS, Olsen JG, Scott TW. A rapid dot immunoassay for the detection of serum antibodies to eastern equine encephalomyelitis and St Louis encephalitis virus in sentinel chicken disease. *American Journal of Tropical Medicine and Hygiene* 1988; **38**: 181–186

Rabbani MW, Iqbal I, Malik MS. A comparative study of cefixime and chloramphenical in children with typhoid fever. *Journal of the Pakistani Medical Association* 1998; **48**: 163–164

Rubin FA, McWhirter PD, Burr D *et al.* Rapid diagnosis of typhoid fever through identification of *Salmonella typhi* within 18 h of specimen acquisition by culture of the mononuclear cell-platelet fraction of blood. *Journal of Clinical Microbiology* 1990; **28**: 825–827

Song J, Cholt, Park MY *et al.* Detection of *Salmonella typhi* in the blood of patients with typhoid fever by polymerase chain reaction. *Journal of Clinical Microbiology* 1993; **31**: 1439–1443

Thomsen LL, Paerregaard A. Treatment with ciprofloxacin in children with typhoid fever. *Scandinavian Journal of Infectious Diseases* 1998; **30**: 335–337

Tong MJ, Youel DB, Cotten CL. Acute pneumonia in tropical infections. *American Journal of Tropical Medicine and Hygiene* 1972; **21**: 50–57

Yap YF, Puthucheary SD. Typhoid fever in children – a retrospective study of 54 cases from Malaysia. *Singapore Medical Journal* 1998; **39**: 260–262

43

Melioidosis

Katherine Kociuba MBBS, FRACP, FRCPA

Microbiology
Presentation
Pathology
Investigations

Treatment
Prognosis and Relapse
References

MICROBIOLOGY

Melioidosis is a disease of animals and humans with an infection caused by the soil saprophyte *Burkholderia pseudomallei* (formerly *Pseudomonas pseudomallei*). Melioidosis was first described in morphine addicts in Rangoon, Burma, in 1912 and had variable clinical manifestations (Whitmore and Krishnaswami 1912).

Melioidosis is endemic in South East Asia with most reports from Thailand, Indo-China and Malaysia and Northern Australia (Dance 1991). Other endemic foci occur most commonly between latitudes 20°S and 20°N. However, there are a few temperate foci believed to be caused by importation of infected animals from tropical endemic foci. In areas of north-east Thailand, melioidosis causes 20% of cases of community-acquired septicaemia and it is the most common cause of fatal bacteraemic community-acquired pneumonia in the tropical Northern Territory (NT) of Australia (Anstey *et al.* 1992).

Melioidosis affects many domestic and wild animals, including goats, wild pigs, cows, horses, camels, dogs, wild cats, dolphins, monkeys, crocodiles, koalas, wallabies and seals (Dance 1991). Movement of infected animals is thought to be an important means of introduction of the organism into a new environment with potential establishment of a new endemic focus. This

is believed to be the cause of an outbreak of melioidosis in zoological gardens, equestrian clubs and racecourses in France in the 1970s when numerous animal infections and two fatal human cases occurred (Dance 1991). Soil contamination persisted for years during that outbreak. An outbreak of melioidosis occurred in cynomolgus monkeys imported to the UK from the Philippines in 1992 (Dance *et al.* 1992).

Molecular typing (ribotyping) of 10 isolates in Western Australia collected between 1966 and 1991 from soil, animals and the human cases from this region demonstrated a single ribotype which differed from all others previously isolated in Australia (Currie *et al.* 1994). This theory of introduction of the organism into an environment with long-term persistence.

Burkholderia pseudomallei is a saprophytic organism found in soil and surface water. It can survive dry periods and exists in the clay layer of soil 25–30 cm below the surface. With rain, the organism migrates to the surface. The peak incidence of disease occurs during the rainy season before November and March in the NT in Australia, and June and September in Thailand.

B. pseudomallei is transmitted by direct contact with soil or water, or by inhalation. Clinical cases often have a history of recent penetrating trauma, or exposure to soil and mud. Outdoor occupations or hobbies such as gardening predispose to the infection. In Thailand, the highest incidence of disease occurs among rice field workers. Males are most often affected, probably related to occupational exposure. The incubation period is between 3 and 21 days (mean 14 days). Sexual transmission of infection has been described in a case where a man with *B. pseudomallei* chronic prostatitis transmitted infection to his wife. Sexual transmission is also suggested by the relatively high incidence (37%) of lower genitourinary tract disease in Aboriginals. Laboratory acquired infection has occurred related to generation of infectious aerosols (and possibly skin contact) (Green *et al.* 1986). Nosocomial transmission has been reported and in one case transmission was linked to bronchoscopy (Markovitz 1979).

Subclinical infection occurs most commonly after exposure as indicated by serologic surveys, and disease usually occurs in immunosuppressed individuals. Once exposed, an individual may carry the organism for prolonged periods (i.e. latent infection) and develop clinical disease years later if immunosuppressed. Seroprevalence in children in north-east Thailand rose to a conversion rate of 24%/year from 12% in children aged 1–6 months and to a plateau of ~80% after age 4 years (Kanaphun *et al.* 1993).

B. pseudomallei was, until recently, classified in the genus Pseudomonas and has been assigned to the new genus Burkholderia with six other species of the previous genus Pseudomonas rRNA homology group II (Yabuuchi *et al.* 1992). *B. pseudomallei* and *B. mallei* may be genetically recognized as a single species but remain separate due to phenotypic and clinical differences (*B. mallei* causes glanders, a disease which usually affects horses, less so other animals and occasionally humans).

B. pseudomallei is a small, mobile, aerobic, non-sporulating Gram-negative rod. It may exhibit bipolar staining creating a 'safety pin' appearance. *B. pseudomallei* grows well on routine culture media and may be overlooked, or overgrown by normal commensals or contaminants. When culturing non-sterile sites, e.g. sputum, throat, soil or wound swabs, a selective medium is preferred. In Ashdown's medium (trypicase soy agar with glycerol, crystal violet, neutral red and gentamicin), the organism produces purple colonies that have a characteristic wrinkled appearance at 48–72 h (Ashdown 1979). The presumptive identification of these as *B. pseudomallei* may be made on the basis of negative Gram stain, positive cytochrome oxidase test and distinctive soil-like

odour. Identification of the organism may be confirmed with commercial biochemical identification systems, e.g. API 20E (Biomerieux, France).

PRESENTATION

Melioidosis manifests in various clinical forms ranging from acute septicaemic illness to subacute and chronic presentations. It may be localized or disseminated and there is a tendency for localized suppuration.

Subclinical infection is the most common form and development of clinically apparent infection is associated with underlying immunosuppressive illnesses such as diabetes mellitus, renal disease, alcoholism, pregnancy, malignancy, malnutrition, tuberculosis, splenectomy (Ashdown *et al.* 1980) and human immunodeficiency virus (HIV) infection (Tanphaichitra 1989). The potential exists for outbreaks of melioidosis in those endemic regions with spreading HIV infection, e.g. Thailand.

Acute septicaemic illness due to melioidosis presents as a profoundly ill patient with a short history of fever. The patient may be in septic shock. There may be no clinical evidence of focal infection. Often there are multiple visceral abscesses in lung, liver, spleen or brain. Bacteraemia complicating pneumonia may present in this way with dyspnoea, cough, and sputum production. Patients usually have a high fever, tachypnoea, tachycardia and skin flushing. Muscle tenderness may be present. The liver and spleen may be palpable. Arthritis and meningitis may be present. Skin lesions may occur and vary from erythematous papules to violaceous abscesses. Neutrophil leukocytosis is usually present. Patients are also more likely to be hyponatraemic, hypokalaemic and have renal impairment compared with other forms of community-acquired sepsis. Abnormal liver function may occur as a result of sepsis or focal abscesses in the liver. The case fatality rate of this type of melioidosis is high – ~60–70% (Puthucheary *et al.* 1992).

Pulmonary infection is the most common presentation either as an acute form (with or without dissemination), or a subacute form similar to tuberculosis. Pulmonary infection may occur directly due to inhalation or due to haematogenous dissemination as described above. Patients are usually febrile, and often have dull or pleuritic chest pain, cough, with expectoration and haemoptysis. They may also complain of weight loss, headache, anorexia, myalgia and pharyngitis. Examination of the chest may be unremarkable or reveal focal signs of consolidation. The mortality rate of pulmonary melioidosis was 40% in a series from the NT and 55% for bacteraemic pneumonia.

Localized, suppurative infection may occur in a variety of sites and carries a lower case fatality rate of ~13% in the NT series. Cutaneous, soft tissue or joint infections may occur at sites of traumatic inoculation. Cutaneous infections may manifest in various ways such as infected wounds, cellulitis, pustules, erythematous papules, ulcers, and chronic granuloma with regional lymphadenopathy. These infections may remain localized or disseminate. Suppurative parotitis is a common manifestation of localized melioidosis in children though uncommonly reported in adults (Lumbiganan and Viengnondha 1995). Suppurative lymphadenitis or osteomyelitis (acute or chronic) also occur. Genitourinary melioidosis may present as pyelonephritis, prostatitis, epididymo-orchitis or renal abscess. The symptoms are non-specific abdominal pain, fever, dysuria, urinary frequency or incontinence. Post-traumatic corneal ulceration with local abscess formation that may lead to aggressive ocular infection has been described (Siripanthong et al. 1991). Pyrexia of unknown origin is another pattern of presentation. Infection of blood vessels may cause aneurysms such as the aorta (Steinmetz et al. 1996).

Melioidosis may present as a brain-stem encephalitis (Woods et al. 1992). Other neurological presentation include aseptic meningitis and peripheral motor weakness (Guillain-Barré-like) that may lead to respiratory failure. Focal neurological signs are often elicited such as cranial nerve palsies, cerebellar dysfunction and hemiparesis.

PATHOLOGY

In the rapidly progressive disease, multiple abscesses may be found in any organ especially in lungs, lymph nodes, liver and spleen showing small well defined yellowish foci consisting of neutrophil including histiocytes and fibrin. The lesions can also be granulomatous with stellate abscesses consisting of central necrosis including caseous type necrosis with Langerhan and foreign body giant cells at the periphery. These simulate tuberculosis, ularaemia, cat scratch disease, lymphogranuloma venereum and sporotrichosis. Causative organisms are rarely demonstrated in these lesions in contrast to the acute suppurative lesions.

INVESTIGATIONS

1. Definitive diagnosis of melioidosis is made by isolation of the organism from blood, sputum or from an abscess.
2. Blood cultures are often the most useful test but requires 3–4 days incubation to become positive (Wuthiekanun et al. 1990). Sputum, urine, swabs of skin lesions or any purulent discharge and aspirated pus from any abscess present should be sent for culture. Throat swab should also be taken.
3. Serology is widely used in the diagnosis of melioidosis. The indirect haemagglutination test (IHA) is the most commonly used test world wide and is sensitive for previous exposure. It is of limited value in the diagnosis of active disease in endemic areas (high titres > 1:320 or 1:640 are more useful). IHA antibodies do not cross the placenta and are thought to be of IgM class. Enzyme-linked immunosorbent assay (ELISA) for the detection of specific IgG to B. pseudomallei is more sensitive than the IHA test (Ashdown et al. 1989). Indirect immunofluorescence assay (IFA) for IgG and IgM is also available. The IgM ELISA and IgM IFA correlate with disease activity and are useful for monitoring progression during therapy (Ashdown et al. 1989). IgG and IgM antibody tests are usually positive when signs and symptoms are present. Serology cannot differentiate B. mallei from B. pseudomallei infection. Monoclonal antibody specific for an exopolysaccharide of B. pseudomallei is available (Steinmetz et al. 1996).
   An enzyme immunoassay for the detection of B. pseudomallei antigen in urine has been described (Desakorn et al. 1994). It was most sensitive in urinary and septicaemic melioidosis and false-positive results were associated with bacteriuria.
4. A method for detection of B. pseudomallei has been developed using PCR and in situ hybridization with a ribosomal DNA probe and may be of use in diagnosis in the future (Lew and Desmarchelier 1994).
5. Chest X-ray may show signs of haematogenous pneumonia – bilateral patchy consolidation, nodular opacities or abscesses, pleural effusion or empyema.
6. CT scan of abdomen and brain may show abscess formation and multiple lesions may give a 'Swiss cheese' appearance.

7. Lumbar puncture reveals mononuclear or polymorphs in cerebrospinal fluid (CSF) with an elevated protein and low or normal glucose levels.
8. MRI scans may show cerebral oedema.

TREATMENT

- Treatment of melioidosis involves prolonged antibiotic therapy that must be adjusted according to the antibiotic sensitivity of the isolate. *B. pseudomallei* is resistant to penicillin, ampicillin, erythromycin, gentamicin, tobramycin and quinolones (Ashdown 1988). It is usually sensitive to kanamycin, piperacillin, tetracyclines, chloramphenicol, amoxicillin clavulanate, third generation cephalosporins, imipenem and trimethoprim-sulphamethoxazole.

Traditional therapy used until the mid-1980s employed combinations of chloramphenicol, tetracyclines, kanamycin and trimethoprim-sulphamethoxazole, however, these had no effect on the high mortality rate of the acute septicaemic form of the disease. Ceftazidime therapy has been shown to halve the mortality rate of severe melioidosis when compared with 'traditional' therapy: 37% from 74% overall; and 43% versus 76% for bacteraemic patients (White *et al.* 1989). Antibiotic resistance may develop during therapy and patients should be monitored carefully for the emergence of resistant strains. In Thailand, emergence of chloramphenicol resistance has been described, usually accompanied by cross resistance to tetracycline, doxycycline, ciprofloxacin, trimethoprim and sulphamethoxazole (Dance *et al.* 1988). Ceftazidime resistance has also been described (Dance *et al.* 1991). Quinolones show poor activity against Australian strains of *B. pseudomallei* (Ashdown *et al.* 1992). Amoxicillin-clavulanate is inferior to ceftazidime and not recommended for Australian cases (Ashdown *et al.* 1992, Suputtamongkol *et al.* 1994). Occasional resistance to trimethoprim-sulphamethoxazole occurs in Australian isolates. Initial therapy for severe disease should be given IV. Ceftazidime is the drug of choice that should be used in combination with another antibiotic, e.g. doxycycline, trimethoprim-sulphamethoxazole or chloramphenicol. Imipenem and ceftriaxone are also useful. Intravenous antibiotics are given for several weeks, then oral therapy for a minimum of 12 weeks (Ashdown *et al.* 1992). Doxycycline 200 mg/day or (trimethoprim-sulphamethoxazole) are suitable oral agents.

- Surgical drainage of abscesses is necessary with debridement of soft tissue infections. Splenic abscesses may necessitate splenectomy

PROGNOSIS AND RELAPSE

High mortality rates still occur in severely ill patients despite prompt treatment. Ceftazidime therapy does not affect mortality rate during the first 48 h of treatment (White *et al.* 1989). Relapse of melioidosis is a serious problem and occurred in 15.3% of survivors/year in a series from Thailand (Chaowagul *et al.* 1993). Relapse was associated with a short course of antibiotic therapy for ~8 weeks and much less likely if ceftazidime was used in initial therapy. The mortality rate with relapse is similar to that of primary infections.

REFERENCES

Anstey NM, Currie BJ, Withall KM. Community-acquired Acinetobacter pneumonia in the Northern Territory of Australia. *Clinical Infectious Diseases* 1992; **14**: 83–91

Ashdown LR, Currie BJ. Melioidosis: when in doubt leave the quinolone alone! [Letter]. *Medical Journal of Australia* 1992; **157**: 427–428

Ashdown LR, Duffy VA, Douglas RA. Melioidosis. *Medical Journal of Australia* 1980; **1**: 314–316

Ashdown LR, Johnson RW, Koehler JM *et al.* Enzyme linked immunosorbent assay for the diagnosis of clinical and subclinical melioidosis. *Journal of Infectious Diseases* 1989; **160**: 253–260

Ashdown LR. An improved screening technique for isolation of *Pseudomonas pseudomallei* from clinical specimens. *Pathology* 1979; **11**: 293–297

Ashdown LR. *In vitro* activities of the newer β-lactam and quinolone antimicrobial agents against *Pseudomonas pseudomallei*. *Antimicrobial Agents Chemotherapy* 1988; **32**: 1435-1436

Chaowagul W, Suputtamongkol Y, Dance DAB *et al.* Relapse in melioidosis: incidence and risk factors. *Journal of Infectious Diseases* 1993; **168**: 1181–1185

Currie B, Smith-Vaughan H, Golledge C *et al. Pseudomonas pseudomallei* isolates collected over 25 years from a non-tropical endemic focus show clonality on the basis of ribotyping. *Epidemiology of Infections* 1994; **113**: 307–312

Dance DAB, King C, Aucken H *et al.* An outbreak of melioidosis in imported primates in Britain. *Veterinary Records* 1992; **130**: 525–529

Dance DAB, Wuthiekanun V, Sputtamongkol Y *et al.* Development of resistance to ceftazidime and amoxicillin-clavulanate in *Pseudomonas pseudomallei*. *Journal of Antimicrobial Chemotherapy* 1991; **28**: 321–324

Dance DAB, Wuthiekanun V, White NJ *et al.* Antibiotic resistance in *Pseudomonas pseudomallei* [Letter]. *Lancet* 1988; **i**: 994–995

Dance DAB. Melioidosis: the tip of the iceberg? *Clinical Microbiology Review* 1991; **4**: 52–60

Desakorn V, Smith MD, Wuthiekanun V *et al.* Detection of *Pseudomonas pseudomallei* antigen in urine for the diagnosis of melioidosis. *American Journal of Tropical Medicine and Hygiene* 1994; **51**: 627–633

Green RN, Tuffnell PG. Laboratory acquired melioidosis. *American Journal of Medicine* 1986; **44**: 599–605

Kanaphun P, Thirawattanasuk N, Suputtamongkel Y *et al.* Serology and carriage of *Pseudomonas pseudomallei*: a prospective study in 1000 hospitalized children in north-east Thailand. *Journal of Infectious Diseases* 1993: **167**: 230–233

Lew AE, Desmarchelier PM. Detection of *Pseudomonas pseudomallei* by PCR and hybridisation. *Journal of Clinical Microbiology* 1994; **32**: 1326–1332

Lumbiganan P, Viengnondha S. Clinical manifestations of melioidosis in children. *Paediatric Infectious Diseases Journal* 1995; **14**: 136–140

Markovitz A. Inoculation by bronchoscopy [Letter]. *Western Journal of Medicine* 1979; **131**: 550

Puthucheary SD, Parasakthi N, Lee MK. Septicaemic melioidosis: a review of 50 cases from Malaysia. *Transactions of the Royal Society of Tropical Medicine and Hygiene* 1992; **86**: 683–685

Siripanthong S, Teerapantinrat S, Prugsanusak U *et al.* Corneal ulcer caused by *Pseudomonas pseudomallei*: report of three cases. *Review of Infectious Disease* 1991; **13**: 335–337

Steinmetz I, Stosick P, Hergenthrother D *et al.* Melioidosis causing a mycotic aneurysm. *Lancet* 1996; **347**: 1564–1565

Suputtamongkol Y, Rajchanuwong A, Chaowagul W *et al.* Ceftazidime vs amoxicillin/clavulanate in the treatment of severe melioidosis. *Clinical Infectious Diseases* 1994; **19**: 846–853

Tanphaichitra D. Tropical disease in the immunocompromised host: melioidosis and pythiosis. *Review of Infectious Diseases* 1989; **11**: S1629–1643

White NJ, Chaowagul W, Wuthiekanun U *et al.* Halving of mortality of severe melioidosis by ceftazidime. *Lancet* 1989; **ii**: 697–700

Whitmore A, Krishnawami CS. An account of the discovery of a hitherto undescribed infectious disease occurring among the population of Rangoon. *Indian Gazette* 1912; **47**: 262–267

Woods ML II, Currie BJ, Howard DM *et al.* Neurological melioidosis: seven cases from the Northern Territory of Australia. *Clinical Infectious Diseases* 1992; **15**: 163–169

Wuthiekanun V, Dance DAB, Chaowagul W *et al.* Blood culture techniques for the diagnosis of Melioidosis. *European Journal of Clinical Microbiological Infectious Diseases* 1990; **9**:

Yabuuchi E, Kosako Y, Oyaizu H *et al.* Proposal of *Burkholderia* gen. nov. and transfer of seven species of the genus *Pseudomonas* homology group II to the new genus, with the type species *Burkholderia cepacia*. *Microbiology Immunology* 1992; **36**: 1251–1275

44

Cholera

Microbiology	Treatment
Presentation	Prevention
Investigations	References

MICROBIOLOGY

Cholera is a toxin-mediated gastrointestinal infection caused by *Vibrio cholerae*, usually serogroup 01 or 0139. *V. cholera* exists as part of the normal, free-living bacteria l. flora in estuaries. Non-01 strains are more often isolated from the environment than 01 strains and can persist in the environment in the absence of known human disease and cause sporadic cases. Surveillance of rivers in Queensland, Australia, between 1977 and 1984 repeatedly yielded toxigenic *V. cholerae* 01 El Tor, Inaba from 13 rivers between Brisbane and Townsville. No human or animal reservoirs were identified. The organism can survive and multiply in the riverine environment. Since 1981, *V. cholerae* 01 has also been isolated from the Clarence and Georges River in NSW and one isolate was non-toxigenic Ogawa subtype. Similar sporadic cases occur on the California coast in the USA, often associated with shellfish ingestion.

V. cholerae may enter a viable but non-culturable state that aids its survival. It produces a clitinase, enabling it to bind to the clitin of the shells of crustaceans. It can also colonize copepods and aquatic plants. Other environmental reservoirs must exist as cholera is endemic in arid and inland areas of Africa. Newly described ecological niches include birds and earthworms (Blake 1993).

Humans with acute cholera excrete 10^7–10^8 *V. cholerae*/g stool, with enormous numbers of organisms being produced as the infected may produce 5–10 litres diarrhoeal stool/day. Although environmental persistence may last for years, in many endemic areas inadequate sanitation and recurrent faecal contamination is responsible for the environmental reservoir (Tamplin and Carillo 1991). Patients excrete vibrios for 1–2 weeks post-illness (El Tor 3–20 days; classical biotype 1–7 days) and occasionally for prolonged periods and even years. Asymptomatic carriage occurs commonly in household contacts of cases, usually lasting < 1 week.

Contaminated water seems the principal route of epidemic spread, particularly in developing countries where high levels of faecal contamination of the water supply occur. Food has been implicated in many studies from countries like Peru in South America. Food may be contaminated by handling (by carriers), washing (e.g. vegetables) or cultivation in contaminated waters (e.g. oysters, mussels).

V. cholerae can multiply in some foods, e.g. cooked rice and neutral sauces such as peanut sauce. *V. cholerae* survives refrigeration, although multiplication is retarded. It thrives in an alkaline environment (pH 7.5–8.5) and acidic foods protect against infection, e.g. tomato sauce, the organism being intolerant of acidic conditions.

The risk of *V. cholerae* infection is higher in household contacts of cases and person-to-person spread may occur; however, multiple household cases are more likely when the index case is a food handler suggesting person-food-person spread. The corpse of a cholera victim is contagious and must be handled with appropriate precautions.

The infectious dose is $\sim 10^{11}$ organisms and neutralization of gastric acidity (e.g. antacids; gastric surgery, etc.) reduces this to 10^3–10^6. Food has a similar effect of reducing the infective dose. Most infections are subclinical resulting in asymptomatic carriage. The ratio of cases to carriers is 1:30–100 for El Tor cholera biotype, and 1:2–4 for classical biotype. The duration of carriage is longer for El Tor.

Susceptibility to cholera varies. Those with blood group O are at risk of more severe disease (El Tor, not classical), gastric hypo-acidity increases susceptibility and breast-feeding confers protection. Cases occur most often during the summer months.

In naive populations, cholera attacks all ages, whereas in areas where cholera is endemic, the highest incidence is in children over the ages of 2 years, due to acquisition of immunity with advancing age (see below).

V. cholerae is a facultative anaerobic asporogenous, comma-shaped Gram-negative rod. It is oxidase-positive, and is motile by a single, polar sheathed flagellum. *V. cholerae* growth is enhanced by addition of 1% NaCl; however, it can grow in NaCl-free media.

V. cholerae will grow on Maconkey's agar and also on non-selective agars, e.g. blood agar, however, over-growth of other flora may be a problem. Isolation is enhanced by the use of an enrichment medium such as alkaline peptone water, and thiosulphate citrate bile salt agar (TCBS) is a widely used selective medium to isolate *Vibrio* spp. from faeces. *V. cholerea* ferments sucrose and appears as smooth yellow colonies.

Biochemical identification of *V. cholerea* may be made with conventional tests or commercially available identification systems.

The serotyping of *V. cholerea* is crucial in identification of epidemic strains. All *V. cholerea* share a common H (flagellar) antigen, and are typed according to the (somatic) O antigen. Colonies from non-selective media must be tested against polyvalent sera raised against the 01 antigen commercially available) and also 0139 antiserums

(held by reference laboratories). All human isolates of *V. cholerea* (01 and non-01) should be sent to a reference laboratory for confirmation of identity.

Epidemic cholera is caused by two serogroups of *V. cholerea*: 01 and 0139. Disease-producing strains produce cholera enterotoxin and occasionally non-pathogenic strains that do not produce cholera toxin may be found, particularly from environmental sources. *V. cholerea* 0139 strains also possess a polysaccharide capsule that is likely a virulence factor. *V. cholerae* 01 strains are divided into two biotypes, classical and El Tor, on the basis of a number of criteria such as Voges-Proskauer reaction, bacteriophage susceptibility and polymyxin B susceptibility. The El Tor biotype was responsible for sporadic cases of cholera until its explosion to cause the seventh pandemic. The Voges-Proskauer test is negative for both classical and El Tor. Inhibition by polymyxin B (50-U disk is positive for classical but negative for El Tor). Agglutination for chicken erythrocytes is positive for El Tor. Lysis by classical bacteriophage (305) and FK bacteriophage 451 is positive for classical and negative for El Tor (Kaper *et al*. 1995).

The 01 serogroup is also further subdivided into three serotypes that have minor differences in the O antigen: Inabe, Ogawa and Hikojima (most rare). Other methods for strain differentiation include bacteriophage typing, examination RFLP of the cholera toxin gene or vibosomal RNA and multilocus enzyme electrophoresis. These are reviewed by Kaper *et al*. (1995)

Sporadic cases of gastrointestinal disease may be caused by *V. cholerae* non-01, non-0139, i.e. serogroups 02-0138. The great majority of these strains do not produce cholera enterotoxin (CT) and are not associated with epidemic diarrhoea. Some strains may produce toxins that may cause disease.

Outbreaks of disease due to these strains have been reported and are often related to shellfish consumption. They have also been isolated from other infections/sites such as wounds, sputum, cerebrospinal fluid (CSF) and urine.

The characteristic diarrhoea of cholera is mediated by the cholera enterotoxin (CT). Blood stream invasion by the organism has been rarely documented. Morris *et al*. reported systemic infection caused by non-0:1 *V. cholerae* (Safrin *et al*. 1988). Of 23 previously reported cases of non-0:1 *V. cholerae* bacteraemia, the case fatality rate was 61.5%, and the majority of known cases have occurred in immunocompromised patients, in particular those with cirrhosis and haematological malignancies. The organism is ingested in contaminated water or food, and passes through the stomach (surviving acidity), colonizing and proliferating in the small bowel. The motility of *V. cholerea* is an important virulence mechanism, enabling it to travel to the mucosal surface and may aid in cellular adhesion. Polysaccharide capsule production, which occurs in 0139 strains, and other non-01 strains may facilitate septicaemia by enabling evasion of host defences. A number of colonization factors have been described which allow adherence to small intestinal cells. The TCP pilus colonization factor has been shown to be important in human disease. Other pili and haemagglutinins may also be important adherence factors.

Cholera toxin binds to the GM_1 ganglioside on the small intestinal epithelial cells and results in activation of adenylate cyclase and increase of intracellular cAMP. This results in increased chloride secretion by intestinal crypt cells and decreased NaCl-coupled absorption by villous cells. The transepithelial osmotic gradient produced causes water flow into the gut lumen. The large volume of water passing through the gut overwhelms absorptic sites in the colon. CT binds tightly and exerts its effect for many hours. CT is thought to also cause increased intestinal motility and release of vasoactive intestinal peptide (VIP) resulting in further secretory diarrhoea. Additional toxins including Zot, Ace, haemolysis/cytolegsin, etc., which may contribute to the disease have also been described.

Immunity after infection is serotype specific. After infection with the classic biotype, near complete immunity to reinfection occurs, lasting at least 3 years (Clemens 1993). El Tor infection, however, does not induce significant immunity. Infection with the 01 serotype does not confer any protection against 0139 serotype infection.

PRESENTATION

The incubation period of *C. vibrio* varies from a few hours to 5 days. The spectrum of infection varies from asymptomatic carriage to severe, rapidly dehydrating diarrhoeal illness that may cause death in 2–3 h without treatment (cholera gravis). Asymptomatic or mild cholera infection is usual, and severe disease uncommon. El Tor infection is less severe than classical *V. cholerea*, rarely causing severe infection. Patients may experience initial anorexia, abdominal discomfort, gurgling bowel sounds and simple diarrhoea. After several motions are passed, the stool becomes pale grey with flecks of mucus and a slightly fishy smell. This is the characteristic 'rice water' stool. Patients may present with abrupt onset of profuse watery diarrhoea progressing from the first liquid stool to shock in 4–12 h, in untreated cases causing death between 18 h and several days. Vomiting often occurs in early disease, starting soon after the diarrhoea. In severe cases, faecal losses may reach 500–1000 ml/h and cause rapid dehydration, coupled with losses of large quantities of electrolytes.

The patients develop signs of hypovolaemia with tachycardia, hypotension, reduced skin turgor, sunken eyes and weak pulses. Most patients remain well orientated despite the severe illness and are restless and thirsty. Hypokalaemia may cause muscle cramps, ileus, muscle weakness and cardiac arrhythmia. Hypoglycaemia occurs, and may be asymptomatic or, particularly in children, cause obtundation and seizures. Patients are generally afebrile, but may have a low-grade fever. Oliguria progressing to renal failure develops if the dehydration is not corrected. Case fatality rates vary, often reflecting local access to appropriate health services. Worldwide the case fatality rate of cholera has fallen during the seventh pandemic from 49.3% in 1961 to 4.8% in 1981 and to 1.8% in 1993 (WHO 1993). Death of a patient from cholera represents a failure of healthcare.

INVESTIGATIONS

1. Definite diagnosis of cholera is made by isolation of *V. cholerae* from infected stool (it is rarely isolated from blood). It is usually present in stool in high numbers (10^7 up to 10^8/ml faeces). Darting vibrios may be seen by direct stool microscopy (dark field or phase contrast).

2. In non-epidemic areas, the isolate must be screened against 01 and 0139 antisera and for production of CT, as these epidemic strains are of public health importance.

3. *V. cholerae* 01 may be detected directly in clinical specimens by various methods. Inhibition of mobility by a specific 01 antibody (sensitivity ~50%, better in cases with higher numbers of organisms); or

a fluorescent labelled 01 monoclonal antibody test can be employed. Commercially available rapid co-agglutination and colovimetric immunoassay tests that use monoclonal antibody against 01 antigen have good sensitivity when used directly on stool specimens. PCR/DNA probe may also detect *V. cholerea* 01 directly in clinical samples. All isolates should be tested for antibiotic susceptibility as increasing resistance is a problem.

4. Detection of cholera toxin is performed in reference centres. Traditional cell culture systems (Chinese hamster ovary or Y-1 adrenal cells) may be used. ELISA test (Ramamurthy *et al.* 1992) and latex agglutination tests for the detection of CT are also available, the latter diagnostic test being less complicated and less time-consuming with specificity and sensitivity of 1.00 and 0.97 respectively (Almeida *et al.* 1990).

5. DNA probes may be used to detect the genes coding for CT. Amplification of the CT gene by PCR has been used successfully in combination with a CT DNA probe. PCR/DNA probes have been used on culture isolates and also directly on stool and food samples.

6. Investigations reveal the effects of dehydration and electrolyte loss with elevation of serum creatinine, serum urea, haematocrit and plasma protein level. Severe acidosis may occur due to stool bicarbonate losses and lactic acidosis, with a depressed blood pH and an increased anion gap. Serum Na^+ and Cl^- usually remain in normal range, although total body NaCl is reduced. Hypokalaemia may occur or the acidosis may result in normal or high potassium levels despite high intracellular losses. Hypoglycaemia may be present.

TREATMENT

- The most essential component of treatment of cholera is to replace losses of fluid and electrolytes by IV solutions or oral rehydration solutions (ORS). In serious cases, rapid IV volume replacement is required early (in adults initially 1 litre/15 min; children 30 ml/kg in the first hour) and when volume losses have been replaced, fluid input is adjusted to the stool losses and level of hydration. Monitor electrolyte level and renal function. The WHO recommends Ringer's lactate as the best commercial IV solution. However, it

needs additional potassium (10 mg/litre). Ringer lactate solution contains 130 mmol Na, 4 mmol K and 109 units Cl^-, and 28 mmol of base, with no glucose. The cholera stool of a child has 105 mmol Na, 25 mmol K, 90 mmol Cl^- and 30 mmol of base; and cholera stool of an adult contains 135 mmol Na, 15 mmol K, 100 mmol Cl^- and 45 mmol of base, when the rate of stool for both child and adult is 50 ml/kg/24 h (Kaper *et al.* 1995).

Normal saline may be used with addition of potassium, bicarbonate and glucose. ORS should be given as soon as possible, and mild-to-moderate cases may be treated by ORS alone. The WHO recommends ORS 50 ml/kg for the first 4 h in mild disease and 100 ml/kg in moderate disease. Stool volume must be closely monitored, and ongoing losses replaced (after initial rehydration) with ORS at a ratio of 1.5:1 for adults (ORS: stool) and 1:1 for children. The upper limit of replacement with ORS for adults is 750 mg/h, i.e. 12 litres/day diarrhoea. IV treatment becomes necessary at this level. The ORS used should be a WHO recommended one. The WHO oral rehydration solution consists of NaCl 2.5 g, $NaHCO_3$ 3.5 g, KCl 1.5 g, glucose 20.0 g dissolved in 1 litre clean drinking water.

- Antibiotics shorten the duration of diarrhoea and reduce the volume of fluid replacement needed. They reduce the duration of bacterial shedding and the potential for contamination of the environment. Appropriate antibiotic therapy must be guided by antibiotic susceptibility results and local resistance patterns. WHO guidelines recommend doxycycline (or tetracycline) for adults and cotrimoxazole for children. Alternatives are furazolidone, erythromycin and chloramphenicol. Treatment should be continued for 3–5 days. *V. cholerae* 0139 is resistant to trimethoprim-sulphamethoxazole but as yet sensitive to tetracycline (WHO 1994). The Rwandan strain is resistant to doxycycline, cotrimoxazole, chloramphenicol and ampicillin (WHO 1994). Tetracycline resistance has been reported also in East Africa, Bangladesh (Albert *et al.* 1993) and parts of India (Takeda *et al.* 1992). Tetracycline prophylaxis may provide protection to close contacts; however, widespread use has been associated with development of resistance and is best avoided.

- Infection control – universal precautions should be practised. Patients should be isolated in a single room. All stool and vomitus should be appropriately sterilized before disposal to prevent possible environmental contamination.

PREVENTION

On a global scale, improvement in sanitation and provision of a clean water supply is needed. For an individual traveller in endemic areas, it is most important that only bottled water is drunk. It is best to avoid uncooked foods that may have been washed in contaminated water. Raw or undercooked shellfish should be avoided, particularly by persons with underlying predispositions, i.e. achlorhydria. (This also applies to achlorhydric patients who have increased risk of other vibrio infections.)

Parenteral vaccines are no longer recommended as they are not very efficacious (~50% protection for 3–6 months) and also cause side-effects producing tenderness and induration at injection sites and, less commonly, fever and malaise. In Australia, a CSL cholera vaccine is available (heat killed V. cholerea 01). Cholera vaccine is not effective against V. cholerea 0139.

Total vaccines consisting of inactivated vibrio with or without B subunit of cholera toxin conferred ~50% protection against cholera for 3 years in Bangladesh (Clemens 1990). Their efficacy is lower in children < 6 years of age and those individuals with blood group O (Levine and Kaper 1993).

Live attenuated cholera vaccines and recombinant live oral vaccines have had some success, however they often have failed to achieve sufficient protection and early vaccines often caused unacceptable rates of gastrointestinal illness. V. cholerea CVD 103-HgR is a live attenuated cholera vaccine that has been shown to provide 82–100% protection against challenge with the classical biotype of V. cholerea 01, and 62–67% after challenge with El Tor. The onset of protection is rapid (8 days) and duration of protection is at least 6 months.

Travellers should not rely on vaccine for protection and must be careful to avoid exposure. At present vaccines are not recommended for use in control of epidemics due to the short duration of protection and limited efficacy. Current vaccines are not effective against V. cholerea 0139, although development of 01/0139 vaccines is underway.

REFERENCES

Albert MJ, Siddique AK, Islam MS et al. Large outbreak of clinical cholera due to *Vibrio cholerae* non-0.1 in Bangladesh. *Lancet* 1993; **341**: 704

Almeida RJ, Hickman-Brenner FW, Sowers EG et al. Comparison of a latex agglutination assay and an enzyme-linked immunosorbent assay for detecting cholera toxin. *Journal of Clinical Microbiology* 1990; **28**: 128–130

Blake PA. Epidemiology of cholera in the Americas. *Gastroenterology Clinic of North America* 1993; **22**: 639–660

Clemens JD, Sack DA, Harris JR et al. Field trial of oral vaccines in Bangladesh. Results from three years follow-up. *Lancet* 1990; **335**: 270–273

Clemens JD, Van Loon F, Sack DA et al. Biotypes as determinant of natural immunizing effect of cholera. *Lancet* 1993; **337**: 883–884

Kaper JB, Morris JG, Levine MM. Differentiation of classical and El Tor biotypes of *V. cholerae* .01[20]. *Clinical Microbiological Review* 1995; **8**: 48–54

Kaper JB, Morris JG, Myson ML. Cholera. *Clinical Microbiology Review* 1995; **8**: 67

Levine MM, Kaper JB. Live oral vaccines against cholera: an update. *Vaccine* 1993; **11**: 207–212

Ramamurthy TS, Battacharya SK, Vesaka Y et al. Evaluation of the bead enzyme-linked immunosorbent assay for detection of cholera toxin directly from stool specimens. *Journal of Clinical Microbiology* 1992; **30**: 1703–1704

Safrin S, Morris G Jr, Adams M et al. Non-0.1 *Vibrio cholerae* bacteremia: case report and review. *Review of Infectious Disease* 1988; **10**: 1012–1017

Takeda Y, Taked T, Pal SC et al. Serovar biotype phage type toxigenicity and antibiotic susceptibility pattern of *Vibrio cholerae* isolated during two consecutive cholera seasons 1989–90 in Calcutta, India. *Journal of Medical Research Section A* 1992; **95**: 125–129

Tamplin ML, Carillo C. Environmental spread of *Vibrio cholerae* in Peru. *Lancet* 1991; **338**: 1216–1217

World Health Organisation. *Cholera in 1993, Part 1: Weekly Epidemiological Record*. Geneva: World Health Organisation, 1994; **69**: 205–212

World Health Organisation. *Cholera Outbreak among Rwandan Refugees. Weekly Epidemiological Records*. Geneva: World Health Organisation, 1994; **69**: 221

Plague

MICROBIOLOGY

It is 106 years to 2000 since the plague bacillus was identified and isolated by Drs Alexandre Yersin and Kitasato. It is an infectious fever caused by bacillus *Yersinia pestis* transmitted by rat fleas. It was referred to as the 'Black Death' in the 14th century. The cycle of spread of plague 'rodent-flea-rodent' is generally enzootic, but under certain environmental conditions it can reach epizootic proportions. The great plague epidemics in London in the 17th century killed more than 70 000 people, nearly one-seventh of the total London population at that time. The alleged epidemic of plague in India in 1994 occurred only among people living in a few, clearly demarcated slums, prompting the Editorial in *The Lancet* in 1994 to comment that 'it is a disease of the poorest of the poor'. However, it was not plague. Plague is endemic in certain parts of India. It is a sporadic disease in many tropical and subtropical countries. In Africa, it has been reported in Tanzania, Malawi, Mozambique, Botswana, Kenya, Zimbabwe and Uganda. Sporadic cases have also been seen in south-western USA, Vietnam, Thailand, Myanmar, South America, Southern China, Mongolia and South East former Soviet Union. Rodents are the natural hosts. The domestic rat, *Rattus rattus*, and

Mastomys natalensis are the commonest rodent species (Kilonzo *et al.* 1992). Domestic dogs can also play a part as plague carriers in some areas as in Tanzania (Kilonzo *et al.* 1993).

Sylvatic plague is caused by > 200 species of wild rodents and is found in Africa, India, Vietnam, Russia and some parts of the USA. There are several species of flea ectoparasites found on the rodents that transmit the disease such as *Xenopsylla cheopis*, *X. brasiliensis* and *Dinopsyllus lypusus* (*The Lancet* 1994).

In the USA, from 1970 to 1991, ground squirrels were the carriers of fleas for transmission of infection and domestic cats played a prominent role in transmission of diseases to humans. Plague existing as an enzootic in wild rodents can be accidentally transmitted to the semi-domesticated brown rat Norwegicus. When the latter dies, the fleas migrate and infect the domestic rat *Rattus rattus*. When the domestic rat dies, the fleas feed on man, causing plague. Sporadic cases generally occur in this manner. The spread of the organism is brought about by blockage of the proventriculus of the flea as a result of multiplication of the bacteria *Y. pestis*. This produces difficulty in ingesting blood from the host, whereby the flea becomes hungry and tries repeatedly to feed, resulting in regurgitation of blood and bacteria to the host. The plague bacilli may also be passed in faeces and can penetrate the skin with rubbing or if the skin is abraded. The rat flea that is not infected lives for 1–2 years. Infected fleas that are not blocked survive for ~2–3 weeks and can continue to transmit the disease. Blocked fleas survive for < 1–2 days.

Person-to-person transmission within ~2 m can take place by respiratory droplets through coughing. It is generally reported that high secondary transmission rates occur where there is poverty and overcrowding. In the USA, person-to-person spread has not been reported since 1925 (Craven 1994). Sporadic cases of human plague occur annually in New Mexico, Arizona and Colorado (Kilonzo et al. 1993) in rural and suburban regions, rarely brought about by droplet transmission from domestic cats with pneumonic plague.

Sylvatic or wild plague is found in rural areas. Plague can occur in those whose work brings them into contact with the reservoir animals. The enzootic in these regions continues from rodent to rodent and man gets infected by handling wild animals and being bitten by their fleas. Surveillance of plague among rodents can be measured by their flea index and their plague antibodies (Kilonzo et al. 1992).

Indiscriminate killing of rodents to minimize destruction of food crops will result in their ectoparasites, the flea, seeking alternative hosts, including man (Kilonzo et al. 1994). Droplet infection occurs where patients with highly contagious pneumonic plague spread the disease from person to person by exhaled droplets and sputum.

Y. pestis is a small, non-mobile Gram-negative rod with bipolar staining. It produces endotoxins causing Gram-negative endotoxin shock. The organism grows well on most media including on non-selective media, in blood culture systems and on MacConkey agar (although some strains may be only pinpoint in size on MacConkey agar at 24 h). Optimal growth occurs aerobically from 25 to 32°C. Y. pestis does not ferment lactose, is indole-negative and does not utilize citrate. Urea hydrolysis is variable. On Kligless Iron agar it produces an alkaline slant and acid bitt.

PRESENTATION

The three distinct forms of plague are bubonic, primary septicaemic and primary pneumonic. Plague is a

treatable disease and responds to antibiotics if diagnosed early. In the initial stages it may present as a non-specific, febrile illness, with symptoms of gastrointestinal or urinary tract infection. It can also present as meningitis (Crook et al. 1992).

Bubonic plague

This is the most common type, sometimes presenting with septicaemia. In the USA, out of a total number of 295 cases of human plague from 1970 to 1991, 89% presented as bubonic or septicaemic plague (Craven et al. 1993). The incubation period is 2–4 days. The illness is acute in onset with chills, rigors, headache and rapid pulse. There is bilateral inguinal lymphadenopathy if the patient is bitten in the lower extremity. Lymphadenopathy can be generalized with the buboes varying in size from 1 to 10 cm. Gastrointestinal symptoms are abdominal pain, bloody diarrhoea with nausea and vomiting. Disseminated intravascular coagulation occurs in ~10% of patients with gangrene and ecchymosis of the skin, fingers and toes. The disease was called the 'Black Death' due to the massive ecchymosis of the skin. If untreated, the disease is complicated by sepsis with hypotension and death within 1 week. In a minor form of bubonic plague with minimal toxaemia and small buboes, the patient may remain ambulatory. Most of these patients who have a minor illness recover fully.

Presentation with painful lymphadenopathy and fever can be confused with syphilis, lymphogranuloma venereum, acute streptococcal, staphylococcal lymphadenitis, cat scratch disease or tularaemia.

Primary septicaemic plague

The flea may introduce the bacilli directly into the blood stream. Most septicaemic plague is secondary to pneumonic or bubonic plague. The clinical presentation in primary septicaemic plague is fever with chills and rigors and sudden in onset. Septicaemic plague may cause endotoxin shock and intravascular coagulation without localized signs of infection (Campbell and Hughes 1995). Meningitis is common. Septicaemic disease is rapidly progressive, resulting in coma and death within 48 h if untreated. Plague meningitis cannot be distinguished from other forms of bacterial meningitis clinically. Meningitis may be a late presentation in patients treated with antibiotics that do not cross the blood–brain barrier.

Sepsis due to *Capnocytophage canimorsus*, a Gram-negative bacterium, has been mistaken for plague. This has been highlighted by the US Center for Disease Control, Atlanta, GA, in their reports (*MMWR* 1993). Sepsis without lymphadenopathy may be mistaken for typhoid. Patients presenting with bloody diarrhoea associated with abdominal pain can be mistaken for dysentery or acute non-infective colitis.

Primary pneumonic plague

Primary pneumonic plague is contracted by inhalation of airborne bacilli from patients with pneumonic plague or from cadavers or carcasses of animals. Plague pneumonia could be secondary to primary bubonic plague, with or without septicaemia. The incubation period in primary pneumonic plague is 24–48 h. The presentation is that of sudden onset of fever with chills and rigors, severe cough and shortness of breath. The sputum is blood stained. Eventually the multilobar involvement leads to respiratory failure. Acute respiratory distress syndrome often complicates pneumonic plague, or may be secondary to plague sepsis. The sputum would be teeming with plague bacilli in pneumonic plague and absent in pure acute respiratory distress syndrome (ARDS) uncomplicated by pneumonia. Auscultation would reveal signs of consolidation with rhonchi and rales. X-ray appearance varies from infiltrates, bronchopneumonic shadows or consolidation. The mortality rate is very high in untreated cases.

Pneumonia has to be differentiated from other bacterial pneumonias, melioidosis and meningitis from other forms of bacterial meningitis.

PATHOLOGY

Infected fleas introduce bacteria through their bites, which migrate to the lymph nodes. Cutaneous lesions are seldom seen at the site of the bite. In the lymph glands the bacteria are taken by up mononuclear cells. The bacteria multiply in the mononuclear cells as they are not killed. The bacteria also multiply intracellularly and develop a capsular envelope. The bacteria produce toxins. This envelope makes the bacillus resistant to phagocytosis by the polymorphonuclear leukocytes. The toxins cause haemorrhagic necrosis of the lymph nodes and also lysis of the macrophages, causing further liberation of bacilli. The lymph nodes are swollen and there is loss of the architecture with necrosis of cells. The associated effusion and haemorrhage makes the lymph node boggy and fluctuant. The organisms spread along lymphatics to other lymph glands. There are petechiae or ecchymosis of the skin due to vascular necrosis by toxins or disseminated intravascular coagulation. The spleen is enlarged with haemorrhagic necrosis. Similar changes are found in the liver. Fibrin casts are found in the glomeruli and the heart is dilated and shows evidence of myocarditis.

Primary pneumonic plague produces a lobular pneumonia with bacilli and exudate in the alveoli. Subsequently there is necrosis of the alveoli and haemorrhage. The changes spread and confluence of the lobular changes produces consolidation. The lungs appear black with large areas of necrosis. There are very few polymorphonuclear cells in the alveoli compared with the number of plague bacilli. In secondary pneumonic plague, the lesions are diffuse in both lungs and the bacilli are found in the interstitial tissue.

Dead rodents should be examined during human infection. They demonstrate enlarged, friable spleens with haemorrhage and organisms can be demonstrated on microscopy. Similar changes are also seen in the liver and adrenal glands.

INVESTIGATIONS

1. Identifying the bacteria makes the positive diagnosis. *Y. pestis* is identified from the following specimens: aspirates of a bubo, sputum, blood, pleural fluid and cerebrospinal fluid (CSF). The techniques available to demonstrate the bacilli are staining with Giemsa stain and cultures of the fluids. CSF will demonstrate polymorphonuclear pleocytosis, an elevated protein, low sugar and Gram-negative coccobacilli.

2. Serology tests for antibodies are passive haemagglutination and passive haemagglutination inhibition tests, indirect immunofluorescent antibody test and complement fixation tests.

   Other modern tests available are the enzyme linked immunosorbent assay (ELISA) and the dot enzyme-immunosorbent assay (Dot-ELISA) to detect IgG antibodies against fraction 1 (F1) antigen of *Y. pestis* (Centers for Disease Control and Prevention 1997). Results from Brazil suggest that Dot-ELISA is a simple and more sensitive test compared with conventional ELISA and haemagglutination tests (De Almeida and Ferreira 1992). The direct immunofluorescence test for rapid presumptive identification of *Y. pestis* F1 antigen to appropriate clinical material, blood films, lymph node isolates are culture isolates.

3. A new method for plague surveillance using polymerase chain reaction to detect *P. pestis* in fleas is by using primers designed from *Y. pestis* plasminogen activator gene. As few as ten *Y. pestis* cells were detected even in the presence of flea tissue (Hinnebusch and Schwan 1995). It gives a rapid and sensitive way to monitor plague in wild animals. Rapid molecular detection techniques based on 16S and 23S rNNA sequence data to identify and differentiate *Yersinia* species from clinical and environmental sources are available (Karlheinz *et al.* 1998).

4. Other ancillary investigations includes white cell count which is generally high > 40 000–100 000 due to increase in polymorphonuclear leucocytes. Occasionally a leukemoid reaction and a low platelet count are seen. The liver enzymes are raised. Coagulation studies for presence of intravascular coagulation. Chest X-ray in pneumonic plague, changes vary from infiltrates to consolidation. In acute cor pulmonale, secondary to pneumonic plague, electrocardiogram shows tall P waves right-axis deviation and arrhythmia, due to myocarditis. In pneumonic plague, blood gases must be regularly monitored. If ARDS is suspected a Swan Gans catheter is used to measure the pulmonary artery wedge pressure and electrolytes.

TREATMENT

- All suspected cases of plague should be isolated and treated in an intensive care setting. The drug of choice for treatment of plague is streptomycin. The management guidelines in Table 45.1 issued by the US Center for Disease Control is recommended. Blood should be collected during a 45-min period before initiation of treatment unless delay is contraindicated. Pencillins and cephalosporins are not effective.

PROPHYLAXIS

Prophylaxis is indicated for medical staff treating patients and for those in close contact. Prophylaxis should be for the duration of the potential exposure and continued for an additional 5–7 days (Campbell and Hughes 1995). Travellers to plague endemic countries are at low risk and therefore prophylaxis is not indicated. Prophylaxis guidelines recommended by Center for Disease Control is outlined in Table 45.2. Chloramphenicol is also effective as a prophylactic drug (Butler 1995).

PREVENTION

The sporadic cases from sylvatic infection of rodents are uncommon and eradication is difficult. In countries like Australia there is no urban or sylvatic source of infection. Measures should be taken when surveillance indicates a probable epidemic. Diminishing rat counts is a good predictive index. Standard epidemiologic techniques should be applied. The magnitude of the problem in urban and semi-urban areas should be assessed. Suspected cases should be under surveillance and prompt action taken to establish a laboratory diagnosis on culture isolation of *Y. pestis* by methods that have been described. Efforts should be intensified to clear up the rat-infested environment at the foci of infection as a priority public health measure. Unlike most other highly infectious diseases, occurrence of plague makes people panic quite out of proportion, both locally and internationally as demonstrated in India in 1994, which was subsequently found not to be plague (Deodhar *et al.* 1998). With effective antibiotics to prevent and treat plague, draconian measures in response to reports of plague are not necessary (Campbell and Hughes 1995). What is essential is a multidisciplinary approach as early as possible which should include clinicians, microbiologists, public health workers, entomologists and mammologists to bring the epidemic under control. Education of workers in rural and semi-urban areas where plague can occur is also necessary. Following the establishment of a control programme, plague cases were reduced from 1092 to zero within 3 years; deaths from 45 to zero in 2 years; and fatality rate from 4.12 to 0% in 3 years in Namibia (Shangula 1998).

REFERENCES

Butler T. *Yersinia* species (including plague). In Mandell GL, Douglas RG, Bennett JE (eds), *Principles and Practice of Infectious Diseases*. New York: Churchill Livingstone, 1995, 2070–2078

Table 45.1 – Treatment of pneumonic, septicaemic and bubonic plague

Drug	Adult dose	Children's dose	Duration of treatment (days)
• Streptomycin	2 g in two equal doses at 12 hourly IMI	30 mg/kg/day in two or three equal doses; 12 or 8 hourly IMI	10
Alternate drugs			
• Gentamicin	3 mg/kg/day in three equal doses 8 hourly IMI or IVI maximum dose 5 mg/kg/day in three equal doses 8 hourly IMI or IVI	6–7.5 mg/kg/day in three equal doses 8 hourly IVI or IMI (not to exceed adult dose)	10
• Oxytetracycline	300 mg/day in two or three doses at 12 or 8 hourly IMI until oral medication is tolerated	Over 9 years 15–25 mg dosage may be divided into two or three equal doses at 12 or 8 hourly IMI until oral medication is tolerated	10
• Tetracycline	2 g/day PO in four equal doses at 6 hourly interval	Over 9 years 25–50 mg/kg/day in four equal doses (not to exceed adult dose)	10
• Chloramphenicol (treatment of choice for plague meningitis)	Loading dose 25 mg/kg IVI subsequently 50 mg/kg/day IVI in four equal doses 6 hourly until oral medication is tolerated	Older children same as adults. Children < 1 year, refer to paediatrician	10

Table 45.2 – Prophylaxis for plague

Drug	Adult dose	Children's dose	Duration of treatment (days)
• Tetracycline	2 g/day in four equal doses 6 hourly orally	Over 9 years 25–50 g/kg/day in four equal doses 6 hourly. Maximum adult dose	7
• Doxycycline	200 mg/day in two equal doses 12 hourly orally	Over 9 years 0.5–1 mg/kg/day in two equal doses at 12 hourly intervals orally. Maximum adult dose	7
• Trimethoprim and general dose (adults and children) sulphamethoxazole	40 mg/kg sulphamethoxazole in two equal doses at 12 hourly intervals		7

Tetracyclines **not** indicated for children < 9 years of age.

Campbell GL, Hughes JM. Plague in India: a new warning from an old nemesis. *Annals of Internal Medicine* 1995; **122**: 151–153

Capnocytophage canimorsus sepsis misdiagnosed as plague – New Mexico 1992. *Morbidity and Mortality Weekly Report* 1993; **42**: 72–73

Centers for Disease Control and Prevention. Fatal human plague – Arizona and Colorado 1996. *Journal of American Medical Association* 1997: **278**: 380–382

Craven RB, Maupin GO, Beard ML *et al.* Reported cases of human plague infection in the United States 1970–1991. *Journal of Medical Entomology* 1993; **30**: 758–761

Craven RB. Plague. In Hoeprich PD, Jordan MC, Ronald AR (eds), *Infectious Diseases: A Treatise of Infectious Processes*, 5th edn. Philadelphia: JB Lippincott, 1994, 1302–1312

Crook LD, Tempest B. Plague. A clinical review of 27 cases. *Archives of Internal Medicine* 1992; **152**: 1253–1256

De Almeida AM, Ferreira LC. Evaluation of three serological tests for the detection of human plague in North East Brazil. *Memorias de Instituto Oswaldo Cruz* 1992; **87**: 87–92

Deodhar NS, Yemul VL, Banerjee K. Plague that never was: a review of the alleged plague outbreaks in India in 1994. *Journal of Public Health Policy* 1998; **19**: 184–199

Editorial. Plague in India: time to forget the symptoms and tackle the disease. *Lancet* 1994; **344**: 1033–1035

Hinnebusch J, Schwan TG. New method for plague surveillance using polymerase chain reaction to detect *Yersinia pestis* in fleas. *Journal of Clinical Microbiology* 1995; **31**: 1511–1514

Karlheinz T, Dga H, Alexander R *et al.* Development of rRNA – targeted PCR and *in situ* hybridization with fluorescently labelled oligonucleotides for detection of *Yersima* species. *Journal of Clinical Microbiology* 1998: **36**: 2557–2564

Kilonzo BS, Gisakanyi ND, Sabuni CA. Involvement of dogs in plague epidemiology in Tanzania. Serological observations in domestic animals in Lushoto district. *Scandinavian Journal of Infectious Diseases* 1993; **24**: 503–506

Kilonzo BS, Makundi RB, Mbize TJ. A decade of plague epidemiology and control in the western Usambara Mountains, North-East Tanzania. *Acta Tropica* 1992; **50**: 323–329

Kilonzo BS, Mbize TJ, Makundi RH. Plague in Lushoto district. Tanzania 1980–1988. *Transactions of the Royal Society of Tropical Medicine and Hygiene* 1992; **86**: 444–445

Kilonzo BS. Importance of intersectoral coordination in the control of communicable disease with special references to plague in Tanzania. *Central African Journal of Medicine* 1994; **40**: 186–192

Shangula K. Successful plague control in Namibia. *South African Medical Journal* 1998; **88**: 1428–1430

Tancik CA, Palmer DL. Plague; bubonic plague. The Black Death. In Conn RB (ed.), *Current Diagnosis*. Philadelphia: WB Saunders, 1991, 181–183

46

Donovanosis (Granuloma inguinale)

Katherine Kociuba MBBS, FRACP, FRCPA

Microbiology
Presentation
Investigations

Treatment
References

MICROBIOLOGY

Donovanosis is a chronic, granulomatous infection caused by *Calymmatobacterium granulomatis*, which usually causes genital ulcerative disease. It is also known as granuloma inguinale, granuloma venereum, granuloma tropicum, granuloma pudendi tropicum, granuloma contagiosa, ulcerating granuloma, sclerosing granuloma and chronic venereal sores. *C. granulomatis* is a Gram-negative bacterium measuring ~1.5 × 0.7 μm, which possesses a thick capsule and is suggested to be related to the genus Klebsiella. *C. granulomatis* is difficult to grow *in vitro* (culture in chick embryo yolk sac and egg based media, cyclohexamide-treated Hep-2 cell monolayers in RPM1 1640 medium has been reported) (Carter *et al.* 1997).

Donovanosis occurs in tropical and subtropical regions including India, Papua New Guinea, (northern and central) Australia, Central America and Africa. Donovanosis is generally reported in Australia from the Northern Territory (NT), North Queensland and the tropical north-west and dry and eastern parts of Western Australia. It is endemic among the Aborigines.

Donovanosis is transmitted by close, often sexual contact and is contagious. Repeated exposures are thought to be needed to transmit infection, and minor trauma at the site of inoculation probably facilitates transmission. Donovanosis may be associated with other sexually transmitted infections such as syphilis and gonorrhoea and may facilitate transmission of HIV infection (Sanders 1998). Poor nutrition, liver disease, ethanol abuse and immunocompromised states may also be predisposing factors. The incubation period is 4 weeks to months.

Molecular methods using polymerase chain reaction (PCR) for diagnosis are currently being developed. Most descriptions focus on the morphologic appearances of the agent, also called Donovan bodies. The organisms are found within the phagosomes of macrophages or histiocytes and rarely in polymorphs. These enlarged infected mononuclear cells are the pathognomonic cells of Donovanosis and when stained with Wright's stain (or Giemsa) they show encapsulated, bipolar staining organisms (with a 'safety-pin' appearance due to prominent bipolar densities), the Donovan bodies. They may be seen as straight or curved dumbbell rods or coccobacillary forms. The capsule of *C. granulomatis* is difficult to see if numerous organisms are present. The organisms reproduce within phagosomes and are liberated on rupture of the infected cell.

PRESENTATION

Donovanosis affects the dermis and subcutaneous tissue, usually of the genital and peri-anal regions. Genital disease occurs in ~80% of cases (usually involving the penis and the labia); inguinal involvement in 10% and anal in 5–10%. Extragenital disease is rare, occurring in ~5% of cases (Brigden and Guard 1980). The patient develops single or multiple, usually painless subcutaneous granulomatous nodules. When these occur in the inguinal region they can mimic lymphadenopathy – 'pseudobubos'. The lesions erode through the skin and slowly expand to form fleshy masses of granulation tissue. These often ulcerate to form enlarging and coalescing ulcers with raised, rolled edges and beefy red, velvety centres. The ulcers are painless, unless secondary infection occurs causing foul smelling necrotic slough with purulent discharge and associated lymphadenopathy. Lymphadenopathy does not usually occur in uncomplicated Donovanosis. The lesions bleed easily on contact, and vary from highly necrotic destructive lesions with exudation to dry and scarred lesions.

Large granulomatous masses may also be seen in the vaginal wall or uterine cervix, which may mimic malignancy and cause vaginal bleeding. Donovanosis lesions may be premalignant and may coexist with squamous cell carcinoma (Sengupta 1981). If left untreated, lesions may progress to cause (pseudo-) elephantiasis of distal tissue such as the labia and penis.

Spread of infection occurs through auto-inoculation, contiguous spread and haematogenous dissemination. Auto-inoculation is the most common means of spread to extragenital sites and is often the cause of disease involving the mouth, face and other sites on the head. Spread from genital lesions can occur by deep contiguous extension to involve pelvic organs and cause faecal fistulae, ureteric obstruction, extensive pelvic inflammation and fibrosis that mimic a frozen pelvis caused by malignancy (Jofre et al. 1976). Haematogenous spread occurs rarely, that affects bones, joints, liver, lungs, spleen and subcutaneous tissue. Multiple osteolytic cortical defects, often with a sclerosing rim or metaphyseal deposits, are seen on X-ray (Paterson 1998). In disseminated or extensive disease, patients present with loss of weight, fever and appear toxic. Blood examination reveals neutrophil leucocytosis and anaemia of chronic disease. Involvement of bladder or ureters may cause haematuria.

The differential diagnosis of Donovanosis includes other genital infective conditions such as syphilitic chancres, condylomata lata, lymphogranuloma venereum, vulval lymphangitis and lymphadenopathy due to other bacterial or parasitic conditions. Malignancy must be excluded, as Donovanosis may mimic or co-exist with cancerous lesions.

INVESTIGATIONS

1. Cytological and histological examination – Diagnosis is made by the identification of the organism in infected mononuclear cells from biopsy material obtained from scraping of the edge of a lesion, a crush preparation made by spreading clean granulation tissue along a glass slide where tissue imprints or smears are examined after staining with giemsa which gives a result in 30 min. In addition formalin fixed biopsy specimens and smears may be stained with Warthin-Starry silver stains which reveals clusters of dark bipolar staining organisms with the 'safety-pin' like appearances (Donovan bodies) within mononuclear cells. Donovan bodies have also been seen in Papanicolaou smears of cervical lesions.
2. Culture of *C. granulomatis* has been reported successfully.
3. PCR and serology – it is hoped that specific PCR testing and the development of serologic tests will assist in the diagnosis of this condition in future.

TREATMENT

- Tetracycline (500 mg PO 6 hourly) is the most frequently used antibiotic, although resistance has occurred
- Doxycycline (100 mg PO twice a day) is also highly efficacious. The duration of therapy is variable – treatment should be continued until the lesions heal completely otherwise relapse is common
- Cotrimoxazole (trimethoprim 160 mg, sulphamethoxazole 800 mg) twice daily for 10 days has also been shown to be effective
- Ceftriaxone (1 g IMI/day) has been used successfully to treat chronic donovanosis with the

duration of therapy varying according to disease severity (7–26 doses) (Merianos *et al.* 1994)

- Azithromycin therapy (1 g PO/week for 4 weeks, or 500 mg/day for 7 days) was recently used with good results, and with better compliance when compared with other oral therapy such as tetracycline or doxycycline in a small series of patients. Medical therapy alone may not cure larger fibrotic lesions and surgical excision of large lesions speeds recovery with cosmetic benefits (Prakash and Radhakrishna 1986). It is also recommended that localized abscesses of bone be surgically drained (Paterson 1998) and multiple peri-anal fistulae surgically treated (Bozbora *et al.* 1998)

- Treatment of donovanosis in pregnancy is more difficult as tetracycline is best avoided and the available data is more limited. Erythromycin (500 mg qid PO 6 hourly) has been used successfully, however combination with lincomycin (2 g/day PO) produced better results. Ceftriaxone is a safe alternative

- Treatment of donovanosis in patients with HIV infection is prolonged. Extensive disease in HIV infected patients has been seen, with failure of standard treatment regimens

REFERENCES

Bozbora A, Erbil Y, Berber E *et al.* Surgical treatment of granuloma inguinale. *British Journal of Dermatology* 1998; **138**: 1079–1081

Brigden M, Guard R. Extragenital granuloma inguinale in North Queensland. *Medical Journal of Australia* 1980; **2**: 565–567

Carter J, Hutton S, Sriprakash KS *et al.* Culture of the causative organism of donovanosis (*Calymmatobacterium granulomates*) in Hep-2 cells. *Journal of Clinical Microbiology* 1997; **35**: 2915–2917

Jofre ME, Webling DD, James ST. Granuloma inguinale simulating advanced pelvic cancer. *Medical Journal of Australia* 1976; **2**: 869, 872–873

Merianos A, Gilles M, Chuah J. Ceftriaxone in the treatment of chronic donovaniasis in central Australia. *Genitourinary Medicine* 1994; **70**: 84–89

Prakash S, Radhakrishna K. Problematic ulcerative lesions in sexually transmitted diseases: surgical management. *Sexually Transmitted Diseases* 1986; **13**: 127–133

Paterson DL. Disseminated donovanosis (granuloma inguinale) causing spinal cord compression: case report and review of donovanosis involving bone. *Clinical Infectious Diseases* 1998; **26**: 379–383

Sanders CJ. Extragenital donovanosis in a patient with AIDS. *Sexually Transmitted Infections* 1998; **74**: 142–143

Sengupta BS. Vulval cancer following or co-existing with chronic granulomatous diseases of vulva. An analysis of its natural history, clinical manifestations and treatment. *Tropical Doctor* 1981; **11**: 110–114

VII

Other Infections

47

Rickettsial Infections

Including Scrub Typhus, Murine Typhus and the Spotted Fever Group

MICROBIOLOGY

Microorganisms of the family Rickettsiaceae are obligate intracellular parasites about the size of bacteria and look like Gram-negative cocco-bacilli. Rickettsial diseases are broadly classified into three categories: the spotted fever group, the typhus group and others.

The Rickettsial diseases of the spotted fever group consist of Rocky Mountain spotted fever, Boutonneuse fever, Rickettsial pox, North Asian tick-borne Rickettsia. The typhus group is made up of scrub typhus, endemic murine typhus, epidemic typhus, Queensland tick typhus and Brill-Zinsser disease and human ehrlichiosis. Other rickettsial diseases are Trench fever and Q fever.

Spotted fever group

Rocky Mountain spotted fever is caused by *Rickettsia rickettsii*, and predominantly found in the western hemisphere. Ticks transmit it. There are two forms of Rocky Mountain spotted fever in North America: eastern and western forms. The Western Rocky Mountain spotted fever is found in the western states of the USA. The vector is a tick, *Dermacentor andersoni* and hosts are the rocky mountain goats, sheep, badger and the black bear. The eastern rocky mountain spotted fever is found in British Columbia, Saskatchewan and Alberta, Canada. The vector is the dog tick *D. variabilis*. Spotted fever occurs in the spring in North America when ticks are found in large numbers. The rickettsial organism infects all cells including the ovaries, resulting in vertical transmission to the larvae.

In the USA the incidence of spotted fever was 5.2 per million in 1981 and due to decreased incidence in the south-east USA has reduced to 2.0 in 1992. Boutonneuse fever is caused by *R. conorii* and found in Africa, Europe, Middle East and India. Ixodid ticks transmit it by their bite. The environments in which these ticks are found are terrains and houses.

Rickettsial pox is transmitted by *R. akari* and found in Russia and the USA. The organism is transmitted by the blood-sucking mite found in house mice and other rodents. The North Asian tick-borne rickettsia fever is caused by the organism *R. siberica* found in Siberia and Mongolia. The ticks are found in wild rodents.

Typhus group

Scrub typhus is transmitted by the larval mites of the genus Leptotrombidium (Trombicula) and the organism is *R. orientalis* (tsutsugamushi). The organism is found in the body cavity of the adult mite and the larval stages are transmitted through their salivary gland. The disease has been described in Japan, China, North East Australia, South East Asia, Taiwan, Papua New Guinea and the Pacific Islands. Scrub typhus occurs where there is a prevalence of rodent hosts and trombiculid mites. Man is an incidental host. Thirty-two newly isolated strains of *R. tsutsugamushi* have been described in Japan (Yamashita *et al.* 1994). A new focus of scrub typhus has been described in remote rain forests region of Northern Territory of Australia. Two near fatal cases with multisystem involvement have been described (Currie *et al.* 1993).

Endemic murine typhus is caused by *Rickettsia typhi*. It is worldwide in its incidence. The rat louse and rat mite transmit the organism from rat to rat similar to louse typhus. The flea *Xenopsylla cheopis* infects man. *Rattus rattus norvegiocus* is the main rodent. Rickettsia-like organisms (ELB agent is named after EL Labs that provided the fleas) have been isolated in blood from human murine typhus (Higgins *et al.* 1994). A high seropositivity among domestic cats and opossums has been found near the residences of patients with murine typhus in Los Angeles and Greece (Chaniotis *et al.* 1994). *Xenopsylla cheopis,* the classic vector of murine typhus was near the residences of cases. Cat flea Chenocephalides has been identified to bite humans.

Epidemic typhus is worldwide in distribution. The organism responsible is *R. prowazeki*. It multiplies in the gut epithelium of the louse. Man gets infected through abrasions in the skin contaminated by mouse faeces or infected louse saliva. Excreta of infected lice can transmit to other lice with death of the infected lice. Brill-Zinsser disease is also caused by *Rickettsia prowazeki*. It is a recurrence of epidemic typhus several years after initial infection. It also occurs worldwide, but is a milder infection and the cause of recrudescence is not known.

South American tick typhus is prevalent in Columbia and Brazil. Tick typhus is also prevalent in north-eastern part of Australia, South East Asia, eastern and western parts of Africa and Siberia. The tick typhus found in north Queensland is a mild form and the organism is *Rickettsia australis* and the tick vector is *Ixodes holocyclus* and *Ixodes tasmanii*. The organism is unique to Australia and its origin is uncertain (Currie 1993). However, it extends outside the tropical area as far south as Sydney in New South Wales. It occurs along a 3200-km span of eastern and coastal Australia from tropical to temperate climates.

Other rickettsial diseases

Trench fever is transmitted by *Rochalimaea quintana* through human body lice. The organisms multiply in the epithelium of the midgut of lice. Feeding on infected humans infects lice. It has been described in Africa, North America and Europe. It was reported in 'epidemic proportions' in Europe during the First World War.

Q fever was first described in abattoir employees in Brisbane in 1937 and the organism was labelled *Rickettsia burnetii*, now called *Coxiella burnetii*. It is spread by ticks *Dermacentor andersoni* and *Ornithodorus tunicata* in western USA. The natural reservoir in Queensland is the bandicoot isoodontorus and *Isoodono besulus*. The tick *Haemaphysalis humerosa* an ectoparasite of the bandicoot is supposed to transmit the rickettsiae organism. Q fever is prevalent worldwide. The rickettsia of Q fever gain entry through the upper respiratory tract by handling infected material or by drinking contaminated milk. In North Africa transovarial transmission of the agent in indigenous ticks has been demonstrated. Epidemics in laboratory workers have also been described. Human to human transmission has not been proved. Q fever essentially is a zoonosis.

Immunity to Rickettsial strains tends to be long-lasting. However, intracellular rickettsiae are usually not entirely eradicated and can remain dormant for months or years. The antibody response that occurs early in the disease does not control the disease quickly. Cell mediated immunity probably plays a dominant role in controlling rickettsia growth.

PRESENTATION

Spotted fever group

Rocky Mountain spotted fever

The incubation period is 3–12 days and is a key epidemiological factor. A history of the tick bite is forthcoming but not always so. The initial symptoms are non-specific and mimic other viral infections. Symptoms are fever, nausea, vomiting, headache, myalgia and anorexia. A rash appears around the fourth day, starting in the wrists and ankles, and then spreads to palms, soles, face and mucous membrane of mouth. Initially, the rash 3–6 mm in diameter blanches on pressure. After 2 or 3 days the rash becomes darker and maculopapular and finally it becomes petechial, and coalesce. The rash tends to disappear after recrudescence of the fever but can remain for a longer period.

Increase in vascular permeability causes hypovolaemia, hypotension and oedema including pulmonary and renal failure. There may be ischaemia in the toes, ears, genitalia and nose. Thrombosis of larger vessels can lead to loss of a limb. Cardiac involvement can lead to ECG abnormalities. Manifestations of central nervous system involvement are insomnia, restlessness, convulsions, tremors and muscle stiffness. In severe cases there may be faecal and urinary incontinence. Liver involvement causes jaundice with elevation of transaminase.

The long-term sequelae of Rocky Mountain spotted fever are neurological including paraparesis, loss of hearing, peripheral neuropathy, bladder and bowel incontinence, cerebellar, motor and vestibular dysfunction and language problems (Archibald and Sexton 1995). Death can occur in ~10–21 days after the onset of the illness. Convalescence can take several weeks to months if there are long standing sequelae. Patients who receive anti-rickettsial therapy within 5 days of the onset of symptoms are less likely to die compared with those who receive treatment after the fifth day (6.5 versus 22.9% respectively) (Kirkland *et al.* 1995).

Rickettsial pox

The incubation period is ~10–21 days. In most patients an eschar develops at the site of the bite. The eschar is initially papular and becomes vesicular and crusted measuring up to 1.5 cm in diameter. The onset of the illness is heralded by fever with chills and rigors. Headache, myalgia and lassitude accompany this. The skin eruption is sparse and appears around days 1–4 on the trunk extremities and mucus membranes. Initially, it is maculopapular and then vesicular with surrounding erythema. The disease is self-limiting with no fatality.

North Asian tick-borne typhus and African tick typhus

The incubation period of this disease is 5–7 days. The illness starts with fever, headache, malaise and conjunctivitis. The primary lesion at the site of the bite is a very small ulcer with a black centre and a red areola with accompanying enlarged regional lymph nodes. The maculopapular rash appears around day 4. It involves palms, soles and face. In severe cases it may be haemorrhagic. fever subsides around the second week. The prognosis is very good except in the debilitated. Complications are unusual.

Queensland tick typhus

The incubation period is 7–10 days. The illness starts with fever, headaches, typhus-like rash and lymphadenopathy. Lymphadenopathy is generally not found in murine typhus in Australia. The rash is maculopapular, non-pruritic and spreads over the whole body. The papules may be up to 10 mm in diameter. There may be an eschar at the site of the bite. One fatal case of Queensland tick typhus has been reported.

Flinders Island spotted fever (Australia)

The illness is abrupt in onset, with high fever, chills and rigors, headaches and myalgia. Joint pains occur without any swelling or tenderness. The fever lasts from 7 to 16 days and is associated with relative bradycardia. The rash appears around the fourth day and persists for ~15 days (Stewart 1991). It is erythematous and maculopapular, non-tender and becomes darker and purplish. The rash gradually fades away without desquamation. A few complications such as thrombocytopenia, non-oliguric renal failure and mildly elevated liver enzymes have been noted.

The clinical presentation is that of fever, severe headache, and myalgia without a rash. Renal failure may be a complication and very ill patients have thrombocytopenia and leukopenia. There is often a history of exposure to ticks. The Weil-Felix test is negative and diagnosis is confirmed by rising titres on the indirect fluorescent antibody test using antigens to *E. canis*.

Human ehrlichiosis (Rickettsia-like)

It was previously thought that ehrlichiosis was restricted to dogs. *E. canis* is an organism of the genus *Ehrlichia* of the family Rickettsiceae. *E. canis* is the cause of canine ehrlichiosis, a worldwide disease which is often fatal. *Rhipicephalus sanguineus*, the brown dog tick, is the common vector. Since 1986, human ehrlichiosis is a newly recognized disease in the USA, ranging from a mild infection to life threatening or fatal disease. The disease may be misdiagnosed as Rocky Mountain spotted fever, murine typhus or Q fever.

Scrub typhus

The clinical disease varies in severity from mild and severe to fatal disease. The incubation period is 7–21 days. A small non-tender papule develops at the site of the bite. The papule increases in size and undergoes central necrosis with crusting to form the eschar. The regional lymph nodes are enlarged and painful. fever sets in with chills and rigors, accompanied by headache, conjunctival injection, generalized aches and pains, and malaise. A rash is not always present (Nagawa *et al.* 1994). During the second week of the disease if untreated complications such as meningoencephalitis with delirium, stupor or coma may occur. The cranial nerves may be involved, and papilloedema can be seen. Cardiac complications due to focal myocarditis, causing cardiomegaly with circulatory failure. Hepatic dysfunction was reported in 77% of patients in Taipei (Yang *et al.* 1995) and some presented with a picture of viral hepatitis. Pleural and pericardial effusions are rare complications. Respiratory complications with bilateral basal infiltrates and severe restrictive defect may occur due to interstitial pneumonitis. The liver and spleen may be palpable. Fulminant *R. orientalis* with haemophagocytic

syndrome has been described with bone marrow aspirates showing proliferation of histiocytes with active haemophagocytosis (Iwasaki *et al.* 1994). The temperature settles after 14 days in untreated patients who survive and recover from most of the complications over several weeks. The unusual presentation of an acute abdomen mimicking acute cholecystitis or acute appendicitis with no abnormal findings at laparotomy has been reported (Chi *et al.* 1997).

Endemic murine typhus

The incubation period of this disease is 6–14 days. Presentation includes fever in all cases and rash in ~20% of cases. The rash is maculopapular over the trunk, appearing on the fifth day after onset of fever. It is associated with non-specific symptoms such as headache, generalized aches and pains. Generally murine typhus is a mild disease similar to louse-borne typhus. It is of a shorter duration, less complicated and has a low mortality rate. However, though uncommon, jaundice, pneumonia, meningitis and renal failure with mortality rate have been reported.

Epidemic typhus and Brill-Zinsser disease

The incubation period is 8–12 days. The disease starts with fever, myalgia and headache, and the latter is generally very severe. Constipation is more common than diarrhoea. The rash appears around the fourth to seventh day. Initially, it is an erythema on the trunk and axillary folds which spreads to the extremities, face, palms and soles. The progression of the rash is related to the severity of the disease. In mild cases it disappears within 48 h. In moderately severe cases it can become maculopapular and in severe cases it transforms to a haemorrhagic or purpuric rash. The rash may also be absent in some cases.

The pulse may be slow compared with the temperature, as in typhoid fever. It becomes more rapid subsequently and the blood pressure tends to drop. In complicated cases there may be thrombosis of vessels. Cranial nerves may be involved with neurological symptoms. The mental state may deteriorate and in severe cases, coma with urinary and faecal incontinence may occur. Cranial nerve palsies lead to dysphagia, deafness and dysphonia. Gangrene of skin, toes and fingers may occur. Secondary bacterial pneumonia may occur. The severity of the disease increases with age. Death from typhus generally occurs in the second or third week.

Trench fever

Trench fever or Wolhynia fever is a 5-day fever. It is hardly recognizable clinically except in certain parts of the world where it is prevalent. Once a person is infected, the organism may be present for variable periods, up to 7 years with or without a relapse. The incubation period is between 2 and 5 weeks. The clinical picture is variable from a very mild disease to a febrile illness. There may be relapses over 2–3 months. The fever may mimic typhoid fever and is associated with non-specific symptoms such as chills, myalgia, headache and joint pain. Some patients develop a macular rash. Mortality is very rare. It may be confused with relapsing fever caused by spirochaetal organism *Borellia* which also is transmitted by body louse, a more serious disease.

Q fever

The incubation period is 2–3 weeks. The disease may go unrecognized. It is a febrile illness associated with myalgia and malaise. Rash is unusual. The common presentation is respiratory with a dry cough and scant mucoid sputum. Fine crepitations may be heard. Radiologic changes are usually in the lower lobes with multiple round homogenous densities. They may be seen around the fourth or fifth day and tend to remain for a longer period when the patient is afebrile. Complications such as pleural effusion and pericardial effusion have been seen. Rarely, the inflammatory lesion may mimic a tumour.

Hepatic manifestations are fairly common in this disease. There may be hepatomegaly due to hepatic granulomas and patient develops jaundice with abnormal liver function tests.

Subacute *C. burnetii* endocarditis is a very serious complication, which is often missed clinically. It is more common with people having abnormal valves. The ordinary blood cultures are negative. The clinical presentation is fever, anaemia and embolic manifestations. There may be splenomegaly. It may be complicated by glomerulonephritis due to deposition of immune complex material. This condition should be considered when blood cultures are negative and vegetations are seen on echocardiography. The initial febrile illness may be forgotten and subacute bacterial endocarditis may manifest several years later.

In the differential diagnosis of Rickettsial disease, meningococcaemia, typhoid fever, malaria, lyme disease and other arboviral diseases such as Dengue, Ross River, Murray Valley encephalitis, Barmah Forest virus and Japanese encephalitis should be excluded depending on the location of the place.

PATHOLOGY

The pathologic changes in the spotted fever and typhus groups are vascular with lesions in the adjacent parenchyma. The most profound changes are found in Rocky Mountain spotted fever. *Rickettsia ricketsii* is an obligate intracellular bacterium that invades vascular endothelium, causing a vasculitis with infiltration of mononuclear cells and neutrophils resulting in occlusive fibrin microthrombi. The rickettsii adhere to endothelial cells and enter by phagocytosis, multiplying within them (Sporn *et al.* 1993). An increase in quantities of TNF-α, IL-6 and IL-8 as well as a marked increase in circulatory ICAM-1 has been described in the blood of a young female who died of multi-organ failure (Sessler *et al.* 1995). The vascular damage occurs in arteries, veins and capillaries with preservation of the anatomy to a large extent. There may be fibrinoid changes in the muscular vasculature. Mononuclear leucocytes, lymphocytes and plasma cells infiltrate the adventitia especially in Rocky Mountain spotted fever.

Thrombosis is relatively uncommon in scrub typhus and murine typhus. However, in cases of multi-organ failure disseminated multi-organ vasculitis of small blood vessels, tubulo-interstitial nephritis, interstitial pneumonitis disseminated intravascular coagulation has been reported in scrub typhus (Chi *et al.* 1997). Myocarditis does occur in Rocky Mountain spotted fever and in scrub typhus. Involvement of kidney with perivascular interstitial nephritis has been described in Israeli Mediterranean spotted fever (IMSF) (Shaked *et al.* 1994).

Rickettsial pneumonitis occurs in Q fever to a lesser extent than in other forms of rickettsial infections. The pneumonitis is patchy with consolidation in alveoli, which are filled with fibrocellular exudate, including lymphocytes, plasma cells, mononuclear cells and very few polymorphonuclear leucocytes. Scrub typhus pneumonitis has been described in open lung biopsy specimens. Vascular typhus nodules also occur in the brain, particularly the midbrain. Perivascular lesions occur in the portal areas of the liver associated with non-specific fatty degeneration.

Coxiella burnetii predominantly affects the reticuloendothelial cells, forming granulomas with multinucleate giant cells. The granulomas may have a surrounding clear area referred to as doughnut granuloma and are found in the liver, lungs and bone marrow.

The members of Rickettsia have common features but their differences account for distinct clinical entities. The disseminated vascular lesion accounts for most of the pathophysiologic changes. There is extravasation of fluid, resulting in hypotension especially in Rocky Mountain spotted fever. Thrombosis of veins can lead to reversible or irreversible skin damage or gangrene. Most lesions resolve without sequelae while others develop minute scars marking the sites of the cutaneous lesions. Severe infections can cause coagulopathy, a major factor contributing to bleeding and death.

INVESTIGATIONS

1. Initial investigations are done to assess the general clinical status of the patients. These include a full blood count, electrolyte status, renal function, liver functions, ECG, coagulation status and lumbar puncture. The more severe the cases, the more of these investigations are warranted, while in mild cases only a few of these investigations are really necessary. The above tests may be abnormal in some but not diagnostic.
2. MRI of the brain in encephalitis secondary to Rocky Mountain spotted fever has shown increased signal intensity in the distribution of perivascular space (Baganz *et al.* 1995).
3. Laboratory diagnoses of Rickettsia are several. Some tests take a longer time to show positive results by which time the patient may have recovered or succumbed to the disease. The tests available are serological, isolation and identification from blood and tissues, immunofluorescence to identify the organism in skin or tissues. Serology tests should be repeated to establish a rise in titre. Scrub typhus can be confirmed serologically by use of a dipstick assay (Watt *et al.* 1995).

Weil-Felix test – one of the earliest serology tests based on similarity of polysaccharide antigens between some rickettsiae and *Proteus* strains. It is an agglutination test that tests strains of *Proteus* OX-2, OX-19 and OX-K strains. Proteus agglutinins may appear as early as the sixth day but generally around the 12th day. A single convalescent titre of 1/160 to 1/320 is considered as diagnostic, a rise in titre is more significant of a recent infection. It is negative in Q fever, Rickettsial pox. OX-K is positive only in scrub typhus. The reactions may be summarized as given in Table 47.1.

Complement fixation test – has been used for a very long time for diagnosis of Rickettsial infection belonging to the spotted fever group or typhus group and Q fever. With group specific antigens the organism can be identified by titre differences. In patients with Q fever complicated by bacterial endocarditis or hepatic granulomas, persisting high titres for phase I antigen suggest chronic infection. It has been used to detect antibodies in population studies as done in inner Mongolia where half the human population showed antibodies to *Rickettsia siberia* (Lin *et al.* 1995).

Indirect immunofluorescent antibody test – is applicable to all Rickettsial infection. It is a very sensitive test for diagnosis of scrub typhus. It may be group specific or species-specific. This test has been used as a surveillance of scrub typhus in Taiwan where it was found that there were serologically positive cases in many counties (Chen *et al.* 1993).

Agglutination test – microscopic agglutination and haemagglutination tests are valuable for identification of rickettsia. Micro-agglutination tests are performed with highly purified rickettsial suspensions and are simple to perform. This test may not distinguish between murine and epidemic typhus.

Table 47.1 – Rickettsial infection

	Proteus strain		
	OX-K	**OX-19**	**OX-2**
Q fever	o	o	o
Scrub typhus	+++	o	o
Rickettsial pox	o	o	o
Typhus group	o	+++	+
Brill-Zinsser	o/+	o/+	o
Spotted fever	o	+++	+

Indirect immunoperoxidase assay – IgG and IgM antibodies are measured in an indirect immunoperoxidase assay using different spots of antigen from *R. orientalis*, *R. typhi* and TT-118 spotted fever group rickettsiae (Strickman *et al.* 1994).

Monoclonal antibodies – detecting antigens of *R. orientalis* has been reported using monoclonal antibodies (Zhang 1993). No cross-reaction was found with antigens of other rickettsia groups including *R. rickettsia*, *R. typhi*, *R. prowazeki* and *R. burnetii*. The method is very sensitive and antigen can be detected early at an antigen level of 6.7 mg/microlitre. It is easy to perform and results can be read by naked eye (Zhang 1993).

Enzyme-linked immunosorbent assay (ELISA) – has been used to detect the 56-kDa protein of *R. orientalis* located on the rickettsial surface, an immunodominant antigen. It has a high diagnostic sensitivity (95%) and a high diagnostic specificity (100%), and has demonstrated the suitability of the recombinant antigen for use as an immunodiagnostic tool (Kim *et al.* 1993).

Dot-blot immunoassay – has been compared with indirect immunofluorescence (IFA) in known positive and negative cases of scrub typhus. It was found that IFA was 99% specific and the dipstick assay was 98% specific. An IFA of 1:64 is either positive or negative may be supported by clinical record dipsticks which are 83% specific and 90% sensitive. This assay will hasten diagnosis especially in areas of high prevalence where the proportion of false-positive results will be low (Weddle *et al.* 1995).

Polymerase chain reaction – more and more cases are now diagnosed by PCR which gives an early diagnosis. Diagnosis of *R. orientalis* DNA in peripheral blood mononuclear cells has been reported before and after therapy (Murai *et al.* 1995). The PCR method is considered to be useful for rapid aetiological diagnosis of spotted fever group rickettsiosis in Japan (Tange *et al.* 1994).

Use of the PCR method has isolated an ELB agent, a recently described typhus-like rickettsia that cannot be distinguished from *R. prowazeki* or *R. typhi* by currently available serologic reagents. Restriction digests of PCR products from fleas revealed ELB infection rates and *R. typhi* infection rates in fleas (Schriefer *et al.* 1994). The first case of ELB agent using PCR facilities in humans has been reported and emphasizes the utility of PCR-facilitated diagnosis (Schriefer *et al.* 1994). PCR has been used on blood clots and urine samples

of patients suspected of Rocky Mountain spotted fever. However, re-amplification was essential in some raising the question of lack of sensitivity as a limitation of PCR as a clinical diagnostic test (Sexton *et al.* 1994). A PCR system for rapid diagnosis of scrub typhus within 6 h has been reported (Sugita *et al.* 1993).

TREATMENT

- Most important, prompt anti-rickettsial therapy. Anti-rickettsial therapy reduces mortality rate and aids speedy recovery. There are two rickettsiostatic drugs that are effective, namely tetracycline and chloramphenicol. Because of occasional blood dyscrasias, tetracycline is preferred unless it cannot be used such as in children or in pregnancy. With the commencement of antimicrobial therapy, the patient responds within 24 h. Fluoro quinolines including ofloxacin have previously been shown to be bacteriastatic against *Rickettsia* spp. and *C. burnetti in vitro*. They are reliable alternatives to tetracycline therapy for Mediterranean spotted fever, scrub typhus and acute Q fever (Maurin *et al.* 1997).

The initial dose of chloramphenicol is 50 mg/kg of body weight and for tetracycline is 25 mg/kg. The subsequent doses of chloramphenical and tetracycline are the same as the initial, given in divided doses 8 hourly. Antibiotics are continued until patient is afebrile for 24 h. For patients where oral therapy is not possible IV preparations may be used initially. Tetracycline and chloramphenicol are effective in human ehrlichiosis.

Long-acting tetracyclines such as doxycycline and micnocycline are used as a single-dose therapy in louse-borne typhus at 100 mg dose. This dose cures most adults. Relapses are uncommon with a dose of 200 mg for adults. A single dose of long acting tetracycline should not be used for murine typhus or Rocky Mountain spotted fever. A single dose of 200 mg doxycycline will cure scrub typhus with occasional recrudescence.

In uncomplicated Q fever, tetracycline or chloramphenicol in the usual dose will cure the disease. Treatment for a longer duration may be necessary for pneumonitis or hepatitis. Treatment of *Coxiella* endocarditis is difficult.

A combination of doxycycline with rifampicin and lincomycin or trimethoprim has been used for months. Valvular replacement may have to be considered in some, although it is controversial as infection in prosthetic valves has been reported. Mortality is high in Q fever endocarditis.

The use of corticosteroids with antimicrobials in severe cases is advocated, as there has been dramatic improvement in coma patients. This is used only for seriously ill patients.

- Supportive measures to reverse pathophysiologic changes such as hypotension with adequate fluid and oxygen therapy
- Prompt treatment of complications such as inotropes in cardiovascular hypotension
- Proper nursing care to prevent bed sores in comatose patients

Treatment of Rickettsial disease includes:

Prophylaxis

Use of insect repellents is advocated for murine typhus, epidemic louse-borne typhus and trench fever. Insecticides such as Lindane are advocated for epidemic louse-borne typhus and trench fever for delousing the patient and the clothing. In murine typhus insecticides are used to reduce the number of fleas. Measures should be taken to prevent tick bite by using insect repellents and avoiding places where ticks are generally found. Ticks should be removed with forceps exerting gentle traction to release the mouthparts intact. Ticks should be removed from house dogs. Poison baits are used to control rodents in spread of murine typhus and control of mites in scrub typhus. Ascarides are used on walls and other mite-infested areas to destroy mites. Animals are screened for Q fever where Q fever is prevalent. QVa (CSL) is a purified, killed suspension of *C. burnetti* and is used for prophylaxis for abattoir, veterinary and laboratory personnel.

REFERENCES

Archibald LK, Sexton DJ. Long-term sequelae of Rocky Mountain spotted fever. *Clinical Infectious Diseases* 1995; **20**: 1122–1125

Baganz MD, Drose PE, Reinhardt JA. Rocky Mountain spotted fever encephalitis: MRI findings. *American Journal of Neuroradiology* 1995; **16**: 919–932

Chaniotis B, Psarulaki A, Chaliotis G et al. Transmission cycle of murine typhus in Greece. *Annals of Tropical Medical Parasitology* 1994; **88**: 645–647

Chen HL, Chen HY, Horng CB. Surveillance of scrub typhus in Taiwan. *Chinese Journal of Microbial Immunology* 1993; **26**: 166–170

Chi WC, Huang JJ, Sung JM, et al. Scrub typhus associated with multi-organ failure: a case report. *Scandinavian Journal of Infectious Diseases* 1997; **29**: 634–635

Currie B, O'Conner L, Dwyer B. A new focus of scrub typhus in tropical Australia. *American Journal of Tropical Medicine and Hygiene* 1993; **49**: 425–429

Currie B. Medicine in tropical Australia. *Medical Journal of Australia* 1993; **158**: 609–615

Higgins JA, Sacci JB Jr, Schriefer ME et al. Molecular identification of rickettsia-like microorganisms associated with colonized cat fleas (*Ctenocephalides felis*). Man is infected by infected flea faeces on abraded skin. *Insect Molecular Biology* 1994; **3**: 27–33

Iwasaki H, Hashimoto K, Takada N et al. Fulminant *Rickettsia tsutsugamushi* infection associated with haemophagocytic syndrome [Letter]. *Lancet* 1994; **343**: 1236

Kim IS, Seong SY, Woo SG et al. High level expression of a 56 kilodalton protein gene (bor 56) of *Rickettsia tsutsugamushi*. Boryong and its application to enzyme-linked immunosorbent assay. *Journal of Clinical Microbiology* 1993; **31**: 598–605

Kirkland KB, Wilkinson WE, Sexton DJ. Therapeutic delay and mortality in cases of Rocky Mountain spotted fever. *Clinical Infectious Diseases* 1995; **20**: 1118–1121

Lin QH, Chen GY, Jin Y et al. Evidence of high prevalence of spotted fever group rickettsial infections in diverse ecologic zones of inner Mongolia. *Epidemiology of Infections* 1995; **115**: 177–183

Maurin M, Raoult D. Bacteriostatic and bactericidal activity of serofloxacin against *Rickettsia ricketsii*, *Rickettsia conorii*, *Rickettsia isreali* spotted fever group rickettsia and *Coxiella bumetti*. *Journal of Antimicrobial Chemotherapy* 1997; **39**: 725–730

Murai K, Okayama A, Horinouchi H et al. Eradication of *Rickettsia tsutsugamushi* from patient's blood by chemotherapy as assessed by the polymerase chain reaction. *American Journal of Tropical Medicine and Hygiene* 1995; **52**: 325–327

Nagawa Y, Hurnie H, Saton H et al. A case of severe tsutsugamushi disease without eruption. [Japanese] *Journal of Japanese Association of Infectious Diseases* 1994; **68**: 1433–1436

Schriefer ME, Sacci JB Jr, Dumler JS et al. Identification of a novel rickettsial infection in a patient diagnosed with murine typhus. *Journal of Clinical Microbiology* 1994; **32**: 949–954

Schriefer ME, Sacci JB Jr, Taylor JP et al. Murine typhus: updated roles of multiple urban components and a second typhus-like rickettsia. *Journal of Entomology* 1994; **31**: 681–685

Sessler CN, Schwartz M, Windsor AC et al. Increased serum cytokines and intercellular adhesion molecule-1 in fulminant Rocky Mountain spotted fever. *Critical Care Medicine* 1995; **23**: 973–976

Sexton DJ, Dwyer B, Kemp R et al. Spotted fever group rickettsial infections in Australia. *Review of Infectious Diseases* 1991; **13**: 876–886

Sexton DJ, Kanj SS, Wilson K et al. The usefulness of a polymerase chain reaction as a diagnostic test for Rocky Mountain spotted fever. *American Journal of Tropical Medicine and Hygiene* 1994; **50**: 59–63

Shaked Y, Shpilberg O, Samra Y. Involvement of the kidneys in Mediterranean spotted fever and Murine typhus. *Quarterly Journal of Medicine* 1994; **87**: 103–107

Sporn LA, Lawrence SO, Silverman DJ *et al.* E selection dependent neutrophil and lesion to RR infected endothelial cells. *Blood* 1993; **81**: 2406–2412

Stewart RS. Flinders Island spotted fever: a newly recognized endemic focus of tick typhus in Bass Strait. *Medical Journal of Australia* 1991; **154**: 94–99

Strickman D, Tanskul P, Eamsila C *et al.* Prevalence of antibodies to Ricketssiae in the human population of suburban Bangkok. *American Journal of Tropical Medicine and Hygiene* 1994; **51**: 149–153

Sugita Y, Yamakawa Y, Takahashi K *et al.* A polymerase chain reaction system for rapid diagnosis of scrub typhus within 6 hours. *American Journal of Tropical Medicine and Hygiene* 1993; **49**: 631–640

Tange Y, Matsumoto M, Okada T *et al.* Detection of DNA of causative agent of spotted fever group rickettsiosis in Japan from the patient's blood sample by polymerase chain reaction. *Microbial Immunology* 1994; **38**: 665–668

Watt G, Strickman D, Kantuipong P *et al.* Performance of a dot immunoassay for the rapid diagnosis of Scrub typhus in a longitudinal case series. *Journal of Infectious Diseases* 1998; **177**: 800–802

Weddle JR, Chan TC, Thompson K *et al.* Effectiveness of a dot-blot immunoassay of anti-*Rickettsia tsutsugamushi* antibodies for serologic analysis of scrub typhus. *American Journal of Tropical Medicine and Hygiene* 1995; **53**: 43–46

Yamashita T, Kasuya S, Noda N *et al.* Transmission of *Rickettsia tsutsugamushi* strains among humans, wild rodents and trombiclid mites in an area of Japan in which tsutsugamushi disease is newly endemic. *Journal of Clinical Microbiology* 1994; **32**: 2780–2785

Yang CH, Hsu GJ, Peng MY *et al.* Hepatic dysfunction in scrub typhus. *Journal of Formosan Medical Association* 1995; **94**: 101–105

Yang CH, Young TG, Peng MY *et al.* Unusual presentation of acute abdomen in scrub typhus: a report of two cases. *Chinese Medical Journal* 1995; **55**: 401–404

Zhang H. Detection antigen of *Rickettsia tsutsugamushi* by using monoclonal antibodies. *Chinese Journal of Epidemiology* 1993; **14**: 49–51

48

Arboviral Infections

Including Dengue fever, Japanese B encephalitis,
Australian encephalitis and Ross River fever

Microbiology
  Dengue Fever Virus
  Japanese B Encephalitis Virus
  Ross River Virus
  Barmah Forest Virus
  Murray Valley Encephalitis and Kunjin Fever
  Virus
  Sindbis Virus
  Kokobera Virus
  Gan Gan and Trubanaman Virus
  Edge Hill Virus
  Stratford Virus
Presentation
  Dengue Fever Uncomplicated
  Complicated Dengue Fever
  Japanese B Encephalitis
  Ross River Virus Infection
  Barmah Forest Infection
  Murray Valley Encephalitis and Kunjin Fever
  Infections
  Sindbis Infection
  Kokobera Virus Infection
  Gan Gan and Trubanaman Infections
Pathology
  Dengue Fever
  Japanese B Encephalitis
  Murray Valley Encephalitis

Investigations
  Dengue Fever
  Japanese B Encephalitis
  Ross River Fever
  Barmah Forest Virus Infection
  Murray Valley Encephalitis and Kunjin Fever
  Sindbis Virus Infection
  Gan Gan and Trubanaman Virus Infection
  Kokobera Virus Infection
Treatment
  Dengue Fever
  Japanese B Encephalitis
  Ross River Fever and Barmah Forest Virus
  Infection
  Murray Valley Encephalitis and Kunjin
  Encephalitis
  Sindbis, Kokobera, Gan Gan, Trubanaman,
  Edge Hill and Stratford Virus Infections
Prophylaxis
  Dengue Fever
  Japanese B Encephalitis
  Ross River Fever
  Barmah Forest Virus Infection
  Murray Valley Encephalitis and Kunjin Fever
References

MICROBIOLOGY

Arboviruses are a group of animal viruses usually transmitted by haematophagus arthropods (mosquitoes and ticks). Birds can also be a source of infection for mosquitoes and infection is transmitted to domestic animals and humans.

Arboviruses are classified into genus orbivirus, phlebovirus, alphavirus, flavivirus, bunyavirus, hantanvirus, filovirus and nairovirus. Australian arboviruses causing disease are mainly of genus flavivirus, namely Murray Valley encephalitis, Kokobera, Dengue fever, Kunjin virus and Edge Hill virus and genus alphaviruses, namely Ross River, Sindbis, and Barmah Forest. The genus bunya virus includes Gan Gan and Trubanaman.

Arboviruses number more than 250 and at least 80 immunologically distinct viruses cause diseases in humans. About 70 arboviruses have been identified in Australia of which nine are pathogenic: Dengue virus, Ross River virus, Barmah Forest virus, Murray Valley encephalitis virus, Kunjin virus, Sindbis virus, Gan Gan virus, Trubanaman virus and Kokobera virus (Boughton 1994).

Dengue fever virus

There are four distinct sero-groups, types I–IV, of Dengue viruses. Epidemics of all four types have occurred. Simultaneous infection with Dengue I and II has been reported (Rocco *et al*. 1998). Each serotype is further divided into distinct genetic subtypes. The Dengue virus is a mosquito-borne virus found in urban and rural areas worldwide between latitudes 30°N and 40°S. Since 1969 Dengue has been endemic in most parts of the tropics and subtropics. Outbreaks have occurred in the Caribbean, Puerto Rico and the US Virgin Islands. It was endemic in coastal North Queensland in Australia until 1955, when the vector was eradicated. The vector is the female of several species of *Aëdes* mosquitoes, the commonest being *A. aegypti*. Infection is transmitted by the bite of the infected mosquito. The breeding activity is maximal in hot, moist conditions. The mosquito becomes infective in 10–12 days after ingesting blood containing the virus and remains infective for the rest of its life. Dengue is not endemic in Australia but produces occasional epidemics.

In areas where the virus circulates constantly, such as in Singapore and Indonesia, the peak incidence is in children.

Females are affected more than males, probably due to the *A. aegypti* being highly domesticated and generally biting females who are generally indoors during the day. Serotype II may be more pathogenic than other serotypes. Epidemiological studies in Thailand and Cuba have suggested that the sequence of infection by Dengue Type I, followed by Type II, is particularly virulent. Over the past 20 years, Dengue has expanded throughout the tropical areas of the world and is the most important arbovirus disease of humans. Over 2 billion people are at risk and millions of cases occur each year.

Dengue haemorrhagic fever is found in South East Asia, in countries such as Thailand, Malaysia, Philippine Islands, China and Cuba. In 1962, in Malaysia Dengue Shock syndrome and haemorrhage was described, occurring mainly in children. Infection by different Dengue serotypes several months after the initial infection is the likely cause of Dengue Shock and Haemorrhagic syndrome. Dengue haemorrhagic fever is believed to be an immunopathological response to secondary infection with a heterologus serotype of Dengue virus (Gagnon *et al*. 1999).

Japanese B encephalitis virus

Japanese B encephalitis, also referred to as Japanese encephalitis, is an infection caused by the Japanese B encephalitis virus that affects the central nervous system. Japanese B virus belongs to the flavivirus group.

Mosquitoes belonging to the genus Culicinae transmit the virus, notably by species *Culex tritaeniorrhynchus*. The vector varies with locality. The disease is endemic and epidemic in Asia, such as Philippines, Japan, Korea, Taiwan, Thailand, Indonesia, Bangladesh, Malaysia, Hong Kong, Mynamar, Laos, Nepal, Sri Lanka, Vietnam, South and Eastern India, Guam and China. About 50 000 human cases occur each year. It is not endemic in Australia. However, cases can occur among travellers. The natural cycle involves Culicinae mosquitoes, vertebrates and wild birds. It is common in swine, while man and equines are incidental hosts. It can cause clinical encephalitis in equines and abortion and stillbirth in swine.

Although the disease can be severe, the risk of contracting the disease is low, particularly for short-term travellers. However, long-term travellers in high-risk areas spending for 1 month are in danger and should be vaccinated. The ratio of overt disease to inapparent infection varies from 1:300 to 1:1000, and fatality ranges from 10 to 30%, with a high mortality rate in children aged 5–9 years (Thisyakorn and Thisyakorn 1994). Transplacental infection from mother to foetus with foetal death can occur.

Japanese B encephalitis is mainly a rural disease associated with paddy fields and pigs. It occurs right throughout the year in the tropics, while in temperate areas, the incidence of Japanese encephalitis is mainly during summer time. Several species of Culicinae vectors have been identified depending on the geography, such as, *Cx. annulus* in Taiwan, *Cx. fuscocephalus* in Thailand and *Cx. vishnui* in India.

Ross River virus

Ross River fever has been reported in Australia, Fiji, Samoa, Cook Island and New Guinea. It is the most common vector-borne disease in Australia. There have been several outbreaks in Australia over the years. Some of the more recent outbreaks were in 1990–91 in the Northern Territory with 368 cases reported (Keat-Song 1993).

The mosquitoes responsible for the transfer of virus are *Aëdes vigilax*, *Aëdes camptorhynchus* during heavy rain that flood the salt marshes, and *Coquillettidia linealis*, *Culex annulirostris* (Skuse), the fresh water-breeding mosquitoes. The virus was also isolated in genus *Tripteroides* in 1992 in Rockingham, Western Australia, as well as from at least ten different species of mosquitoes.

Ross River fever is a zoonoses. There are two virus cycles: animal-vector-human and human-vector-human. The animals are native as well as animals introduced such as marsupials.

The Ross River virus can remain in the desiccation-resistant eggs of *A. vigilax* and *A. tremulus* for long periods of drought. Thus, there can be vertical transmission of the virus in arid regions when virus activity commences after heavy rains (Lindsay *et al.* 1993).

Barmah Forest virus

This is a viral infection unique to Australia, causing epidemic polyarthritis. Barmah Forest virus that has been discovered recently belongs to the alphavirus genus of the family Togaviridae. It is now known to cause infection in humans. It was known to cause clinical disease in humans in the mid-1980s on the South coast of New South Wales.

The mosquito vectors isolated were *A. vigilax* in salt marsh breeding places during high tides, and in the inland areas *A. normanensis*, *A. eidsvoldensis*, *Cx. annulirostris*, *Anopheles amictus*, *Coquillettidia linealis* and *A. camptorhynchus*.

The vertebrate hosts of Barmah Forest virus are not definitely known; however, serology studies so far suggest marsupials, such as wallabies and kangaroos as possible hosts.

The male/female ratio of the infection is 1.5:1 in Queensland and New South Wales, Australia. The age group most susceptible to the virus is between 30 and 60 years.

Murray Valley encephalitis and Kunjin fever virus

Two mosquito-borne flavivirus cause Murray Valley encephalitis (MVE) and Kunjin fever with or without encephalitis. These viruses cause Australian encephalitis (Hall *et al.* 1995). MVE is a severe and sometimes fatal illness, while Kunjin viral infection is relatively mild. The Kunjin virus is prevalent in some summers and may cause occasional encephalitis. Culex mosquitoes transmit it, the principal vector being *Cx. annulirostris*.

MVE is a severe disease in young Aboriginal children in Australia due to exposure early in life (Mackenzie *et al.* 1993). There are only a few reports of MVE occurring in Queensland (Newland *et al.* 1991). However, MVE is endemic in the Northern part of Western Australia and to a lesser extent in the top end of the Northern Territory (Smith *et al.* 1993).

Sindbis virus

Sindbis virus first isolated in Africa in 1952 and named after a village in the Nile Delta was subsequently found in Australia, Malaysia and India. Antigenic differences have been noted between the strains of Sindbis virus from Australia, Africa and Asia. The strain in Australia (C-377) is distinct from the prototype Sindbis virus (Lundstorm 1993). There are several species of mosquitoes carrying the virus but mainly *Cx. annulirostris*. The principal host is the bird. Wild cattle, wallabies, dogs and man could also be infected.

Kokobera virus

Kokobera virus was isolated in 1960 from *Cx. annulirostris* mosquitoes trapped in the Mitchell River area of north Queensland, Australia. There is occasional human infection with Kokobera virus in Queensland and New South Wales, Australia.

Gan Gan and Trubanaman virus

Sero-epidemiological study carried out on human sera from all regions of New South Wales, Australia demonstrated neutralizing antibodies in titres up to 1280 to Gan Gan and 640 to Trubanaman viruses, with a prevalence of 4.7 and 1.4% respectively (Boughton *et al.* 1990). Gan Gan virus is pathogenic for man and results in an acute polyarthritis-like illness.

Gan Gan virus was isolated in the Gan Gan Army Camp at Nelson Bay and Port Stephens Peninsula from *A. vigilax* in Australia. It was also isolated at the Mitchell River Mission. Antibodies to Trubanaman were reported in human sera, marsupials and domestic animals.

Edge Hill virus

Doggett *et al.* (1995) in their study on arbovirus and mosquito activity on the south coast of New South Wales, Australia, using monoclonal antibodies, have identified Edge Hill (EH) virus in mosquitoes. EH virus isolates were from *A. vigilax* mosquitoes, mainly in Bateman's Bay of New South Wales. One case of EH (presumptive) was reported with symptoms of arthralgia, myalgia and muscle fatigue (Aaskov *et al.* 1993). It is worthwhile requesting for EH serology when screening for fever and polyarthritis, along with other viruses such as Ross River and Barmah forest virus.

Stratford virus

Stratford virus was isolated in a lesser number of mosquitoes, also from Bateman's Bay in N.S.W. a study by Doggett *et al.* (1995). Few documented cases had similar symptoms as Edge Hill virus infection, such as fever, arthritis and lethargy (Phillips *et al.* 1993).

It is very likely that some of these cases are missed and serology be looked at for STR infection in epidemics of polyarthritis and fever.

PRESENTATION

Dengue fever uncomplicated

The incubation period is usually 5–9 days. It manifests suddenly with a temperature ~40°C, chills, headache, conjunctival infection, pain in the eyes on movement and severe muscle ache in the lumbar region, legs and joints. There is loss of appetite with nausea and vomiting. The pulse is relatively slow for the temperature (Faget's sign). Photophobia is often present with puffiness of the eyelids. The lymph glands are enlarged. Fever lasts for ~2–4 days, followed by a rapid defervescence with marked sweating. After an afebrile period of ~1 day, a second temperature follows, producing the 'saddle back' temperature curve. It is at this stage that an itchy maculopapular rash develops generally spreading from the extremities to the trunk, to involve the whole body except the face. The palms and soles may be red. The 'Dengue triad' refers to the fever, headache and rash. The second febrile period may not manifest always. Epistaxis and petechial haemorrhages without haemoconcentration is unlikely to be due to Dengue haemorrhagic fever. There is virtually no mortality rate in uncomplicated cases. Convalescence can take several weeks or months.

In the investigation of fever, rash and arthralgia, other non-arboviral infections should be considered. These include measles, rubella, Epstein-Barr virus, cytomegalovirus and protozoal infections such as toxoplasmosis. Bacterial infections should be considered in acutely ill patients such as meningococcal sepsis.

Infection with a particular Dengue serotype confers long-lasting homotypic immunity while heterotypic immunity lasts a brief period and patients are susceptible to another serotype (Thisyakorn *et al.* 1994). Dengue haemorrhagic fever is linked to maternal Dengue antibodies.

Uncomplicated Dengue fever is a mild illness in children, while older children and adults have a more severe illness with symptoms lasting for longer.

The prognosis is excellent in classic Dengue. However, recovery may be prolonged. The mortality rate is high in Dengue haemorrhagic fever and Dengue shock syndrome, especially if not treated in an intensive care unit. The mortality rate varies from 10 to 30%.

Development of profound disseminated intravascular coagulation can lead to fatal haemorrhages in patients with severe and prolonged shock.

Complicated Dengue fever

Dengue shock syndrome

This sets in once the temperature has settled, around the fifth day, during the critical period of the illness. There is a sudden drop in blood pressure coinciding with the state of shock. The extremities are cold and clammy with weak thready pulse and cyanosis of lips. The patient is quite restless. Cerebral oedema associated with Dengue shock syndrome may be fatal (Janssen *et al.* 1998).

Dengue haemorrhagic fever

Haemorrhage, purpura, petechiae or ecchymoses generally accompany shock. Haematemesis, melaena, epistaxis and subarachnoid haemorrhage may also occur during this phase. Bronchopneumonia is a secondary complication. Myocarditis and central nervous system manifestations may occur without permanent sequelae. Women may present with menorrhagia or septic shock syndrome. Mortality from Dengue haemorrhagic fever ranges from 10 to 30%. Dengue haemorrhagic fever mostly affects children, 14 years or below, who are well nourished. It is rarely seen in malnourished children (Thisyakorn and Thisyakorn 1991). However, Dengue haemorrhagic fever has been diagnosed in primary Dengue. The clinical criteria for diagnosis of Dengue haemorrhagic fever are sustained fever of acute onset, haemorrhagic manifestations, thrombocytopenia of $< 100 \times 10^9$ and rise in haematocrit of 20%.

Japanese B encephalitis

The incubation period is from 5 to 15 days. It is a febrile illness with headache, malaise and other non-specific chest and abdominal symptoms. After 2–5 days, acute encephalitic features appear with signs of meningeal irritation, altered levels of consciousness, muscular rigidity, convulsions, hemiparesis, cranial nerve palsies, cerebellar ataxia and involuntary movements. Patients with minimal neurological features improve by the sixth or seventh day and neurological features disappear at the end of the second week. Most severe cases with cardiorespiratory complications and coma die about the tenth to 12th day. Patients who recover with severe disease have late sequelae after fever has subsided and may show mental impairment, aphasia, emotional lability and permanent weakness.

Poor prognostic features are severe central nervous system (CNS) manifestations such as convulsions, a high protein content in cerebrospinal fluid (CSF), presence of the virus in CSF, low levels of JE-specific IgG, IgM in CSF and serum as well as sensory deficit (Thisyakorn and Thisyakorn 1991). The fatality rate is 25% in encephalitis and 30% of cases that recover have permanent neurological deficiencies (Beecham *et al.* 1997).

Ross River virus infection

The incubation period of Ross River fever is ~12 days (range 5–19 days). The common presentation is fever, headache, arthritis, arthralgia, followed by rash, which is more marked in the elderly. Most have more than one joint involved, the commonest being the wrists, fingers, ankles and knee, although any joint can be affected. Other clinical manifestations are stiff neck, myalgia, nausea and anorexia, lymphadenopathy, giddiness and paraesthesia. Meningitis has been rarely reported. The signs and symptoms suggestive of CNS involvement are headache, paraesthesia, stiff neck, photophobia and high fever. CSF abnormalities have not been reported except in one case where the cerebrospinal fluid showed raised white blood cells, predominantly lymphocytes, with normal glucose and protein levels. Nephritis presenting with haematuria has been reported. The period of incapacitation varies from a few days with mild subclinical infection up to 7 or 8 weeks. While most of the affected recover in 8–12 weeks, a small percentage continues to have persisting arthritic pains while others develop chronic fatigue syndrome which can persist for years (Boughton 1994). The main symptoms of these chronic cases are pain and morning joint stiffness lasting ~1–2 h.

Barmah Forest infection

The common clinical presentation is fever, headache, swollen, inflamed joints, myalgia, sweating, fatigue and weakness. Skin rash is also a predominant feature and it may be vesicular or non-vesicular. The joints commonly affected are those of the feet, ankles, hips, elbows and thumbs. The disease may last for a prolonged period, and once the acute symptoms have subsided, difficulty in concentration and irritability is commonly seen. The illness in Barmah Forest virus is probably less severe than Ross River virus illness and resolution is quicker (van Buynder et al. 1995). A few symptoms that are uncommon in other arboviruses have been observed in Barmah Forest viral infection. These include rash with blisters, vomiting and abdominal pain.

Murray Valley encephalitis and Kunjin fever virus infections

The incubation period of these two viruses is not clearly defined. However, from clinical cases of MVE, the incubation period is probably from 7 to 28 days. Subclinical infections are much more common than actual clinical illness as with most arbovirus infections. The majority of human infections with Kunjin virus follow this pattern. Non-encephalitic Kunjin virus infection is commoner than encephalitic infection. However, there is, so far, no evidence demonstrating that MVE can cause a non-encephalitic illness. The non-encephalitic form of Kunjin viral infection is very non-specific. The first case, reported in a 32-year-old female virologist, showed mild fever, lymphadenopathy and a mixed pattern with macular, papular and vesicular skin rash and the second case had a febrile illness with nausea, anorexia, lethargy and tremor.

The encephalitic patients in both diseases can be mild, moderate, severe or fatal. The disease may have a prodromal symptom that lasts 1–4 days and consists of fever, vomiting, nausea, headache and dizziness.

In mild disease patients present with headache, drowsiness, confusion, disorientation, irritability and delirium. Most recover fully with minimal residual disability such as emotional lability and impaired motor coordination. The neurological changes improve from the fifth to tenth day on.

Patients with moderately severe disease show fever and altered mental state, convulsions and neck stiffness.

Prodromal symptoms such as vomiting, diarrhoea and respiratory symptoms may precede it. The patients subsequently develop definite neurological signs. The CNS involvement may be diffuse or localized to the cerebral cortex, brain stem, cerebellar or spinal cord. The EEG shows diffuse, slow wave activity (Mackenzie et al. 1993).

Intention tremors may be generalized or confined to one side, with limb hypertonicity and hyperreflexia. The prognosis is generally good with almost full but with prolonged recovery. A few patients may have residual neurological manifestations.

The severe disease is common in children, mainly Aboriginal, and especially with Murray Valley encephalitis. They present with convulsions, headaches, fever, confusion, coma and progress to respiratory failure. There may be bilateral cranial nerve palsies with absent gag and palatal reflexes. Cerebral oedema may cause hydrocephalus. The limbs may be hypotonic initially with areflexia, followed by hypertonicity, hyperreflexia and extensor plantar reflexes. The prognosis is poor in these patients. Patients who recover may have residual disabilities such as paraplegia, quadriplegia, facial palsy, Parkinson's disease, defective cognition and speech disorders.

In fatal disease, CNS involvement can be very severe with rapid progression to coma and respiratory failure due to brain stem involvement with resultant pharyngeal paralysis and quadriplegia. The availability of intensive care facilities has reduced the mortality rate.

Australian encephalitis has no specific clinical features that distinguish it from other viral encephalitis which are common in Australia and overseas, such as herpes encephalitis, enteroviral encephalitis or post-measles, mumps and chicken pox encephalitis.

Sindbis infection

Most Sindbis virus infections are subclinical. The disease is mild compared with the South African Sindbis viral infection. Clinical presentation is fever and rash. The rash progresses from macules, papules, vesicles to pustules, mimicking chicken pox. The duration of the illness is ~4–6 days. The rash is maximally on the face, ears, palms, arms and legs. An unusual case of haemorrhagic manifestations with Sindbis infection was reported with long duration and recurrences of the rash. The reported cases of Sindbis virus in South Africa had headaches, sore throat, muscle and joint pains, lymphadenopathy and maculopapular sometimes vesicular rash. Patients with mild jaundice have been reported in Uganda and the virus has been isolated from blood.

Kokobera virus infection

Very few serologically proven cases of Kokobera virus infection have been reported. Polyarthritis is a common symptom in the reported cases. It can affect all joints. Lethargy is another common symptom that can last for some time. Fever or rash may be seen in some but not all cases. The rash desquamates but can recur, accompanied by shooting pains in the joints. Neck pain with difficulty in moving is also a feature described. Symptoms of chronic fatigue syndrome can last for long periods.

Gan Gan and Trubanaman infections

Few cases have been reported with Gan Gan and Trubanaman viral infections. In the 1983/84 outbreak of acute epidemic polyarthritis, three patients living in the Griffiths and Murrumbidgee irrigation area in New South Wales, Australia, with a febrile illness, rash, conjunctivitis, myalgia and malaise were positive for Gan Gan antibodies and negative for Ross River virus.

PATHOLOGY

Dengue fever

The Dengue virus multiplies in the regional lymph nodes and is subsequently disseminated through the lymph and blood to other organs and tissues such as the reticuloendothelial system and skin. The microscopic changes seen in the skin are perivascular oedema, mononuclear cell infiltration and swelling of the endothelial cells. Biopsies of specimen from purpuric lesion may demonstrate lymphocytic vasculitis with T-cell dominance and without immunoglobulin or complement deposition around the blood vessels (Ishikawa *et al.* 1999). Councilman or apoptotic bodies in the liver, glomerulonephritis and minor haemorrhages may be seen in the soft tissues. Pleural effusion and ascites has been noted. Fatal cases with cerebral oedema have shown loss of integrity of cerebral vascular endothelium and involvement of complement activation (Janssen *et al.* 1998).

In Dengue shock and haemorrhagic fever, there is generally a capillary leak of intravascular fluid. The exact mechanism is not clear. Activation of C_3 and C_5 components of complement results in dissociation of low molecular weight fragments of C_{3a} and C_{5a} which degranulate mast cells and release histamine. Complement activation can also initiate disseminated intravascular coagulation. The levels of C_3 correlate with the severity of the disease (Malasil 1987).

The possibility of an immune elimination response, mediated by T lymphocytes has been proposed. The T lymphocytes activate Dengue-infected monocytes that release a variety of factors such as thromboplastin, vascular permeability factor and complement activating factors.

Japanese B encephalitis

With the introduction of the virus through a mosquito bite, the virus multiplies in extraneural tissues and invades the blood stream. The virus then crosses the blood-brain barrier and may cause the pathologic changes of encephalitis. JE involves many portions of the supratentorial and infratentorial compartments including brain stem, hippocampus thalamus, basal ganglia and white matter (Abe *et al.* 1998). The brain is oedematous with focal haemorrhages in the brain tissue and in the meninges. Microscopically, there is necrosis of neurones, neuronophagia occurring in basal ganglia, cerebellum and cerebral cortex, with perivascular cuffing with mononuclear cells.

Murray Valley encephalitis – pathological changes

The brain is oedematous and shows widespread viral activity with destruction of neurones in the cerebrum, the spinal cord and in the Purkinje cells of the cerebellum. There is infiltration of the meninges with lymphocytes and perivascular lymphocyte cuffing in the brain substance. Neuronal degeneration and proliferation of glial cells are commonly seen. Glial plaques are found in the grey and white matter. In some cases, areas of the cortical neurones disappear with conspicuous gliosis. Strains of MVE virus have been isolated from brain specimens of fatal cases of encephalitis. The virus was isolated from brain tissue in patients who died within a fortnight of onset of illness but has not been isolated in those who died after a prolonged illness.

INVESTIGATIONS

Dengue fever

1. White cell count – leucopenia with reduction of polymorphs
2. Urine – albuminuria and few casts
3. Haematocrit – in Dengue shock syndrome, haematocrit > 50; platelet count < 100×10^9
4. Tourniquet test – generally positive with peticheae below the tourniquet. This sign alone is not sufficient to diagnose Dengue haemorrhagic fever
5. Coagulation disorders – abnormalities in prothrombin time, partial thromboplastin time, reduced fibrinogen factors II, V, VII, IX and X.
6. Electrolyte abnormalities – seen in Dengue shock syndrome, with metabolic acidosis, a rise in urea and creatinine occurs in renal failure
7. Serology – rise in haemagglutination inhibition test, complement fixation test and neutralizing antibody in appropriately time paired sera. Titres should be done 10–14 days after convalescence. Enzyme-linked immunosorbent assay (ELISA) for Dengue antibodies offers an improvement over previous haemagglutination tests. Culture of serum in *Aedes albopictus* C6/36 cell line with immunoperoxidase staining method in a microtitre plate format (Gleeson et al. 1999)
8. Culture – may be done by isolation of virus from serum and inoculation of cell cultures
9. Saliva for rapid screening by detecting specific immunoglobulin M antibodies. It has a high positivity rate > 80%, 5 days after onset of disease (Artimos de Oliveira *et al.* 1998)

Japanese B encephalitis

1. Leucocytosis and neutrophilia is seen in the peripheral blood
2. CSF is usually clear, with normal sugar and raised protein and a variable number of lymphocytes
3. Diagnosis can be confirmed by demonstration of JE-specific IgM antibodies in CSF as ~80% of cases will have these antibodies at the time of admission. This is measured by an ELISA

4. Haemagglutination-inhibiting and neutralizing antibodies may be demonstrated during the first week and complement-fixing antibodies during the second week. However, the ELISA test on CSF is more reliable and quicker
5. In patients who die early, the virus may be isolated from brain and viral antigen can be demonstrated by immunofluorescence. CT scan may show hypodense areas in the basal ganglia
6. Culture from serum and CSF
7. Magnetic resonance imaging – demonstrates lesions of JE as hyperdense on T2-weighted images and hypodense on T1-weighted images. Haemorrhagic transformation has been shown. However, differential considerations are broad (Abe *et al.* 1998)

Ross River fever

1. ELISA using monoclonal antibodies is a more recent test (Mackenzie *et al.* 1993) and IgM antibodies
2. Culture from serum – generally paired sera, one in acute phase and another in convalescent phase, must be tested together to obtain comparable results. The acute phase is within 7 days of onset of symptoms. Early convalescent phase is 8–14 days of onset of symptoms and late convalescent within 15–28 days of onset of symptoms.

Interpretation of serology tests

Different tests have different specificity and cross-reactivity with different arboviruses.

Generally, a 4-fold rise or fall of antibody titre is an acceptable positive diagnosis. IgM antibody assay is a more rapid diagnostic test, as it is detected in serum soon after infection with arboviruses but may remain elevated. IgG is detected later in the infection and remains for a considerable period. IgM antibodies are more specific than IgG antibodies, however, as cross-reactions may occur interpretation may be difficult. Detection of IgM antibody in cerebrospinal fluid is a very useful diagnostic tool in flavivirus encephalitis. IgM assay is done by the IgM antibody capture-ELISA (Mac-ELISA).

One has to be cautious in interpreting IgM antibody as it can remain elevated for months in flavivirus infections or for several years as in Ross River virus. Serology reports are classified into:

1. Confirmed infection with a 4-fold rise or fall in antibody titres.
2. Presumptive of infection when an acute phase serum available with IgM antibody and low titres for other tests. If the antibody titre rises in 10–14 days the classification may be changed to a confirmed case.
3. Inconclusive infection where only an acute phase serum demonstrates negative IgM and negative other tests. If a second specimen after 10–14 days shows a diagnostic rise, the classification may be changed to a confirmed case.

Barmah Forest virus infection

The investigations are similar to Ross River fever. Serological diagnosis is along the lines of all arbovirus infections as described in detail under Ross River fever. Barmah Forest virus is serologically closer to Sindbis virus than Ross River virus.

Murray Valley encephalitis and Kunjin fever

1. Haematology – white cell count is generally elevated > 15 000/mm³ with neutrophilia
2. CSF – non-purulent, protein is elevated and non-specific with white cells varying from 40 to 200 × 10⁶/litre and predominantly lymphocytic (~70%). The glucose level is normal. The virus is hardly ever isolated from the CSF
3. EEG – non-specific, generalized, slow wave activity compatible with diagnosis of encephalitis
4. Cerebral CT scan – non-specific. Occasionally there may be flattening of the lateral wall of the right ventricle suggestive of encephalitis. Other findings on cerebral CT are oedema and hydrocephalus (Mackenzie et al. 1993)
5. Serology – tests available are as described for Ross River fever and investigations are similar. However, CSF should also be examined in addition to the serum for specific MVE IgM or specific Kunjin IgM. This could be done using a blocking enzyme immunoassay (EIA), such as a monoclonal antibody. Serology/CSF should be sent to a reference laboratory
6. Culture from serum and CSF

Sindbis virus infection

Diagnosis is confirmed by serology as for other arboviruses. Blood should be sent to a standard reference centre.

Gan Gan and Trubanaman virus infection

As for other arboviral infections, demonstration of antibodies such as specific IgM, haemagglutination test as described under Ross River fever.

It is essential to include Gan Gan and Trubanaman in the panel of antigens used by arbovirus diagnostic laboratories (Boughton et al. 1990).

Kokobera virus infection

For serological diagnosis refer to Ross River virus infection. The serological diagnosis is based on haemagglutination-inhibition antibodies, ELISA antibody class capture-IgM, on paired serum. Monoclonal antibodies, which are specific for KOK, have been identified, and can be applied to arboviral surveillance (Hall et al. 1991).

TREATMENT

Dengue fever

- The management of classic Dengue is symptomatic. Acetaminophen is prescribed for the fever with plenty of oral fluids and rest
- Management of Dengue shock syndrome and haemorrhagic fever is more complicated. The patients should be treated in intensive care setting. They should be monitored for pulse, blood pressure, haematocrit, coagulation studies, renal function, urine output and arterial blood gases
- In Dengue shock syndrome, IV colloids or crystalloids are indicated to maintain a normal blood pressure. In countries where this complication is seen, proper hydration from the beginning is important in all cases of Dengue fever
- Oxygen should be administered to patients in shock and haemorrhage. The acid-base status should be monitored, as there is both respiratory alkalosis and metabolic acidosis. Sodium

- bicarbonate should be administered in profound acidosis
- In case of disseminated coagulation and intractable bleeding fresh blood, platelets and fresh frozen plasma is indicated and IV infusion of heparin after consultation with the haematologist
- There is no beneficial effect from corticosteroids
- Once the haematocrit is ~40%, one should be cautious of fluid overload, as fluid is absorbed from the interstitial compartment during recovery. A drop in haematocrit with good maintenance of blood pressure is not a sign of haemorrhage

Japanese B encephalitis

- There is no specific antiviral drug that is beneficial. Treatment is mainly supportive. Patients with serious disease should be treated in an intensive care setting
- There is no beneficial effect from corticosteroids (Hoke *et al*. 1992)
- Interferon-α has been used in Thailand with encouraging results

Ross River fever and Barmah Forest virus infection

- Treatment is only symptomatic, with rest, adequate fluids, antipyretic agents and anti-inflammatory agents for arthritis

Murray Valley encephalitis and Kunjin encephalitis

- Treatment of Australian encephalitis is symptomatic. Patients with Australian encephalitis should be treated in an intensive care unit to maintain the airways. Some patients may require intubation, artificial respiration or even tracheostomy
- Corticosteroids have been used to alleviate intracranial pressure
- Acutely ill patients require monitoring of blood gases and electrolytes
- Watch out for bacterial complications in the lung and urinary tract and prophylactic antibiotics

may be used. Patients who are comatosed or have brainstem involvement require IV fluids
- The mortality rate in severe cases can only be reduced by life support

Sindbis, Kokobera, Gan Gan, Trubanaman, Edge Hill and Stratford virus infections

Treatment is symptomatic.

PROPHYLAXIS

Dengue fever

Reducing the vector population, by eliminating breeding sites and use of insecticides should prevent outbreaks of Dengue fever. At present there is no proper vaccine available. The vector of Dengue virus was eradicated from the Northern Territory of Australia in the 1950s. Vigilant entomological surveillance has prevented reintroduction of the mosquito (Communicable Disease Bulletin 1994).

Surveillance of the mosquito *A. aegypti* has been assessed by two indices. The Breteaux Index (BI) refers to the number of containers breeding *A. aegypti* per 100 houses, ascertained by house-to-house survey. The World Health Organisation considers a BI > 5 as the hypothetical lower limit required for the transmission of yellow fever, a limit also applied to Dengue fever (Communicable Disease Bulletin 1994). The Premise Condition index is a score from 3 to 9 assigned to properties based on a relative condition of the house and yard and on the degree of shade. A high score is assigned to a property with dilapidated house, untidy yard and much tree shade (Tun-Lin *et al.* 1995). Analysis of Dengue fever spread in French Polynesia confirmed that Dengue transmission occurs primarily in the house. Therefore control campaigns should incorporate insecticide spraying and systematic daily use of insecticides in homes (Dopans *et al.* 1998).

Japanese B encephalitis

Immunization of all people at risk. Primary immunization consists of 3 doses of 1.0 ml each over 3 years given subcutaneously on days 0, 7 and 30. Children 1–3 years should have 0.5 ml on days 0, 7 and 30. If no contraindications booster dose of 1.0 ml (0.5 ml for children) may be given after 2 years. Adverse reactions to the vaccine have been reported, more common in those who have had other vaccines within a 1–9-day period, rather than concurrent with JE vaccine and in those consuming large amounts of alcohol within 48 h after vaccination (Tilman 1994). Therefore, concurrent administration of other vaccines and avoidance of alcohol after vaccination is recommended (Robinson *et al.* 1995). Because of adverse reactions to the vaccine, the Commonwealth of Australia withdrew the vaccine at one time. Pseudoephedrine containing drugs should not be used (Franklin 1999). For travellers to countries where JE is prevalent, the National Health and Medical Research Council in Australia recommends vaccination if they spend 1 month or more in rural areas or 12 months or more in urban areas.

Preventive measures include public health measures such as vector control and protection of animal reservoirs, and measures to prevent mosquito bites, such as use of insect repellents, proper clothing, footwear and insecticide impregnated mosquito nets. Immunization of pigs has been advocated. Larvicides such as *S*-methoprene pellets and insecticides to kill adult mosquitoes such as pyrethrum preparation (Drift) are advocated.

Ross River fever

Mosquitoes transmit the arboviruses, hence mosquito control measures such as effective water drainage and larval control is essential as an important public health measure. In an impending epidemic, control measures should be taken early.

Travellers should take personal preventive measures such as wearing proper clothing and using insect repellents such as 20% diethyltoluamide (DEET). DEET should not be used on very small children, as high levels of DEET causes neurological symptoms. Mosquito nets impregnated with mosquito repellents used indoors after dusk can, to a large extent, prevent being bitten by mosquitoes.

Surveillance of arbovirus infections by using human sentinels is a new public health system in operation (Weinstein 1994). The antibodies in humans are monitored for Ross River virus. Surveillance of arbovirus infections can be done by using sentinel chicken flocks. These are bled four times a year for antibody conversion rates as determined by the haemagglutination tests.

Barmah Forest virus infection

Prevention and surveillance are along lines similar for all arboviral infections as described in the chapter on Ross River fever. Public awareness of arboviral infections and their prevention should be stressed, as such infections can affect not only tropical Australia, but also the more temperate regions.

Murray Valley encephalitis and Kunjin fever

Personal care should be taken by visitors to prevent mosquito bites where Australian encephalitis has been described. Construction of homes in such areas should include adequate screening against mosquitoes. Awareness of the mosquito-borne virus and better methods of recognition will require research into the incidence of both apparent and clinically significant illness. Surveillance of sentinel chickens converting to positive Murray Valley encephalitis serology which were negative is a warning sign for occurrence of human cases in the same region.

REFERENCES

Aaskov JG, Phillips DA, Weimers MA. Possible clinical infection with Edge Hill virus. *Transactions of the Royal Society of Tropical Medicine and Hygiene* 1993; **87**: 452–453

Abe T, Kojima K, Shoji H. Japanese encephalitis. *Journal of Magnetic Resonance Imaging* 1998; **8**: 755–761

Artimos de Oliveira S, Rodrigues CV, Camacho LA *et al.* Diagnosis of Dengue infection by detecting specific immunoglobulin M antibodies in saliva samples. *Journal of Virology Methods* 1998; **77**: 81–86

Beecham HJ, Pock AR, May LA *et al.* A cluster of severe reactions following improperly administered Takeda Japanese encephalitis vaccine. *Journal of Travel Medicine* 1997; **4**: 8–10

Boughton CR, Hawkes RA, Naim HM. Arbovirus infection in humans in New South Wales. Seroprevalence and pathogenicity of certain Australian Bunyaviruses. *Australia and New Zealand Journal of Medicine* 1990; **20**: 51–55

Boughton CR. Arboviruses and disease in Australia. *Medical Journal of Australia* 1994; **160**: 27–28

Doggett S, Russell R, Cloonan M *et al.* Arbovirus and mosquito activity on the South Coast of New South Wales 1994–95. *Communicable Diseases Intelligence Australia* 1995; **19**: 473–475

Dopans X, Roche C, Murgue B *et al.* Possible Dengue sequential infection: Dengue spread in a neighbourhood during 1996/97 Dengue-2 epidemic in French Polynesia. *Tropical Medicine and Internal Health* 1998; **11**: 868–871

Franklin QJ. Sudden death after typhoid and Japanese encephalitis vaccine in a young female taking pseudoephedrine. *Military Medicine* 1999; **164**: 157–159

Gagnon SJ, Ennis FA, Rothman AL. Bystander target cell lysis and cytokine production by Dengue virus – specific human CD_4 (+)cytotoxic T-lymphocyte clones. *Journal of Virology* 1999; **73**: 3623–3629

Gleeson C, McBride J, Norton R. Culture-amplified detection of Dengue virus from serum in an outbreak of Dengue fever. *Journal of Medical Virology* 1999; **57**: 212–215

Hall RA, Broom AK, Hartnell AC *et al.* Immunodominant epitopes on the NS1 protein of MVE, and KUN viruses serve as targets for blocking ELISA to detect virus specific antibodies in sentinel animal serum. *Journal of Virology Methods* 1995; **51**: 201–210

Hall RA, Burgess GW, Kay BH *et al.* Monoclonal antibodies to Kunjin and Kokobera viruses. *Immunology and Cell Biology* 1991; **69 (pt 1)**: 47–49

Hoke CH, Vaughan DW, Nisalak A *et al.* Effect of high dose dexamethasone on the outcome of acute encephalitis due to Japanese encephalitis virus. *Journal of Infectious Diseases* 1992; **165**: 631–637

Ishikawa H, Okada S, Katayama I *et al.* A Japanese case of Dengue fever with lymphocytic vasculitis. *Journal of Dermatology* 1999; **26**: 29–32

Janssen HL, Bienfait HP, Jansen A *et al.* Fatal cerebral oedema associated with primary Dengue infection. *Journal of Infectious Diseases* 1998; **36**: 344–346

Keat-Song T, Whelan PI, Patel MS *et al. Medical Journal of Australia* 1993; **158**: 522–525

Lindsay MD, Broom AK, Wright AE *et al.* Ross River virus isolations from mosquitoes in arid regions of Western Australia: implication of vertical transmission as a means of persistence of the virus. *American Journal of Tropical Medicine and Hygiene* 1993; **49**: 686–696

Lundstrom JD, Vene S, Saluzzo JF *et al.* Antigenic comparison of Ockelbo virus isolates from Sweden, and Russia with Sindbis virus isolates from Europe, Africa and Australia. Further evidence for variation among alpha virus. *American Journal of Tropical Medicine and Hygiene* 1993; **49**: 531–537

Mackenzie JS, Broom AK, Calisher CH *et al.* Diagnosis and reporting of arbovirus infections in Australia. *Communicable Diseases Intelligence, Australia* 1993: **17**: 202

Malasil P. Complement and Dengue haemorrhagic fever shock syndrome. *South East Asian Journal of Tropical Medical Public Health* 1987; **18**: 316–320

Newland J, Phillips D, Wiemers M *et al.* Murray Valley encephalitis virus infections in Queensland. *Communicable Disease Intelligence, Australia* 1991; **15**: 447–448

Northern Territory Communicable Disease Bulletin, Australia 1994; **2**: 17

Phillips DA, Sheridan J, Aaskov JG *et al.* Epidemiology of arbovirus infection in Queensland 1989–92. In Uren MF, Kay BH (ed.), *Arbovirus Research Australia, Proceedings of the Sixth Symposium 1992*, 7–11 December, Brisbane. Brisbane: Queensland Institute of Medical Research, 1993, 245–248

Robinson P, Ruff T, Kass R. Australian care-control study of adverse reactions to Japanese encephalitis vaccine. *Journal of Travel Medicine* 1995; **2**: 159–164

Rocco IM, Barboas MC, Kanomata EH. Simultaneous infection with Dengue 1 and 2 in a Brazilian patient. *Review Institute Medical Tropico Sao Paulo* 1998; **40**: 151–154

Smith D, Mackenzie JS, Broom D *et al.* Preliminary report of Australian encephalitis in Western Australia and the Northern Territory 1993. *Communicable Diseases Intelligence, Australia* 1993; **17**: 209–210

Thisyakorn U, Thisyakorn C. Diseases caused by arboviruses – Dengue haemorrhagic fever and Japanese B encephalitis. *Medical Journal of Australia* 1994; **160**: 22

Thisyakorn U, Thisyakorn C. Studies on flavivirus in Thailand. In Miyaki, KT, Ishikawa E (eds), *Progress in Clinical Biochemistry*. Proceeding of the 5th Asian Pacific Congress of Clinical Biochemistry, 1991; 29 September-4 October

Tilman AR. Japanese B encephalitis vaccine. Time for reappraisal? [Letter]. *Medical Journal of Australia* 1994; **161**: 511

Tun-Lin W, Kay BH, Barnes A. Understanding productivity, a key to *Aëdes* (Stegomyia) *aegypti* (Linnaeus) Diptera (Chlicidae) immatures in Queensland with special reference to improved surveillance. *Commercial Disease Intelligence* 1995; **19**: 366–369. Dissertation, University of Queensland, Brisbane, 1992

Van Buynder P, Sam G, Russell R *et al.* Barmah Forest virus epidemic on the South Coast of New South Wales. *Communicable Diseases Intelligence, Australia* 1995; **19**: 188–191

Weinstein P, Worswick D, MacIntyre A *et al.* Human sentinels for arbovirus surveillance and regional risk classification in South Australia. *Medical Journal of Australia* 1994; **160**: 494–519

49

Rabies

Microbiology	Pre-exposure Prophylaxis (Primary)
Presentation	Post-exposure Prophylaxis
Pathology	Immunization in Pregnancy
Investigations	Side Effects of Immunization
Treatment	**Prevention**
Immunization	**References**

Oh Lord, don't stay away from me!
Come quickly to my rescue!
Save me from the sword;
Save my life from these dogs.

(Psalm 22: 19, 20)

Three thousand years after the Psalmist prayer, physicians still have no cure for the victims of rabies. Rabies is one of the oldest known diseases and man has been combating it for many centuries. Rabies in Latin means 'rage' or 'madness'. With the increase in the modern day worldwide travel, physicians all over the world should have an understanding of the disease rabies and its prevention. They should be able to advise travellers on immunization when indicated or to follow up on immunization commenced overseas, on their return home.

MICROBIOLOGY

Rabies is worldwide except in a few countries. With law enforcement, it has failed to get a foothold in countries like Australia and Hawaii. In developed countries, by proper public health measures, it has almost been completely wiped out in humans. Nevertheless, it is a serious public health problem in South East Asia, Philippines and in tropical South America. Rabies kills > 25 000 people each year in India and almost half a million people have received prophylaxis after exposure each year. In parts of India, one in 500 hospital admissions is due to bites by rabid dogs. In Bangkok, one in ten dogs caught was found to carry rabies. More than three cases of rabies/100 000 persons/year were reported in India and Sri Lanka in the 1970s. According to World Health Organisation (1994), countries free of rabies in America are Bermuda and many of the Caribbean Islands (excluding Cuba, Granada, Haiti, Puerto Rico and Trinidad) and Europe are Denmark, Finland, Gibraltar, Greece, Iceland, Ireland, Malta, Monaco, Norway (excluding islands of Svalbard), Portugal, Spain (continental), Sweden and the UK.

There are two epidemiological forms of rabies, the urban and the sylvatic or wild. In the urban form unimmunized dogs or cats propagate the disease. In the sylvatic form it is propagated by bats, foxes, wolves, racoons, skunks, monkeys and mongooses. However, there can be a spill over from sylvatic to domestic forms. About 2–20% of wild carnivores in the USA are rabid and 3–20% of bats tested are positive. However, transmission to humans is extremely rare. Hence, it is important to know the enzootic statistics in a particular geographic area when a decision has to be made whether to immunize or not after exposure to rabies. The principal wildlife vectors of rabies include the mongoose and jackal in Africa, the fox in Europe, Canada, the Arctic and Sub-Arctic regions, the wolf in Western Asia and vampire bat in Latin America.

By far the commonest mode of infection in humans is through the bite of dogs in most endemic areas and in the USA rare cases occur through bites of cats. The virus does not penetrate the normal skin unless there is a break. In fact mucous membranes can transmit the virus. Rabies can also be transmitted by corneal transplants, from rabid patients, or in laboratory workers dealing with rabies virus, attendants of rabid patients, through handling of infected dog carcasses, and from bat-infested caves presumably from aerolized saliva. In Yon-An Hospital in China, of 64 patients treated for rabies, 61 were exposed to dogs and two were involved in the handling of dog carcasses used for meals in rural areas.

There is a theoretical possibility of the virus being introduced into open cuts or wounds in the skin or mucous membrane through infected secretions such as saliva through person to person.

Rabies virus belongs to the family Rhabdoviridae, which includes over 200 bullet-shaped viruses that infect plants and animals. It belongs to the genus Lyssa virus family Rhabdoviridae that includes rabies and five rabies-related viruses.

Rabies is a bullet-shaped virion with one rounded and one flat end, measuring 180×75 μm. It has a bilayered lipid envelope (derived primarily from host cell membranes) with protruding spikes, surrounding a nucleocapsid core.

During replication, the virus attaches to muscle cells via the glycoprotein spikes and enters the host cell by endocytosis. Uncoating occurs within lysosomes to release the nucleocapsid. Endoserous viral RNA-dependent RNA polymerase initiates transcription. Proteins are synthesized within the cell and the nucleocapsid is assembled, with M protein and G protein associating with the plasma membrane (and internal membranes) of the host cell as the virus buds through to create an enveloped version.

The rabies virus is a negative-stranded RNA virus and the 12 000 base-locus genome has been sequenced. It encodes five polypeptides: N (nucleocapsid, Lyssa virus group specific antigen), NS (associated with nucleocapsid), M (envelope-associated), G (glycoprotein) and L (viral polymerase). The G (glycoprotein) is the major component of surface projections, which cover the viral surface (except the flattened end). It is also highly antigenic and induces viral neutralizing antibodies. Antinucleocapsid antibodies are used in an immunofluorescent technique to identify Negri bodies and the intracellular rabies inclusions made up of nucleocapsid.

The rabies virus is thermolabile, surviving ~4 h at 4°C and 35 h at 60°C. It will survive ~24 h in moist saliva in temperate areas and may survive indefinitely when frozen at –70°C. It is inactivated by pH < 4 or > 10 detergents, quaternary enzymes, ether; oxidizing agents, desiccation, UV and X-irradiation.

Rabies is a neurotropic virus that first replicates at the site of initial bite probably in muscle cells in acetyl choline receptors. After the incubation period, it invades peripheral nerves and travels to the central nervous system by passive transport in the axoplasm at 12–24 mm/day. Nerve endings in the olfactory neuro-epithelium are easily infected and this may explain aerosol transmission in bat-infested caves or in laboratory accidents.

When the concentration of incubated virus is sufficient it enters the nervous system through unmyelinated sensory and motor terminals. If organs are secretory, the viruses would be found in the secretions such as the saliva. The virus has been demonstrated in the chromaffin cells of the adrenal medulla, epidermal cells of the skin root sheath cells of hair follicles and corneal epithelial cells. Hence, the presence of viral antigens in extraneural tissues is a potential risk to certain occupational groups where transmission is not from a bite. The antigen titres are high in the salivary glands and low in nasal glandular cells and in the adrenal gland (Balachandran and Charlton 1994). The virus has also been demonstrated in kidney, lung, liver, skeletal muscle and cornea. Once the virus is sequestered from the immune system infection can no longer be halted by immunization.

PRESENTATION

The incubation period is variable, ranging from 10 days to > 7 years, the mean is 4–8 weeks. The incubation period is determined by the ferocity of the bite, the quantity of viruses introduced, site of the bite and the host defence mechanisms. A bite on the head will have a shorter incubation period compared with a bite in the periphery. A bite in the leg will have a longer incubation than a bite in the arm. The clinical presentation of rabies is so variable and the clinical features of 'furious rabies' or clinical hydrophobia or aerophobia may not be seen in all patients. There are two clinical types of rabies. The commonest is furious rabies or classical rabies (80%) and paralytic rabies (20%).

The clinical course of 'furious' rabies passes through the stages of incubation, prodromal symptoms, neurological manifestations and coma. Prodromal symptoms are non-specific and last for 1–4 days. There may be headache, anorexia, nausea, myalgia, sore throat or gastrointestinal symptoms. In ~70% of patients there is pain, paraesthesia and pruritus at the site of the bite. This is probably secondary to multiplication of virus in the dorsal root ganglion of the sensory nerve supplying the bitten site.

At this stage, the neurological manifestations are excessive motor activity, anxiousness, agitation and uneasy behaviour. The breathing becomes rapid with sighing respiration. The patient becomes confused, has hallucinations with alternating periods of extreme aggression and extreme lucidity. Increased motor activity results in muscle spasms brought on with minimal stimulation such as a gentle touch or a mild breeze (aerophobia). If patient is brought close to a fan it stimulates immediate muscle spasm. Muscles of respiration, diaphragm, accessory muscles, pharynx and larynx go into spasms even at the thought of swallowing liquids. Hence, the term hydrophobia. It is found in ~50% of patients, there is excessive salivation and froth from the mouth due to difficulty in swallowing. Muscle spasms become generalized resulting in generalized seizures with opisthotonos and cessation of breathing. The patient experiences panic and terror during these episodes. Autonomic disturbances result in dilated pupils, excessive salivation and postural hypotension.

Clinical examination reveals weakness of one or more limbs. There may be upper motor or lower motor involvement of the brainstem, causing cranial nerve palsies and diplopia due to involvement of the ocular nerves. The temperature is generally elevated, partly due to muscle spasms. The pulse may be irregular or there is tachycardia.

Priapism and spontaneous ejaculation is secondary to involvement of amygdaloid nucleus (Dutta 1994). Pneumomediastinum is a known complication towards the end of the illness but can present early. Gagging with inspiratory muscle spasm producing interstitial leak of air causes it. The episodes of violent behaviour become less due to muscle paralysis and patient lapses into the stage of coma.

During the comatose phase, the pupils are dilated, brainstem reflexes gradually diminish with progressive deterioration in EEG responses and finally there is cessation of respiration and death.

Recovery is most unusual. However, there are a handful of case reports of patients who actually recovered from rabies. A 6-year-old boy with rabies treated in an intensive care unit had a slow recovery taking 6 months (Hatwick et al. 1972) and a 45-year-old woman where encephalitic symptoms persisted for 75 days, took 13 months for full recovery (Porras et al. 1978). In paralytic rabies the prodromal symptoms are similar to those of furious rabies. This is followed by ascending paralysis, which may be symmetric or asymmetric. Hydrophobia is generally not seen. The clinical cause is slower, up to ~1 month without intensive care management. The disease mimics Guillain-Barré syndrome or acute immune-mediated polyneuritis.

Rabies should be considered in the differential diagnosis of acute encephalitis, delirium tremens, toxic psychosis, tetanus, psychiatric disorders and hysteria. A clue to the diagnosis as opposed to other forms of viral encephalitis is the early involvement of brainstem dysfunction and rapid, downhill course. Non-rabies Lyssavirus human encephalitis from fruit bats has been reported in Australia. It causes meningoencephalitis with neuronal intracytoplasmic inclusions similar to Negri bodies of rabies (Samaratunga et al. 1998).

Tetanus can be excluded by a history of tetanus immunization. A tetanus-prone wound, presence of risus sardonicus and intermittent muscle spasms are features of tetanus. In addition, tetanus patients are quite conscious and cranial nerve involvement or brainstem dysfunction are not features of tetanus.

The differential diagnoses of paralytic rabies are Guillain-Barré syndrome, post-vaccinal neuroparalytic reactions and poliomyelitis.

PATHOLOGY

The autopsy of brain in humans and dogs shows diffuse meningoencephalitis with hyperaemia, oedema and small haemorrhages. Histologically, it resembles other viral diseases of the central nervous system with perivascular infiltration by lymphocytes and plasma cells. There is microglial infiltration with destruction of nerve cells. The ganglion cells are swollen, vacuolated with eccentric nuclei. Destruction of Purkinje cells of the cerebellum, the peripheral nerves and anterior horn cells are seen. Negri bodies are found in the cytoplasm of nerve cells, mainly in Ammon's horn, cerebral cortex, brainstem and hypothalamus. Negri bodies are lamella eosinophilic cytoplasmic inclusions. They may also be found in the endoneurocytes in the sympathetic nerves of face and in trigeminal ganglion. They may not be found in all cases of rabies and their absence does not exclude rabies. Negri bodies may not be found in dogs if they are killed prematurely.

Extraneural lesions, especially myocarditis and pancreatitis can be found. Myocarditis with round cell infiltration in ~20% of patients (Hoffman *et al.* 1992) has been reported.

INVESTIGATIONS

Definitive laboratory diagnosis depends on the detection of the rabies antigen, antibody or isolation of the virus. The materials used are highly innervated skin biopsies of the back of neck, saliva, corneal impression smears, brain biopsy, cerebrospinal fluid and serum.

In Australia, the samples should be sent to the Commonwealth Scientific and Industrial Research Organisation, the Australian Animal Health Laboratory, Geelong, Victoria, and outside Australia, to the US Center for Disease Control (Rabies Laboratory) in Atlanta, GA.

1. Neck skin biopsies, corneal impression smears and smears of saliva can be stained for antigen using a fluorescent antibody. The skin biopsy is positive in 50–60% of patients and may be diagnostic before serological tests are positive.
2. Brain biopsies are important to exclude a treatable condition such as Herpes simplex encephalitis. The specimens of brain are examined histologically including immunoperoxidase studies. Mouse inoculation tests, electron microscopic examination and brain neutralizing antibody tests can also be carried out.
3. Cerebrospinal fluid (CSF) or serum for antibodies. Antibodies appear in the serum between the sixth and 15th day. It appears in the CSF 1–7 days after its appearance in the serum. The tests available are neutralizing antibody, rapid fluorescent inhibition test, mouse neutralization test and ELISA test (Pandit *et al.* 1991). Antibody titres in serum using neutralizing antibody tests in patients with rabies may be as high as 1:200 to 1:100 000. Patients who have had antirabies vaccine rarely develop antibodies in CSF. From available data, serum neutralization titres > 1:5000 are seen in association with clinical rabies and not after vaccination alone. CSF shows white cells, mainly monocytes.
4. Dipstick dot enzyme immunoassay for detection of rabies antigen. This test was compared with fluorescent antibody test on brain tissue in rabies-suspected dogs, cattle, horses, cats and goat and was very reliable without false positives (Jayakumar and Padmanaban 1994).
5. Polymerase chain reaction (PCR). PCR has been used in Thailand where the incidence of rabies is high. As little as 8 pg rabies virus RNA can be detected by this technique, which has its application at busy rabies diagnostic centres as an added confirmatory test (Kamolvarin *et al.* 1993). It is very useful when the serology is positive but virus cannot be cultured.

    Inability to culture rabies in brain specimens in otherwise proved cases of rabies has been documented. This is probably due to the development of high levels of serum neutralizing antibodies (Parker and Stary 1966). This phenomenon is called autosterilization whereby the antibody neutralizes the virus.
6. White cell count is normal, slightly elevated, or very high, up to 35 000 cells/microlitre. There may be thrombocytopenia.
7. Electrolytes – owing to inappropriate secretion of antidiuretic hormone there is hyponatraemia.
8. Electroencephalograph may show wave activity consistent with diffuse encephalitis or electrical status epilepticus, poor development of normal sleep pattern and poor arousal.
9. Electrocardiographic monitoring for cardiac arrythmias.
10. Intraventricular catheter for monitoring CSF pressure and removal of CSF if required.

11. CT scan and magnetic resonance scanning shows hardly any diagnostic changes.

TREATMENT

- Patients are admitted to intensive care for management in an isolated section. The patients who have recovered are few
- Treatment of cases should be designed to maximize the chance of recovery from rabies. They are prevention of hypoxia by tracheostomy and ventilation at the first sign of respiratory compromise and careful management of the tracheostomy, monitoring arterial PO_2 and careful suctioning of trachea regularly, prevention of increases in intracranial pressure by close monitoring and shunting if required, anticonvulsants to control focal seizures and prevention of secondary infections
- There is no antiviral agent available for rabies. Human rabies immunoglobulin is of no value once the disease has progressed
- Patients caring for rabies patients must take proper precautions according to strict infectious diseases guidelines to avoid needle stick injuries and contamination of mucous membranes or wounds from patient's body fluids. They should wear protective gowns, face cover and rubber gloves
- Dog bite wounds should be attended to at the earliest opportunity. The wound should be scrubbed with soap and water for at least 20 min. Chemical agents such as 1% cetrimonium bromide or 4% benzalkonium inactivates the rabies virus, or use 40–70% alcohol or tincture of iodine. If a decision is made to treat as a post-exposure rabies case, pour the antirabies serum into and around the wound. Tetanus immunization and antibiotic cover are recommended

IMMUNIZATION

1. Passive immunization – for post-exposure is human rabies immunoglobulin (HRIG). Immunoglobulin (rabies) CSL 150 IU/ml antirabies IgG, thimerosal 0.01% concentrated sterile solution (refer to MIMS 1994)
2. Active immunization (human diploid cell vaccine) – vaccine available is Mérieux an inactivated rabies vaccine – inactivated rabies vaccine 2.5 IU/ml with neomycin 100–150 μg: 1.0 ml single dose of vial of lyophilized vaccine with accompanying diluent. The two rabies vaccines currently available in the USA are human diploid cell vaccine (HDCV) (ImovaxRabies) and rabies vaccine adsorbed (RVA)

Other preparations available are passive immunization – equine antirabies immunoglobulin. This causes serum sickness-like reaction and rarely anaphylaxis. For active immunization (vaccines) include duck embryo vaccine, purified Vero cell vaccine, purified chick embryo cell rabies vaccine (PCEC) and Fuenzalida vaccine. Purified Vero cell vaccine has been tested pre-exposure in children. Intradermal and IM comprising of three doses of either 0.1 ml intradermal or 0.5 IM administered during 28 days and a booster at 1 year with satisfactory antibody levels (Sabchareon et al. 1998).

The original vaccines were made from infected brain tissues. They need to be given daily for ~2 weeks. They are still used in developing countries because of low cost. However, side-effects occur such as peripheral neuritis, ascending myelitis due to sensitization reaction to animal brain tissue so that they are no longer used in developed countries and should be avoided if possible.

Pre-exposure prophylaxis (primary)

Pre-exposure immunization is recommended for people at high risk such as veterinarians, laboratory workers handling rabies virus, cave explorers and persons handling animal carcasses in endemic areas of rabies.

Three injections of HDCV or RVA (active immunization) is recommended the first (day 1), the second 8 days later (day 9) and the third 28 days later (day 29). The injections are given IM to the Deltoid in a 1 ml dose of the vaccine, or 0.1 ml HDCV or RVA in skin over the deltoid area on days 1, 9 and 28 (Dreeson and Hanton 1998) only special intradermal syringe Imovax Rabies, 1D should be used.

Check antibody titres every 6 months in laboratory workers dealing with live rabies vaccine and in others every 2 years.

Boosters if antibody level falls is administered generally every 2 years. HDCV or RVA (1 ml) in the deltoid area IM or 0.1 ml HDCV or RVA in the skin over the deltoid region.

Do not use chloroquine with vaccine as the level of antibody does not reach the maximum response. Do not give rabies vaccine in the gluteal region due to poor absorption (Wilde *et al.* 1994).

Post-exposure prophylaxis

A decision has to be made whether post-exposure prophylaxis should be administered and, if so, as early as possible. A dog bite suffered in an endemic area should be considered serious. The WHO recommendation is to observe the animal for 10 days and if the dog appears to be ill, post-exposure prophylaxis must be carried out, the animal killed and the brain examined for rabies. It is often difficult to keep a dog under quarantine and dogs can recover from rabies and may continue to secrete the virus through saliva as chronic carriers (Wilde *et al.* 1994). Dogs have survived for a long period when their victims have died. Two immigrants to the USA died of rabies after they were bitten by their pet dog in their native countries Laos and Philippines (Smith *et al.* 1991) and the dog survived for at least 1 month. Post-exposure prophylaxis should therefore be given in all cases of bites (suspected for transmission of rabies) including contamination of mucous membranes where even minor transdermal wounds at any site have caused rabies (Wilde *et al.* 1991).

There are grey areas of possible transmission where there is a history of touching or feeding of animals where they have licked intact skin (Wilde *et al.* 1994). In these cases the decision to give a pre-exposure course of immunization should be left to the attending physician.

- Passive immunization post-exposure – the prophylaxis in full consists of a single dose of HRIG (human rabies immunoglobulin) 20 IU/kg body weight mass. Half the dose should be infiltrated to the wound and half given IM (NHMRC Australia 1994). Prophylaxis should be commenced immediately and within 72 h for the best results (Groleau 1992) but may be given up to the eighth day (NHMRC Australia 1994). This is recommended in the USA. Rabies immunoglobulin should not be given in previously vaccinated people and a documented history of antibody response
- Active immunization post-exposure – the vaccine recommended is HDCV Mérineux given in

a 1 ml dose to the deltoid IM at intervals of 1, 3, 7, 14 and 28 days. Those previously vaccinated and documented history of antibody response 1.0 ml HDCVA is given IM on days 1 and 3.
In children, anterolateral aspect of thigh is acceptable. If HRIG is administered, use the other arm for HDCV.

- If a patient returns to their home, and within 10 days or less, it is recommended that the antirabies antibody level be determined and full course of five doses of HDCV or RVA be given according to schedule and for those returning after 10 days, if the antibody titre shows active immunity, then two booster doses should be given 12 days apart (NHMRC Australia 1994) or else the full course. Those who show active immunity HRIG is not essential
- Pre-exposure vaccinated people exposed to rabies require two doses of HDCV or RVA on days 1 and 3, even though rabies neutralizing antibody is present. If antibodies are very low or absent, they require a full course
- If the person did not receive the full course of HDCV or RVA pre-exposure or there is an uncertainty of the immune states, full course of HDCV or RVA plus HRIG (before 8 days) is recommended. In the meantime, antibody level should be assessed
- Many countries follow the recommendations of the WHO which has approved the use of a number of tissue culture-derived rabies vaccine in the five dose IM regimens and two abbreviated post-exposure regimens that reduce the cost of post-exposure treatment. One, an IM regimen on days 1 and 9, and 21 or intradermal regimen 0.1 ml on days 1, 4, 7 and booster 0.1 ml on days 30 and 90. The USA has not approved abbreviated regimen

Immunization in pregnancy

There is no contraindication for immunization in pregnancy following a rabid animal bite. Two patients were reported to be immunized with Vero cell vaccine and fuenzalide vaccine respectively in second and third trimester of pregnancy without any complications (Figueros *et al.* 1994). Twenty-four patients who were pregnant and subsequently exposed to rabies virus were immunized with equine rabies immunoglobulin and/or purified Vero cell vaccine or duck embryo vaccine, and one case with human rabies immunoglobulin and human diploid cell vaccine, without any adverse effects (Chabola *et al.* 1991).

Side-effects of immunization

HDCV

Side-effects to HDCV are uncommon. Hypersensitivity reactions such as urticaria can occur and mild systemic reactions such as nausea, headache and fever in a small percentage of people. Neurological illness resembling Guillain-Barré syndrome has occurred but has resolved completely in 12 weeks (Boe *et al.* 1980).

Booster doses can rarely produce immune complex-like reactions associated with angioedema and arthritis. It is not life threatening (NHMRC Australia 1994).

Human rabies immunoglobulin

The side-effects are at the injection site pain and fever. Very rarely angioedema and anaphylaxis can occur. Adequate precautions should be taken for those who have had allergic manifestations in the past. Immunization should not be discontinued because of rare side-effects (Groleau 1992), as patients' risk of developing rabies must be weighed carefully. Adequate precautions to treat any serious side-effects should be undertaken.

Equine rabies immunoglobulin

There are serious adverse reactions such as anaphylaxis and sensitivity reactions.

Rabies vaccines prepared from nerve tissue

Nerve tissue vaccines may cause serious average neuroparalytic complications and has a lower efficacy (5–50%) (Centre for Disease Control 1991).

Other non-human diploid cell vaccines

Other non-human diploid cell vaccines such as duck embryo rabies vaccine is rarely associated with neurological complications, an incidence of 0.3/10 000 (Hatwick

et al. 1972). Encephalitogenic protein in vaccines, if present, can produce allergic encephalitis in animals.

PREVENTION

Avoid all direct animal contact with dogs and cats while overseas in countries where rabies is endemic. People at high risk should have pre-exposure prophylaxis. Medical staff attending on rabies patients should take full infectious diseases precautions. In endemic countries, immunization of dogs and cats should be enforced by law and the immunization status should continue.

Rigid enforcement of quarantine regulations and control of domestic dog population. Australia has strict quarantine regulations to maintain its rabies-free status. There are only certain countries from where one can import dogs and cats such as Hawaii or the UK, and there is a quarantine period of 9 months after importation. The Australian Quarantine and Inspection Services permits importation of controlled urban pets from areas where rabies is prevalent provided immunization is done 6 months before importation and should have rabies antibody of not < 0.15 IU/ml within 30 days before export and also 120 days of quarantine.

The public should be educated about handling the carcasses of stray dogs. Oral vaccination of animals at risk (enzootic) has been a success in Europe where it has contributed to the elimination of fox rabies (Blancou 1993).

Post-exposure prophylaxis together with the presently available non-toxic immunoglobulins and vaccines has contributed to the prevention of rabies developing in exposed persons. Further, experimental research is being conducted with rifampicin. Rifampicin (30–70 mg/kg) inhibited reproduction of the fixed rabies virus in the brain of infected animals. The drug did not interfere with synthesis of virus neutralizing antibodies after vaccination. Rifampicin and antirabies gammaglobulin had a marked synergistic effect. Hence, the use of rifampicin during incubation period with antirabies immunoglobulin and vaccine may be worth considering at an early stage of the infection.

REFERENCES

Australian Immunization Procedures Hand Book 1994; 5 (NHMRC): 93–95

Balachandran A, Charlton K. Experimental rabies infection of non-nervous tissues in skunks (*Mephitis mephitis*) and foxes (*Vulpes vulpes*). *Veterinary Pathology* 1994; **31**: 93–102

Blancou J. Recent development in the epidemiology and prevention of rabies. *Bulletin de l'Academie Nationale de Medicine* 1993; **177**: 1221–1231

Boe E, Nyland H. Guillain-Barré syndrome after vaccination with human diploid cell rabies vaccine. *Scandinavian Journal of Infectious Diseases* 1980; **12**: 231

Centres for Disease Control. Rabies prevention – United States 1991, recommendations of the Immunisation Practices Advisory Committee (ACIP). *Morbidity Mortality* 1991; **40**: 1–19

Chabola S, Williams M, Amunta R *et al.* Confirmed rabies exposure during pregnancies. Treatment with human rabies immunoglobulin and human diploid cell vaccine. *American Journal of Medicine* 1991; **91**: 423–424

Dreeson DW, Hanlon CA. Current recommendations for the prophylaxis and treatment of rabies. *Drugs* 1998: 801–809

Dutta JK, Dutta TK, Das AK. Human rabies – modes of transmission. *Journal of the Association of Physicians of India* 1992; **40**: 322–324

Dutta JK. Rabies presenting with priapism [Letter]. *Journal of the Association of Physicians of India* 1994; **45**: 430

Figueros DR, Oritz IFJ, Arredondo GJL. Post exposure antirabies prophylaxis in pregnant women. *Ginecologia y Obstetricia de Mexico* 1994; **62**: 13–16

Groleau G. Rabies environmental emergencies. *Emergency Medicine Clinics of North America* 1992; **10**: 361–368

Hatwick MAW, Thomas T, Weis MD *et al.* Recovery from rabies. A case report. *Annals of Internal Medicine* 1972; **76**: 931–942

Hoffman P, Bourhy H, Michiels JF *et al.* Rabies encephalomyelitis with myocarditis and pancreatitis. Report on a case recently imported into France. *Annales de Pathologie* 1992; **12**: 339–346

Jayakumar R, Padmanaban VD. A dipstick dot enzyme immunoassay for detection of rabies antigen. *Internal Journal of Microbiology, Virology, Parasitology and Infectious Diseases* 1994; **280**: 382–385

Kamolvarin N, Tirawatnpong T, Rattanasiwamoke R *et al.* Diagnosis of rabies with nested primers. *Journal of Infectious Diseases* 1993; **167**: 207–210

Pandit V, Joseph LW, Veerabandran JS *et al.* Rapid fluorescent focus inhibition test for rabies. Antibody estimation using murine neuroblastoma cell line. *Indian Journal of Medical Research* 1991; **93**: 67–70

Parker RI, Stary RK. Development of rabies inhibiting substance in skunks infected with rabies. *Public Health Review* 1966; **81**: 941–944

Porras C, Barboza JJ, Eduardo FDVM *et al.* Recovery from rabies in man. *Annals of Internal Medicine* 1978; **85**: 44–48

Sabchareon A, Chantavanich P, Pasuralertsakul S *et al.* Persistence of antibodies in children after intradermal or intramuscular administration of pre-exposure primary and booster immunisation with purified Vero cell rabies vaccine. *Paediatric Infections and Diseases Journal* 1998; **11**: 1001–1007

Samaratunga H, Searle JW, Hudson N. Non-rabies Lyssavirus human encephalitis from fruit bats: Australia bat Lyssavirus (pteropid Lyssavirus) infection. *Neuropathology Applied Neurobiology* 1998: 331–335

Smith JS, Fishbein DB, Rupprecht CE *et al.* Unexplained rabies in three immigrants in USA. *New England Journal of Medicine* 1991; **324**: 205–211

Wilde H, Chutivongse S, Hemachudha T. Rabies and its prevention. *Medical Journal of Australia* 1994; **160**: 83–87

Wilde H, Chutivongse S, Tepsumethanon W *et al.* Rabies in Thailand – 1990. *Review of Infectious Diseases* 1991; **13**: 644–652

VIII

Emergency Room Presentation of Tropical Infectious Diseases

INTRODUCTION

There are three categories of patients that present to an emergency department with parasitic or tropical diseases.

1. Patients who have acquired an endemic disease in one's own country, e.g. Ross River fever, melioidosis, Murray Valley encephalitis, Donovanosis as in Australia.
2. Migrants who have acquired the disease in their country of origin, e.g. schistosomiasis, leishmaniasis, *Loa loa*, onchocerciasis, as in African countries.
3. The traveller who acquired the infection abroad, e.g. malaria, typhoid fever or diarrhoea.

Patients presenting to the emergency room should be assessed clinically and a decision should be made with reference to the urgency of the case so that adequate investigations and treatment are commenced accordingly. This is not different from the normal triaging process in an emergency room.

The diseases described in detail in this book may be broadly classified according to the severity of the disease (Table 1). Some of the parasitic diseases are not lethal but it can affect one organ that will cause life-long disability such as parasitic diseases of the eye, e.g. toxocariasis, onchocerciasis (river blindness) and acanthamoebic keratitis. In some diseases that have been present for some time, the presentation can become more acute, e.g. ruptured hydatid cyst of the liver. For more detailed information on the clinical conditions mentioned refer to appropriate chapters in the text. This chapter deals with presentation in emergency room, with a guide to assessment, investigation and treatment.

Severity of parasitic and tropical diseases (graded 1–5) (Table 1)

1. Life-threatening, e.g. falciparum cerebral malaria, plague, visceral leishmaniasis and rabies
2. Acute infection – may be lethal if treatment not promptly given, e.g. visceral leishmaniasis, typhoid, cholera, dengue haemorrhagic fever, encephalitis, melioidosis, trichinosis, scrub typhus and plague
3. Acute infections generally not life-threatening, e.g. Ross River fever, Barmah Forest fever, uncomplicated dengue fever
4. Chronic debilitating disease, e.g. helminthic diseases, leprosy, schistomiasis, tuberculosis and lymphatic filariasis
5. Chronic non-debilitating disease, e.g. skin infections, pediculosis and scabies

A detailed description is given in the text and these life-threatening diseases are described briefly (Table 2).

PROTOZOAL INFECTIONS (LIFE THREATENING)

Malaria

Malaria is the most common life-threatening parasitic infection seen in some parts of the world. It may be missed at the initial presentation. There may be a history of malarial prophylaxis that has been inadequate or inappropriate for that particular geographical area, or the patient's compliance has not been satisfactory. All patients who return from overseas where malaria is endemic and present with fever should be screened for malaria.

Visceral leishmaniasis

Visceral leishmaniasis should be suspected in individuals who have travelled from or resided in endemic areas. It may present as fever, anorexia, weight loss, hepatosplenomegaly, lymphadenopathy, anaemia, darkening of feet, hands and face. The onset of the disease may be acute or insidious. Frank visceral leishmaniasis may be fatal in a few weeks. However, it may be insidious in onset in some infectious species. Definitive diagnosis of visceral leishmaniasis or Kala-azar is made by demonstration of the amastigotes in lymph nodes, liver biopsy or bone marrow biopsy. Splenic aspirates yield a high rate of positive specimens but at considerable risk to the patients.

Trypanosomiasis

Trypanosomiasis may be acquired in Central and West Africa. The presentation is generally that of a chancre at the site of bite which resolves spontaneously in a few days. This is followed by fever, lymphadenopathy, commonly of the posterior cervical lymph nodes (Winterbottom's sign) and erythematous rash, suggestive of erythema multiform, lasting a few hours. This is followed by the 'sleeping sickness' stage due to invasion of the central nervous system, which is more rapid in *Rhodesiense trypanosomiasis*. The clinical features are those of meningoencephalitis which progresses to coma and death.

Diagnosis is made by demonstration of trypanomastigotes that are highly infectious and those handling the specimens should take special precautions. The parasite may be detected in lymph node aspirates, blood or cerebrospinal fluid. Multiple daily examinations of the blood may be necessary.

Primary amoebic encephalitis

Primary amoebic encephalitis (PAM) is caused by *Naegleria fowleri*. It is a fulminant and rapidly fatal disease that mainly affects young adults and children. Generally the patients are healthy and the symptoms are fever, vomiting, neck stiffness, mental confusion and coma. PAM may resemble bacterial meningitis. The nasopharyngeal mucosa may show ulceration. Diagnosis is made by exclusion. A definitive diagnosis can be made if amoebae are identified in the cerebrospinal fluid. Computed tomography with contrast may

demonstrate basal arachnoiditis that is highly suggestive of *N. fowleri* infection.

Acanthamoeba meningoencephalitis

Acanthamoeba meningoencephalitis is more a subacute or chronic disease. The primary site may be the lung or skin and transmission through water is less well established. It also causes keratitis. Diagnostic procedures are similar to *N. fowleri* encephalitis. Cysts may also be seen in the cerebrospinal fluid.

NON-PARASITIC TROPICAL DISEASES (LIFE THREATENING)

These tropical diseases are caused by bacterial, viral or rickettsial organisms. Infections indigenous to Australia are Murray Valley encephalitis and Kunjin virus encephalitis. Both of these have been reported in the Northern Territory and are caused by flaviviruses (Table 3). Dengue haemorrhagic fever seen in some parts of South East Asia may sometimes be a life-threatening condition.

Dengue fever

Dengue haemorrhagic fever is caused by one or more of the four viruses Dengue 1, 2, 3 or 4. They are different serotypes with no cross immunity (Russell 1993). All four dengue serology types can cause dengue haemorrhagic fever and dengue shock syndrome. Dengue haemorrhagic fever in Asia is a childhood disease. The illness is abrupt in onset with fever, pharyngitis, petechiae in the forehead and distal extremities. Haematemesis, melaena, shock and coma are poor prognostic signs. Fatalities occur on the fourth or fifth day. The illness is quite different from ordinary dengue fever, which is non-fatal. The platelet count is low. It is an immunologically mediated disease and diagnosis is made by serological examination, such as immunoblot kit or IgM ELISA (Kuno *et al.* 1998). Cerebral oedema may be fatal (Misra *et al.* 1998).

Yellow fever

Yellow fever is very rarely seen nowadays as a result of successful immunization of travellers to endemic areas such as some parts of South America and Africa. The illness manifests as high fever and marked bradycardia

(Faget's signs), epistaxis and gingival bleeding. In the more malignant form, the manifestations are copious haemorrhage, jaundice and delirium. Death occurs in such cases on the fourth or fifth day. Diagnosis is made by the travel history and serology where yellow fever IgM antibodies and antigens are detected by the ELISA method.

Murray Valley encephalitis

Murray Valley encephalitis may be fatal and residual disability may persist in those that recover.

Japanese B encephalitis

The terminology is now revised to Japanese encephalitis. The mortality rate is high and the clinical manifestations are fever, headache or encephalitis. Diagnosis is made by a positive travel history. The prognosis depends on age, degree of coma, decerebration or decortication, cerebrospinal fluid changes and neurophysiological changes (Janssen et al. 1998).

Cholera

The clinical presentation is sudden with painless, watery diarrhoea associated with very large fluid loss. The stools described as 'rice water' stools are slightly cloudy with no blood and have a sweet, inoffensive odour. The symptoms correspond to the quantity of volume depletion. Diagnosis is made from the history and identification of the organism in the stools.

Plague

Travel during the incubation period to or from an endemic area and exposure to rodents is significant points in the history. The clinical presentation depends on the type of plague:

1. Bubonic plague presents with painful, enlarged lymph glands, fever, rigors, cutaneous petechiae as well as abdominal symptoms such as pain and bloody diarrhoea.
2. Septicaemic form presents with fever, chills, rigors, headache, vomiting and delirium.

Death occurs as early as 48 h after development of symptoms without treatment.

Pneumonic plague with multilobular consolidation presents with rapidly progressive cough, fever and tachypnoea. It is rapidly progressive, complicated by adult respiratory distress syndrome, which is often fatal. Diagnosis is made from the history. In bubonic plague, diagnosis is made by needle aspiration of lymph nodes with fluorescent antibody staining for the organism and in other types, cultures of blood, sputum, cerebrospinal fluid, staining and serology. Microscopic examination of peripheral blood buffy coat smear may demonstrate the organism.

Rabies

Rabies is invariably a fatal disease. The incubation period of rabies ranges from 10 days up to 7 years. Hence, there is always the possibility of the disease in a person who was bitten by a rabid dog many years previously. During the prodromal phase there may be fasciculations and paraesthesia at the site of inoculation of the virus. Transmission can occur through corneal transplants and from aerosols in caves contaminated by bat rabies virus. During the encephalitic stage there is hyperexcitability with increased motor activity to the slightest stimulation such as touch, fanning or noise. There is difficulty in swallowing and even the thought of drinking (hydrophobia) causes involuntary contraction of the muscles of respiration and pharynx. The mental status varies from confusion to lucid intervals. Diagnosis is made from a history of exposure and the clinical presentation. Serological methods are available for infected secretions such as the saliva, cerebrospinal fluid or brain biopsy.

Melioidosis

Melioidosis is the commonest fatal community acquired sepsis in the Northern Territory of Australia (Currie 1993). It can cause acute fulminant sepsis with pneumonia or may exist in a subclinical form and reactivate later. Abscesses can also form in skin deep tissues and in internal organs such as the spleen (Currie 1993). Diagnosis is made by the history and microscopic demonstration of small Gram-negative rods in exudates.

Typhoid and paratyphoid fever

Typhoid and paratyphoid fever should always be considered in a returned traveller with fever and without an obvious diagnosis, the other diseases being malaria and dengue fever. It is a relatively uncommon disease in travellers. However, if it is not diagnosed there can be complications and even a fatal outcome. The clinical presentation is that of fever, preceded by a severe headache and constipation. The spleen may be palpable. Blood shows a leukopenia. Rose spots may be present in the skin and diagnosis is made by culture of blood, urine, stools and bone marrow and by serological investigations.

Tuberculous meningitis

Tuberculous meningitis can present with headache, fever, malaise and meningism. There is often a cognitive decline which is mostly the result of miliary tuberculosis and the patient appears very ill with fever, anorexia, weight loss, night sweats and rigors. Tuberculosis should be considered in the differential diagnosis of all suspected cases of meningitis in overseas settlers from developing countries. Diagnosis is made by examination of cytocentrifuged samples of cerebrospinal fluid for acid-fast bacilli and new and quicker methods such as PCR and DNA probes.

Angiostrongylus cantonensis

A. cantonensis presents with headache and paraesthesia. Other presentations are neck stiffness, convulsions, weakness of limbs and facial paralysis. Eye involvement presents with pain and visual impairment. Diagnosis is made from a history of having eaten uncooked or partially cooked crabs, fresh water prawns, slugs and snails. Peripheral eosinophilia, eosinophils and larvae in the spinal fluid, ELISA (serologic) test for larval antibodies help to make the diagnosis.

Trichinosis

Trichinosis infection occurs by consumption of the nematode in uncooked or partly cooked pork. Often the symptoms are mild. However, with a large worm burden, gross muscle damage can affect chewing, swallowing or breathing. The most severe clinical feature is myocarditis, which can be fatal. Invasion of the central nervous system causes Trichinella encephalitis. The clue to the diagnosis is the history, a marked eosinophilia and high ESR. Muscle biopsy will confirm the diagnosis.

EOSINOPHILIA

Having excluded a life-threatening parasitic or tropical disease, one should now have a systematic approach based on symptoms and/or a laboratory finding, such as eosinophilia, which is common to a large number of parasitic diseases.

The list of parasitic diseases where eosinophilia is a characteristic feature is listed in Table 4.

Parasitic eosinophilia should be distinguished from other causes of eosinophilia such as drug induced, eosinophilic fasciitis, eosinophilic gastritis, hypereosinophilic syndrome, allergic angiitis and granulomatosis of Churge and Strauss with asthma.

IMMUNOCOMPROMISED PATIENTS

When patients present with severe, acute illnesses such as pneumonia, gastroenteritis, meningoencephalitis, the possibility of compromised immunity with an opportunistic parasitic infection must be considered. Immunocompromised patients following splenectomy, HIV patients, patients with malignant diseases, transplant patients on therapy with cytotoxic drugs, alcoholics, patients on radiotherapy and corticosteroids are all more prone to such infection.

PRESENTATION WITH NEUROLOGICAL SIGNS AND SYMPTOMS

There are some parasitic diseases that are insidious in onset, that affect the central nervous system. The presentation may be headache, convulsions, visual disturbances and localizing signs such as paralysis with cerebral manifestations. In such a clinical setting the following parasitic conditions should be considered:

Toxocariasis

The larvae can invade the central nervous system to produce granulomatous lesions. Rarely seizures or behavioural disorders may be seen. Eosinophilia is a clue to the diagnosis. Diagnosis is made by serology.

Hydatid disease

About 3% of *Echinococcus granulosus* infections can affect the central nervous system. Presentation may be headaches, epilepsy and localizing signs. Cerebral computerized tomography will demonstrate an indistinct solid mass with central necrosis and plaque-like calcification. Serology would be helpful in the diagnosis.

Cysticercosis

Cysticerci of the brain are probably the most common parasitic infection in immunocompetent patients. A common presentation is epilepsy. Adults who present with epilepsy (especially among immigrants) who have no family history of epilepsy, cysticercosis should be considered (Medina et al. 1990). Diagnosis is made by computed tomography or magnetic resonance imaging. However, it is not specific for cysticercosis. Serology and immunoblot serology for neurocysticercosis may be useful. Diagnosis is made by the demonstration of *T. solium* antigen in cerebrospinal fluid.

Toxoplasmosis

Symptoms of congenital toxoplasmosis of the central nervous system may not appear until many years later. In infants the symptoms are mental retardation, epilepsy, hydrocephalus, microcephalus and retinochoroiditis. Radiology may show cerebral calcification. Central nervous system involvement is uncommon if the infection is acquired postnatally, except in immunocompromised patients where it is usually fatal. Diagnosis is made by serology.

Schistosomiasis japonicum

Cerebral schistosomiasis is a distinct syndrome attributed to *S. japonicum*. Central nervous system involvement can produce focal neurological signs or an encephalitic picture. Computed tomography will demonstrate multiple enhancing lesions. Diagnosis is made by demonstrating ova in the faeces.

Gnathostomiasis

Gnathostoma spinigerum can rarely affect the central nervous system through larval migration along a peripheral nerve to the spinal cord and then to the central nervous system. Symptoms are epilepsy, paralysis, coma and even death. The cerebrospinal fluid is xanthochromic. There may be skin lesions. Definitive diagnosis is made by identification of the larva. A history of consuming raw fish is a useful pointer to the diagnosis.

Sparganosis

Clinical presentation is epilepsy with localizing signs such as hemi-anaesthesia or paralysis. A useful aid to diagnosis is a history of eating raw frogs, snakes, mammalian flesh or fowl. Diagnosis is made by computed tomography and magnetic resonance imaging that may demonstrate a focal lesion. Definitive diagnosis is made by demonstrating the characteristic sparganum.

Loa loa

The adult Loa (African eye worm) migrates actively in subcutaneous tissue. The loa microfilariae enter the blood stream and may be found in different organs. Patients treated with diethylcarbamazine, a drug that penetrates the blood–brain barrier, can cause destruction of microfilariae in the brain causing encephalitis (Carme *et al.* 1991).

Cerebral paragonimiasis

Cerebral invasion of the larvae is the most serious of its complications and is found in the younger age group. The cerebral manifestations are headache, nausea and vomiting, fever, epilepsy and localizing signs such as motor weakness and paralysis. The disease can be fatal. Diagnosis is made from a history of eating raw or undercooked crab or crayfish. Serology and detection of Paragonimus antigen in the cerebrospinal fluid should be looked at. Computed tomography and magnetic image resonance should be performed.

Microsporidiosis

Encephalitozoon cuniculi can affect the central nervous system. The neurological presentations are headaches, fever, vomiting and convulsions. There may be altered levels of consciousness. The disease can affect immunocompromised patients and diagnosis is made by isolation of spores in cerebrospinal fluid and urine.

Trypanosomiasis

Trypanosomes invade the central nervous system to produce the stage of sleeping sickness and behavioural changes such as apathy, confusion, somnolence and fatigue, eventually leading to coma and death if untreated.

Trichinosis

Neurological manifestations are present in ~10–20% of patients with trichinosis. In untreated patients mortality rate is ~50% (Nickolic *et al.* 1998). For non-parasitic tropical diseases such as tuberculosis, rickettsial, viral encephalitis of the central nervous system, refer to the appropriate chapter in the text.

PRESENTATION WITH OCULAR SYMPTOMS

Acanthamoeba

Acanthamoeba can cause keratitis, uveitis and corneal ulceration. It is common among wearers of soft contact lenses. Corneal abrasions can lead to ulceration, iritis, scleritis and loss of vision. The patients should be referred to an ophthalmologist for corneal scrapings and identification of organism.

Onchocerciasis

It is a major cause of blindness. The ocular lesions are the result of immunological response to the microfilariae. Presentation varies from conjunctivitis, photophobia, punctate keratitis, anterior uveitis to chorioretinal lesions and finally optic atrophy. Diagnosis is made from skin snips for microfilariae, and serology.

Toxoplasmosis

Eye complications are common in congenital infection and may be present at birth. In immunocompromised patients it may develop later in life or can be acquired in adulthood. Immunosuppressed patients are very vulnerable to developing fulminant chorioretinitis. The ocular manifestations in others are granulomatous lesions and chorioretinitis. Patients present with blurred vision, photophobia and scotomata. Macular involvement results in loss of central vision. Diagnosis is made by serology for IgG and IgM antibodies. In ocular toxoplasmosis, the serum titres may not correspond to the acute eye lesions and may be low.

Loa loa

Microfilariae may be seen migrating through the conjunctiva through slit lamp examination. It does not cause blindness.

Toxocariasis

Eosinophilic granulomatous lesions may be seen in the posterior pole of the retina and may mimic retinoblastoma. Other lesions are endophthalmitis, chorioretinitis and uveitis. The common presenting symptoms are unilateral visual disturbances, pain and strabismus. Eosinophilia is not common in pure ocular toxocariasis. Diagnosis is by detection of antibodies in the aqueous humour. The antibody titres in serum are low in ocular lesions.

Sparganosis

The symptoms are pain, lacrimation, pruritus and oedema of the eyelids. Diagnosis is made by identifying the worm from a skin lesion.

Microsporidiosis

Microsporidiosis produces several eye infections in AIDS patients and is caused by *Encephalitozoon hellem* (Didier *et al.* 1991). The lesions in HIV patients are confined to the superficial epithelial layers of the cornea or conjunctiva. Ocular microsporidiosis caused by *Nosema* sp. causes keratitis or corneal ulcers in healthy people.

PRESENTATION WITH PULMONARY SYMPTOMS

The symptoms and signs of pulmonary disease in parasitic and tropical diseases are pneumonia and its complications, asthma, pneumonitis, cough and haemoptysis.

Pulmonary tuberculosis

This disease should be always considered in immigrants from South East Asian countries. The chapter on pulmonary tuberculosis deals with this condition in detail.

Melioidosis

Patients from the Northern Territory of Australia, Vietnam and Thailand who present with pneumonia, melioidosis should be considered in the differential diagnosis. Fever, tachypnoea and productive cough are prominent symptoms. Chest X-rays show upper lobe consolidation or thin walled cavities which may mimic pulmonary tuberculosis (refer to the chapter on melioidosis).

Dirofilaria immitis

Humans are infected when bitten by mosquitoes carrying microfilaria of the dog heart worm *D. immitis*. Symptomatic patients present with fever, cough and sometimes haemoptysis. X-rays show pulmonary opacities resembling coin lesions and the patients have moderate eosinophilia.

Pneumocytosis

It is the most common pulmonary infection in patients with AIDS and may be life-threatening. It is rare in immunocompetent patients, however, infection in normal people have been reported (Jacobs *et al.* 1991). Clinical presentation is non-productive cough, fever, tachypnoea, diffuse rales and diminished ventilatory capacity with hypoxia (for diagnosis, refer to the chapter on pneumocystosis).

Toxoplasmosis

This has been reported rarely in HIV patients. It may or may not be associated with neurotoxoplasmosis. Clinical presentation is fever, cough, shortness of breath, febrile illness and abnormal chest X-ray (Schnapp et al. 1992) (for diagnosis, refer to the chapter on toxoplasmosis).

Paragonimiasis

This is essentially a lung fluke where a fibrotic capsule forms around the worms once the larva migrates from the intestine, to mature in the lung. The cyst contains purulent fluid and can perforate into the bronchioles, liberating eggs and necrotic material. The clinical presentation is cough with blood–stained expectorant, chest pain and shortness of breath. It may be mistaken for bronchitis. Diagnosis is made from the history of eating uncooked crabs or crayfish, cysts in the sputum and serology.

Hydatid disease

Of all patients with hydatid disease, the general incidence of hydatid disease in the lung is ~30%. Children have a higher percentage of lung infection compared with the liver. Presenting features are chest pain, cough, malaise and haemoptysis. Diagnosis is made by X-ray showing rounded opacities that are avascular on pulmonary angiography. Serology is available for diagnosis (refer to the chapter on hydatid disease).

Pneumonitis and asthma

Helminthic infections in lung can produce hypersensitivity reactions in bronchial mucosa. Transient migration of larvae such as toxocara, ascaris, ancylostoma and strongyloides can produce transient eosinophilic 'pneumonitis'. Often they are asymptomatic with pulmonary infiltrates that are generally transient. Previous infections and the larval load determine the allergic reaction. Patients with heavy infections of strongyloides develop cough, fever and wheezing with transient pulmonary infiltrates. Larvae may be found in the sputum (Chu *et al.* 1990). Use of steroids in such patients can be disastrous. Allergic ascaris pneumonitis can manifest with dyspnoea, dry or productive cough, wheezing and fever with transient pulmonary infiltrates. These infections are associated with eosinophilia in the blood. Inhalation of antigens from *Anisakiasis simplex* is in those who handle fish and fish flour (Armentia *et al.* 1998).

Tropical eosinophilia

This is a distinct entity caused by larvae of filarial species infiltrating the lung from the peripheral blood to produce an allergic inflammatory reaction. The adult filarial worms are *Wuchereria bancrofti* and *Brugia malayi* found in South East Asian countries. The presentation is paroxysmal cough, worse at night, and wheezing. X-ray may be normal or show mottled opacities in the mid- and lower lung zones. Tropical eosinophilia is associated with peripheral eosinophilia (for diagnosis of the helminthic infection, refer to the appropriate chapters in the text).

PRESENTATION WITH GASTROINTESTINAL SYMPTOMS

Several protozoan and helminthic parasites may infect mainly the small intestines, liver and biliary tract and a few, the large bowel. Tropical diseases such as tuberculosis and typhoid can affect the large bowel and small bowel respectively. Typhoid bacillus has a predilection for the gallbladder causing a carrier state. Melioidosis in the acute suppurative stage can affect abdominal viscera, forming abscesses in organs like the spleen (Tables 5 and 6).

Protozoal and helminthic infections of small intestine have a broad spectrum of presentation from asymptomatic to abdominal pain, diarrhoea and weight loss. Diagnosis cannot be made by clinical examination alone and history is important. Diarrhoea in HIV and immunocompromised patients can be severe due to some of the newly described protozoan organisms. There are some markers that indicate intestinal parasitic diseases such as eosinophilia, mainly from nematode and cestode helminthic infections such as hookworm, *T. trichiura* and malnutrition. Hydatid disease of the liver does not produce symptoms until very late and they are non-specific. However, with abdominal trauma they may rupture and produce acute symptoms.

Flukes such as *Fasciola hepatica*, *Clonorchis* and *Opisthorchis* presents with right hypochondrial pain, jaundice and fever which may mimic gallbladder disease with ascending cholangitis. A history of dietary habits may give a clue to the diagnosis.

The following infections may mimic malignancy of the large bowel or chronic inflammatory bowel disease (refer to appropriate chapters in text), *Schistosomiasis mansoni* and *japonicum* infestation, amoebiasis or amoeboma, tuberculosis of caecum or colon and *Trichuriasis*.

Acute abdomen

Some parasitic diseases of the small intestine can present rarely as an acute abdomen mimicking acute appendicitis, intestinal obstruction, intestinal perforation or obstructive cholangitis.

Eosinophilic gastroenteritis is caused by *Anisakiasis*, mimics acute appendicitis or inflammatory bowel disease (Gomez *et al.* 1998). Ascariasis can cause obstructive perforation and common bile duct obstruction, *Angiostrongylus costaricensis* may produce a palpable mass in right hypochondrium. Human eosinophilic enteritis secondary to *Ancylostoma caninum* causes abdominal pain, tenderness and diarrhoea, and massive *Strongyloides stercoralis* infection causes intestinal obstruction and septicaemia. *Enterobis vermicularis* (pin worm) infestation can cause symptoms of acute appendicitis (Ajao *et al.* 1997).

PRESENTATION WITH GENITOURINARY SYMPTOMS

Parasitic and tropical diseases such as schistosomiasis due to *S. haematobium* and genitourinary tuberculosis can present with haematuria.

Schistosomiasis

In schistomiasis infection, haematuria may be at the end of micturition, and is associated with frequency. Symptoms develop 3–6 months after the infection (for diagnosis, refer to the chapter on schistosomiasis).

Male genital tract

Tuberculosis can present with an abacterial urinary tract infection or rarely, haematuria. Genital infection secondary to urinary tract infection manifests with beading of epididymis and enlarged irregular testes.

Female genital tract

In females, genital tuberculosis leads to primary or secondary amenorrhoea.

TRAVELLER'S DIARRHOEA

One of the common presentations to the Emergency Room is traveller's diarrhoea. The aetiology is manifold, the predominant cause being enterotoxigenic *E. coli* rather than a parasitic disease. Among other pathogens are *Entamoeba histolytica* and *Giardia lamblia*. Most patients with traveller's diarrhoea have an exacerbation of prior irritable bowel syndrome or post-acute diarrhoea variant that settles with time.

DERMATOLOGICAL PRESENTATION

Skin manifestations are common presentations to the Emergency Room. Often the diagnosis is missed, as in early leprosy. The skin manifestations are described in detail in the relevant chapters in the text. For the list of parasitic and tropical disease with skin manifestations, see Table 7.

Tropical ulcer

These are found in certain parts of the tropics including Papua New Guinea. It is frequently caused by *Fusobacterium ulcerans*. Tropical ulcers occur mostly on exposed parts such as the limbs, particularly the leg and also on fingers. It generally starts as an itchy papule that ulcerates, expands and may be as wide as 8–10 cm in diameter. The ulcer spreads rapidly and its margins are elevated and edges may be undermined. The ulcer is foul smelling and its surface sloughy. The ulcer may heal completely in a few weeks or may spread deeper and become chronic. When it heals, the skin is very thin and delicate. These ulcers should be differentiated from primary lesion of yaws that grow slowly with a positive Wassermann serology and from mycobacterial ulcers which contain acid-fast bacilli. Treatment is by parenteral penicillin and proper dressings. Metronidazole is effective.

Erythema nodosum

These are painful, dusky red, elevated plaques in the skin. It is a vasculitis in the deep dermis and subcutaneous fat. Malaise, joint pains and fever are associated with this condition. Tropical diseases associated with erythema nodosum are tuberculosis and leprosy. The other causes of erythema nodosum are bacterial such as streptococcal infections and brucellosis, viral infections, mycoplasmal rickettsial, chlamydial and fungal infections. Drug-induced diseases, systemic diseases such as sarcoidosis, Crohn's disease and ulcerative colitis can also cause erythema nodosum.

COMMON FUNGAL INFECTIONS OF SKIN (SUPERFICIAL)

Tinea capitis

The fungi causing these lesions are of the species *Microsporum* and *Trichophyton*. *Trichophyton schoenleinii* is a common cause. Patients present with a partially bald head or bald patches, which are scaly. These may be a kerion that is a boggy granulomatous mass that causes alopecia and scarring. Diagnosis is made by scrapings from the lesion for microscopy. Wood's ultraviolet light will demonstrate fluorescence with the *Microsporum* spp. Treatment is with terbinafine for 4 weeks, taken PO and local application of econozole or miconozole or terbinafine hydrochloride.

Tinea corporis and cruris

Tinea corporis and cruris are caused by all three species of fungi, *Microsporum*, *Trichophyton* and *Epidermophyton*. The lesion in tinea corporis is a small, red macule that spreads with a border and scaly central part. The lesions are often circinate and multiple. Inflammation can cause vesiculation and form crusted patches.

Tinea cruris usually affects males. The lesions are itchy, red, scaly plaques in the genitocrural folds and on the inner aspect of the thighs and scrotum. Older lesions are flat and scaly. Diagnosis is made from scrapings for fungal mycelia and spores. Treatment is with local antimycotic creams such as terbinafine hydrochloride.

Tinea pedis

This is caused by a variety of *Epidermophyton* and *Trichophyton* species. It appears as deep seated vesicles in between the toes, hollow of the sole and interdigital clefts. The lesions are itchy and become secondarily infected. Treatment is with topical antifungal agents and oral terbinafine – the latter if there is no response to local treatment.

Tinea unguium

Tinea unguium (onychomycosis) is usually associated with fungal skin lesions elsewhere. It is a slow and chronic infection and resistant to treatment. The affected nails are discoloured, friable and thickened. The distal end of the nail flakes off and the surface is pitted.

Treatment is a long, oral course of terbinafine for 6–12 weeks and the infected nail should be filed daily.

Tinea imbricata

This is common in the South Pacific, Indochina, Malaysia and New Guinea. It starts as small light brown papulovesicles that extend to produce concentric scaly rings. The infection is widespread. Treatment is with local terbinafine and the relapse rate is high.

Chromomycosis

Several types of fungi cause this. The fungi penetrate the skin through a trauma site. The lesions are nodular and develop into verrucous plaques that expand in size. Diagnosis is made by biopsy that demonstrates the fungus. Treatment is itraconazole for 1 year (Borelli 1987).

Sporotrichosis

This is caused by the fungus *Sporothrix schenckii* that lives as a saprophyte on plants in many countries including Australia. The fungus enters through a breach in the skin and forms a painless red papule. It spreads through adjacent lymphatic channels, forming nodules in adjacent skin. It can also affect joints of the elbow, knee, wrist and ankle. They may eventually produce sinuses over the joints. Diagnosis is made by culturing of pus, joint fluid or by skin biopsy. Treatment is potassium iodide as a saturated solution PO over 6–8 weeks (Barnetson 1993). Side-effects are acneiform rash over the neck and face. Itraconazole is effective in some patients (Restrepo *et al.* 1986) and is also effective in lymphocutaneous and extracutaneous sporotrichosis.

Pityriasis versicolor

This is caused by *Malassezia furfur* that is a part of the normal human skin flora. It appears as hyper- or hypopigmented macules in upper trunk and arms. It generally has a border but confluence of lesions make it difficult to demarcate the lesions. Diagnosis is made by scrapings of the lesions and microscopy. Treatment is with oral ketaconazole supplemented by local application of selenium sulphide or Selsun, and a shower after 10 min of the application.

Table VIII.1 – Severity of parasitic or tropical infections (graded 1–5 in decreasing grades of severity)

Acanthamoeba	1	Melioidosis	2
Angiostrongyliasis	1 → 3	Murray Valley encephalitis	2
Anisakiasis	3	Mycobacterium (HIV)	2
Ankylostomiasis	4	Mycobacterium tuberculosis	2, 3, 4
Ascaris lumbricoides	4	Myiasis	5
Atypical mycobacteria	3	*Naegleria fowleri*	1
Atypical mycobacteria (HIV)	2	Neurocysticercosis	1
Atypical mycobacteria skin	5	Onchocerciasis	5
Barmah Forest virus	3	Onchocerciasis to eye alone	1
Coenurosis cerebral	1	Paragonimiasis	4
Coenurosis skin	4	Paragonimiasis cerebral	1
Cryptosporidiosis	2 (in HIV), 3	Pediculosis	5
Cyclospora (HIV)	2	Plague	1
Cysticercosis	4	Pneumocystosis in HIV	2
Dengue fever	3	Ross River fever	3
Dengue haemorrhagic	1	Scabies	5
Dirofilariasis	4	Schistosomiasis	4
Donovanosis	4	Schistosomiasis cerebral	1
Enterobiasis	5	Scrub typhus	2
Erythema nodosum leprosum	2	Sparganosis cutaneous	5
Fascioliasis	4	Sparganosis neurological	1
Filariasis lymphatic	4	Sparganosis others	4
Fungal infections organs	2	Strongyloidiasis	4, 5
Fungal infections skin	4, 5	Taeniasis	4 or 5
Giardiasis	4	Tick typhus	2, 3
Hydatid disease	4 → 1	Toxocariasis	3
If immunosuppressed or HIV	1	Toxoplasmosis cerebral	2
Japanese B encephalitis	1	Toxoplasmosis congenital (foetus)	1, 2 or 3 → more
Leishmaniasis (cutaneous)	4	Trichinella	2, 3
Leishmaniasis (visceral)	2	Trichuriasis	4
Leprosy	4	*Trypanosoma cruzi*	3
Loa loa (filarial)	4	*Trypanosoma gambiense*	2
Malaria falciparum complicated	1	*Trypanosoma rhodesiense*	2
Malaria other species	3	Tungiasis	5
Mansonella perstans	4	Typhoid	2

Table VIII.2 – Life threatening diseases (parasitic)

1. Life threatening parasitic diseases.
   - falciparum cerebral malaria
   - visceral leishmaniasis
   - *Trypanosoma gambiense* and *Trypanosoma rhodesiense* infections (sleeping sickness)
   - primary amoebic encephalitis
   - *Angiostrongylus cantonensis*
   - other cerebral parasitic diseases
   - Trichinosis

2. In HIV patients and immunocompromised patients, parasitic infections caused by the following opportunistic organisms may be life threatening:
   - fulminant *Strongyloides stercoralis*
   - Coccidiosis
   - *Isospora belli*
   - Microsporidiosis
   - *Pneumocystis carinii*
   - *Toxoplasma gondii*
   - Cryptosporidiosis

3. Parasitic helminths
   - *Angiostrongylus cantonensis*
   - Trichinosis

Table VIII.3 – Life threatening diseases (viral and bacterial)

A) Viral or Bacterial
   Haemorrhagic Dengue Fever
   Yellow Fever
   Japanese B Encephalitis
   Cholera
   Plague
   Rabies
   Melioidosis
   Typhoid and Paratyphoid Fever
   Tuberculous Meningitis

Table VIII.4 – Parasitic diseases causing eosinophilia

1. Protozoa
   The only protozoan disease which may produce infrequent and mild eosinophilia is malaria.

2. Helminths
   a) Intestinal nematodes
      Ascariasis – transient eosinophilia during migration phase with chest X-ray suggestive of viral pneumonia.
      Ankylostomiasis – eosinophilia during migratory phase.
      Enterobiasis – eosinophilia may or may not be present.
      Trichuris trichura – eosinophilias of up to 15%.
      Strongyloidiasis – low eosinophil counts occur in chronic cases.
   Tissue nematodes
      Trichinosis – can vary from 20–90% of eosinophils.
      Visceral larva migrans. Toxocariasis – eosinophil count of up to 90%. There is no eosinophilia in ocular larva migrans.
      Ankylostomiasis. *Ankylostoma caninum* causes eosinophilic enteritis in man (Carme *et al.* 1991).
      Angiostrongylus cantonensis and *costaricensis* cause up to 80% eosinophils.
      Gnathostomiasis. *Gnathostoma spinigerum* – an eosinophilia between 30–75% is reported in patients with cutaneous involvement.
      Anisakiasis cause up to 10% eosinophils.
   Filarial nematodes
      Loa loa can cause up to 30% eosinophils
      Bancroftian and Malayan filaria causes tropical eosinophilia and is characterized by hyper eosinophilia up to 30% with cough and wheezing
      Dirofilaria immitis infection causes high or low eosinophilia
      Mansonella perstans causes eosinophils up to 50%
      Onchocerca volvulus causes up to 13% eosinophils
   b) Trematodes
      Schistosomiasis up to 30% eosinophils
      Fascioliasis up to 30% eosinophils
   c) Cestodes
      Sparganosis – most patients have leucocytosis and eosinophilia
      Diphyllobothrium latum – mild leukocytosis with eosinophilia
      Cysticercosis – cerebrospinal fluid eosinophilia
      Hydatid disease – 20–25% eosinophils
      Taenia solium – low grade eosinophilia under 15%

Table VIII.5 – Protozoal and helminthic infection of the small intestines and large intestine

Protozoal Infections
Small Intestine
      Giardia lamblia
      Cryptosporidium parvum
      Coccidian like bodies (cyclospora)
      Isospora belli
Large Bowel
      Entamoeba histolytica
      Trichuris trichiura (caecum and ascending colon)
Bacterial Infection of Small Bowel
      Cholera vibrio
      Typhoid bacillus
      Enteropathogenic *E. coli*
      Salmonellosis
Helminthic Infections
Small Intestine
      Ascaris lumbricoides
      Ancylostomiasis
      Strongyloides stercoralis
      Angiostrongylus costaricensis
      Trichinella spiralis
      Capillaria philippinensis
      Anisakis
      Taenia saginata
      Taenia solium
      Schistosomiasis
      Fasciolopsis buski

Table VIII.6 – Protozoal and helminthic infections of the liver and gallbladder

Visceral leishmaniasis	Presents with fever, loss of weight, diarrhoea, hepatosplenomegaly, lymphadenopathy and occasionally acute abdominal pain. Visceral leishmaniasis should be considered in immigrants from endemic areas presenting with hepatosplenomegaly
Intestinal amoebiasis	The clinical presentation is pain in the right hypochondrium, enlarged liver with tenderness in the right hypochondrium. *Entamoeba histolytica* causes abscesses in the liver.
Malaria	Hepatomegaly and mild icterus
Hydatid disease	Cysts in the liver which gradually enlarge
Opisthorchiasis	Affects the bile-ducts and gall bladder and *O. viverrini* causes cholangiocarcinoma, cholecystitis and cholelithiasis Clonorchiasis
Fascioliasis	*Fasciola hepatica* lives in the bile ducts causing biliary obstruction
Schistosomiasis	Fibrosis of the liver
Toxocariasis	Liver involvement may mimic hepatitis

Table VIII.7 – Parasitic and tropical diseases with skin manifestations

Viral Infections
1. Rashes – acute in onset. These are found in viral infections such as Ross River fever, Barmah Forest fever, dengue fever, Murray Valley encephalitis and Kunjin fever. Tick Typhus and Scrub Typhus – maculopapular rashes appear early with fever (refer to appropriate chapter in text).

2. Bacterial
   - Tuberculosis
   - Leprosy and erythema nodosum leprosum
   - Typhoid
   - Buruli ulcer (Barnsdale ulcer)

3. Mites
   - Scabies
   - Pediculosis
   - Pyemote mites

4. Helminthic infections
   - Enterobiasis (perianal dermatitis)
   - *Loa loa* (Calabar swellings)
   - Onchocerciasis (onchocercomas)
   - *Mansonella streptocerca*
   - Schistosomiasis (cercarial itch)
   - Strongyloides (larva migrans)
   - *Toxocara canis*
   - *Lymphatic filariasis, Brugia malayi, Wuchereria bancrofti*
   - Sparganosis
   - Gnathostomiasis

5. Protozoal infections
   - *Cutaneous leishmaniasis*
   - *Cutaneous amoebiasis*

6. Myiasis
   - *Dermatobia hominis*
   - *Cordylobia anthropophaga*

7. Fungal infections

8. Tropical ulcers (phagadenic ulcers)

REFERENCES

Ajao OG, Jastamiah S, Malatani *et al. Enterobis versicularis* (pin worm) causing symptoms of appendicitis. *Tropical Doctor* 1997; 182–183

Armentia A, Lombardero M, Callego A. Occupational asthma by *Anisakis simplex. Journal of Clinical Immunology* 1998; **102**: 831–834

Barnetson R. Skin diseases in the tropics. *Medical Journal of Australia* 1993; 159

Borelli D. A clinical trial of itraconazole in the treatment of deep mycoses and leishmaniasis. *Review of Infectious Diseases* 1987; **9**: 557–563

Carme BJ, Boulesteix J, Boutes J *et al.* Five cases of encephalitis during treatment of loiasis with diethylcarbamazine. *American Journal of Tropical Medicine and Hygiene* 1991; **44**: 684–690

Chu E, Witlock WL, Dietrich RA. Pulmonary hyperinfection syndrome with *Strongyloides stercoralis. Chest* 1990; **97**: 1475–1477

Currie B. Medicine in tropical Australia. *Medical Journal of Australia* 1993; **158**: 609–615

Didier PF, Didier ES, Orenstein JM *et al.* Fine structure of a new human microsporidium *Encephalitozoon hellem* in culture. *Journal of Protozoology* 1991; **38**: 502–507

Gomez B, Tabor AI, Tunon T *et al.* Eosinophilic gastroenteritis and anisakis *Allergy.* 1998; **53**: 1148–1154

Jacobs JL, Libby DM, Winters RA *et al.* A cluster of *Pneumocystis carinii* pneumonia in adults without predisposing illness. *New England Journal of Medicine* 1991; **324**: 246–250

Janssen HL, Bienfait HP, Jansen CL *et al.* Fatal cerebral oedema associated with primary dengue infection. *Journal of Infection* 1998; **36**: 346–346

Kuno G, Cropp CB, Wong-Lee J *et al.* Evaluation of an IgM immunoblot for dengue diagnostics. *American Journal of Tropical Medicine and Hygiene* 1998; **59**: 757–762

Medina MT, Rosas E, Rubico-Donadien *et al.* Neurocysticercosis as the main cause of late onset epilepsy in Mexico. *Archives of Internal Medicine* 1990; **450**: 325–327

Misra UK, Kalita J, Srivastava M. Prognosis of Japanese encephalitis: a multivariate analysis. *Journal of Neurological Sciences* 1998; **161**: 143–147

Nickolic S, Vujosevic M, Sang M *et al.* Neurologic manifestations in trichinosis. *Serbian Archives* 1998; **126**: 209–213

Restrepo A, Robledo J, Gomez I *et al.* Itraconazole therapy in lymphangitic and cutaneous sporotrichosis. *Archives of Dermatology* 1986; **122**: 413–417

Russell RC. Vector-borne diseases and their control. *Medical Journal of Australia* 1993; **158**: 681–685

Schnapp LM, Geaghan SM, Campagna A *et al. Toxoplasma gondii* pneumonitis in patients with the human immunodeficiency virus. *Archives of Internal Medicine* 1992; **152**: 1073–1077

Appendix

Species of parasitic protozoa and helminths for comparison

a. *Lamblia (Giardia) intestinalis,* cyst
b. *Entamoeba coli,* 8-nucleate cyst
c. *Entamoeba histolytica,* 4-nucleate cyst
d. *Schistosoma mansoni,* egg containing a miracidium
e. *Paragonimus westermani,* egg
f. *Fasciolopsis buski,* egg
g. *Opisthorchis felineus,* egg
h. *Clonorchis sinensis,* egg
i. *Enterobius vermicularis,* egg
j. *Trichuris trichiura,* egg
k. *Ancylostoma duodenale,* egg
l. *Ascaris lumbricoides,* egg
m. *Strongyloides stercoralis,* larva
n. *Taenia saginata,* embryophore
o. Erythrocyte of man (diameter about 7 μm): as an object for comparison

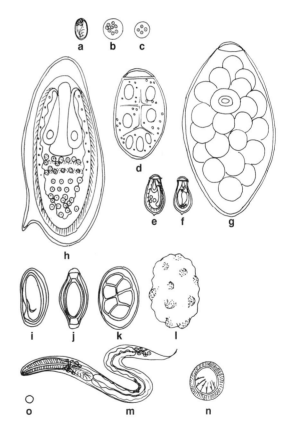

Index

Trichinella spiralis nativa 103, 104
Trichinella spiralis nelsoni 103
trichinosis 103–5
  presentation 104
    emergency 303, 305
  treatment/prevention 105
Trichophyton 308
Trichophyton schoenleinii 308
trichostrongyliasis 93–4
  investigations 94
  treatment/prevention 94
Trichostrongylus colubriformis 93
Trichostrongylus orientalis 93
Trichostrongylus spp. 93
trichuriasis (whipworm) 95–6
  treatment 96
Trichuris trichiura 77, 95, 307
  life cycle 95, 96
triclabendazole
  fascioliasis 153
  paragonimiasis 157
trophozoite 3
tropical pulmonary eosinophilia
    306–7
  lymphatic filariasis 127
tropical ulcer 52, 308
Trubanaman virus infection 280,
    282
  investigations 287
  presentation 285
  treatment 288
Trypanosoma 3
Trypanosoma brucei gambiense 59
  life cycle 59–60
Trypanosoma brucei rhodesiense 59
  life cycle 59–60
Trypanosoma cruzi 63
  life cycle 61–2
Trypanosoma rangeli 63
trypanosomiasis *see* African
    trypanosomiasis (sleeping
    sickness); American
    trypanosomiasis (Chagas'
    disease)
tuberculides 213, 216, 219
  treatment 225
Tuberculin test 217, 219–20
tuberculoma 211
  management 225
tuberculosis 207–30
  active 209
  adrenal 213, 216, 219, 225
  AIDS opportunistic infection
    214, 219, 225, 226

antituberculous drugs 220–1
  chemoprophylaxis 227
  extrapulmonary disease
    226–7
  hypersensitivity 225–6
  pregnant patients 227
  resistance 226
BCG vaccination 227–8
  contraindications 225
bone 212, 216, 219, 225, 227
central nervous system 211, 215,
    218, 224–5, 227
cutaneous
  primary 212–13, 216, 219,
    225
  tuberculides 213, 216, 219,
    225
disseminated non-reactive 214
empyema 209–10, 217–18
endobronchial 210, 218
epidemiology 208
erythema nodosum 308
gastrointestinal tract 211, 216,
    218, 225, 227, 307
genital tract
  female 210, 215, 218, 227,
    307
  male 211, 215, 218, 227, 307
inactive 209
investigations 216–20
laryngeal 210, 218
lymph nodes 210, 215, 218, 224,
    227
meningitis 211, 215, 218, 303
  chemotherapy 224–5, 227
  emergency presentation 303
miliary 213, 215, 216, 219, 225,
    227
non-tuberculous drug treatment
    224
ophthalmic 213, 225
pathology 214–16
pericarditis 210, 215, 218, 224,
    227
peritonitis 211–12, 216, 218–19,
    225, 227
pleural effusion 209, 214,
    217–18, 224, 227
prevention 227–8
pulmonary
  post-primary (adult type)
    209
  primary 209, 214, 216–17,
    306

subacute (cryptic miliary) 214,
    225
  surgical treatment 227
  transmission 208
  treatment regimens 221
    disease grading 220
    intermittent supervised
      chemotherapy 221, 223
  Tuberculin test 217, 219–20
  urinary tract 210, 215, 218, 224,
    227, 307
tuberculosis cutis orificialis 212,
    213, 216
tuberculosis paronychia 212, 213
tuberculous complex 212
tumbu fly (*Cordylobia
    anthropophaga*) 183, 184, 185
Tunga penetrans 195, 196
tungiasis 195–6
  septic complications 195–6
  treatment 196
typhoid 239–42
  chronic carriage 239, 240, 242,
    307
  complications 240, 242
  epidemiology 239
  investigations 241
  pathology 240–1, 307
  presentation 239–40
    emergency 302–3
  transmission 239
  treatment 241–2

U

urogenital myiasis 185
Uta ulcer 51

V

Vibrio cholerae 251–2
  asymptomatic carriage 252
  cholera toxin 252, 253, 254
  classical biotype 251, 252, 253,
    255
  El Tor biotype 251, 252, 253,
    255
  environmental reservoirs 251
  01 serotype 251, 252, 253, 255
  0139 serotype 252, 253, 255
  systemic infection 252–3
  virulence factors 253
visceral larva migrans 100
  treatment 101